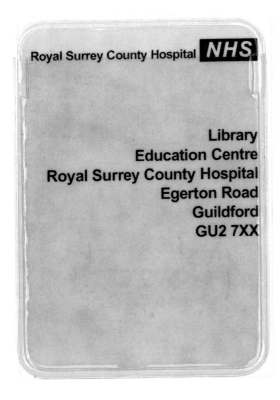

R. Bruening · A. Kuettner · T. Flohr (Eds.)

Protocols for Multislice CT

Second Edition

R. Bruening · A. Kuettner · T. Flohr (Eds.)

Protocols for Multislice CT

Second Edition

With 202 Figures

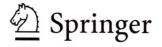 Springer

Roland Bruening, M.D.
Department of Neuroradiology
Institute of Clinical Radiology
Clinic of the University of Munich
Marchioninistr. 15
81377 Munich
Germany

Axel Kuettner, M.D.
Department of Diagnostic Radiology
University Clinic Erlangen
Maximiliansplatz 1
91054 Erlangen
Germany

Thomas Flohr, Ph.D.
Siemens Medical Solutions
Computed Tomography
Siemensstr. 1
91301 Forchheim
Germany

ISBN-10 3-540-27271-2   Springer Berlin Heidelberg New York
ISBN-13 978-3-540-27271-7   Springer Berlin Heidelberg New York

ISBN-10 3-540-43040-7 1st edition   Springer Berlin Heidelberg New York

Library of Congress Control Number: 2005930324

Springer is a part of Springer Science + Business Media

springeronline.com

© Springer-Verlag Berlin Heidelberg 2003, 2006
Printed in Germany

Editor: Dr. Ute Heilmann, Heidelberg
Desk Editor: Dörthe Mennecke-Bühler, Heidelberg
Cover design: Frido Steinen-Broo, eStudio Calamar, Spain
Typesetting: SDS, Leimen
Production: LE-TEX Jelonek, Schmidt & Vöckler GbR, Leipzig

21/3150 – YL – 5 4 3 2 1
Printed on acid-free paper

Preface to the Second Edition

The development of Multislice (multidetector row) computed tomography (CT) have had a deep impact on the general use of CT. Ct is now again being increasingly used as compared to other modalities, especially magnetic resonance imaging (MRI). Consequently, the interest in practical aspects of the method must keep pace. While in recent years the questions included when and how to use the systems, dedicated protocols are now requested for each important medical indication.

To address the more and more dedicated examinations, the second edition of *Protocols for Multislice CT* has become a multiauthor volume, the contributors being well-known experts in their fields. Their chapters provide structured up-to-date information on all routine protocols used for multislice CT. Also, the en bloc display is aimed to enable rapid appreciation of the indications and the necessary scanner settings.

New medical indications for computed tomography, such as cardiac CT, are established. There are six chapters in this volume addressing this important and fascinating application. Children are increasingly referred for an investigation using a multislice CT since the technique is fast, reliable, and only a small radiation dose is involved. A dedicated chapter addresses the special protocol and contrast material regimen necessary. Mulislice CT scanners are also increasingly used to guide interventional procedures; the most common are described in four chapters to enable fast appreciation.

The way the CT examination is planned and carried out has been substantially changed. Instead of individual axial slices, there is a thin-collimation acquisition of a volume. Subsequent reconstructions in different planes are becoming more and more routine and are indispensable for many protocols. Thin-collimation acquisition has also been recognized as being useful for minimizing artifacts.

However, care must always be taken so as not to increase the patient radiation dose unnecessarily. A chapter has been dedicated to this important topic. According to recent recommendations, and whenever possible, the mAs must be reasonable even at thin collimation. Also, the scanned volume must be restricted, especially since multiphase whole-body scans are easily performed. Last, but not least, the indication for examination must be established. The increased speed of multislice CT also suggests a change in the use of intravenous contrast agents. While the different injection doses, velocities, and concentrations are currently under investigation, both theoretical considerations and practical protocols for each body part are included in this book.

In the first edition, most protocols were optimized for Siemens scanners. In this second edition, however, the protocol layout and the data presented were intentionally changed so that they can be employed for all systems regardless of the manufacturer. Also, all protocols were adapted to accommodate all scanner generations, including the latest available 64-slice generation from all manufacturers. While we made substantial effort to adjust the protocols according to current knowledge, preferences change quickly and may vary from site to site. Therefore, if the reader has any comments or suggestions for variations of these protocols, please do not hesitate to contact any of us. Please note that despite careful editing, there can be no liability on the part of the authors for the use of any of these protocols.

We would like to express our sincere thanks to all the contributors and to all who supported us. After the first volume sold out, Springer and LE-TeX kindly supported the idea of publishing this second edition and again provided us with invaluable assistance. We hope that everyone enjoys reading this book.

Roland Bruening   Munich
Axel Kuettner   Erlangen
Thomas Flohr   Forchheim

Preface to the First Edition

The radiology community has seen a substantial technical innovation with the development of multislice computed tomography (CT). The introduction of multiple parallel detectors is undoubtedly one of the most important technical improvements in the field of CT. Moreover, the new advantages of CT may also have an impact on the general use of CT and magnetic resonance imaging (MRI).

Multislice CT is becoming increasingly available in industrialized countries. Consequently, interest in practical aspects of the method is also growing. Common questions include when and how to use the systems. While the initial scanners were equipped with two or four detector rows, current advances have led to scanners with up to 16 rows becoming available for clinical use. And there is still more to come.

As these multislice CT systems maintain the general advantages of CT, i.e. reliability and short examination times, their ability to investigate large areas of the body in a very short time with improved transverse resolution has broadened the potential medical applications of CT. Thus, new medical indications for CT, such as cardiac CT, have emerged. Some questions in diagnostic imaging, e.g. a non-invasive neck study for suspected carotid stenosis, may in future be solved more frequently with multislice CT than with MRI. Other indications such as the staging of rectal or laryngeal cancer may see a higher sensitivity and specificity with multislice CT than with single-slice systems.

There is also a substantial change in the way the examination is planned and carried out. Instead of individual axial slices, there is a thin-collimation acquisition of a volume. Subsequent reconstructions are becoming more and more important. In some protocols, such as the cranial sinuses, only the coronal reconstructions are read at our institution, while the axial data are not used.Thin-collimation acquisition is also useful for minimizing artefacts. It is here that reconstructions are made in thicker slices to minimize image noise.

Care must be taken so as not to increase the patient radiation dose unnecessarily. Therefore, whenever possible, the mAs must be adapted and reduced, the scanned volume must be restricted and last but not least the indication for the examination must be established. The increased speed of multislice CT suggests a change in the use of intravenous contrast agents. While the different injection doses, velocities and concentrations are currently under investigation, the protocols in this book include a subjective recommendation for use.

This book includes a personal selection of protocols for application with four-row or 16-row scanners. These protocols have been optimized for Siemens scanners; however, the protocol layout and the data presented can also be employed with different bands. While we made substantial effort to adjust the protocols to the current knowledge, prefereces on the use of protocols change quickly and also vary from site to site.Therefore, if the reader has any comments or suggestions for variations of these protocols, they should not hesitate to contact us. Please note that despite careful proofreading, there can be no liability on the part of the authors for the use of any of the protocols.

We would like to express our sincere thanks to all the contributors and to the local CT technicians. We gratefully acknowledge Prof. Maximilian Reiser, who enabled and encouraged this early clinical experience with multislice CT in Großhadern by his personal patronage and vision. Springer kindly supported the idea of publishing this volume and provided us with invaluable assistance. We hope that everyone interested in the technique of multislice CT finds this book useful.

R. Bruening   Munich
T. Flohr   Forchheim

Contributors

Katharina Anders
Institute for Diagnostic Radiology (IDR)
Friedrich-Alexander University
Erlangen–Nürnberg
Maximiliansplatz 1
91054 Erlangen
Germany

Andrik J. Aschoff
Department of Diagnostic Radiology
University of Ulm
Steinhövelstr. 9 (Klinikbereich Safranberg)
89075 Ulm
Germany

Ulrich Baum
Institute for Diagnostic Radiology (IDR)
Friedrich-Alexander University
Erlangen–Nürnberg
Maximiliansplatz 1
91054 Erlangen
Germany

Gunnar Brix
Federal Office for Radiation Protection
Department of Radiation and Health
Division of Medical Radiation Hygiene
and Dosimetry
Ingolstätter Landstr. 1
85764 Oberschleissheim
Germany

Roland Bruening
Dept. of Radiology
General Hospital Barmbek (AKB)
LBK Hamburg GmbH
Rübenkamp 148
22291 Hamburg
Germany

Stephan Clasen
Department of Diagnostic Radiology
Eberhard-Karls University
Hoppe-Seyler-Str. 3
72076 Tübingen
Germany

Florian Dammann
Dept. of Radiology
Klinikum am Eichert
Eichertstr. 3
73035 Göppingen
Germany

Roger Eibel
Institute of Clinical Radiology
Clinic of the University of Munich –
Innenstadt
Ziemssenstr. 1
80336 Munich
Germany

Birgit Ertl-Wagner
Institute of Clinical Radiology
Clinic of the University of Munich –
Großhadern
Marchioninistr. 15
81337 Munich
Germany

Roman Fischbach
Department of Clinical Radiology
University of Münster
Albert-Schweitzer-Str. 33
48149 Münster
Germany

Dominik Fleischmann
Department of Radiology
Stanford University Medical Center
300 Pasteur Dr., Room S-072
Stanford
California 94305-5105
USA

Thomas Flohr
Siemens Medical Solutions
Computed Tomography
Siemensstr. 1
91301 Forchheim
Germany

Thomas Helmberger
Clinic of Radiology
University of Lübeck
Ratzeburger Allee 160
23538 Lübeck
Germany

Peter Herzog
Institute of Clinical Radiology
Clinic of the University of Munich –
Großhadern
Marchioninistr. 15
81337 Munich
Germany

Martin Heuschmid
Department for Diagnostic Radiology
University of Tübingen
Hoppe-Seyler-Str. 3
72076 Tübingen
Germany

Martin Hoffmann
Department of Diagnostic Radiology
University of Ulm
Steinhövelstr. 9 (Klinikbereich Safranberg)
89075 Ulm
Germany

Ralf-Thorsten Hoffmann
Institute of Clinical Radiology
Clinic of the University of Munich –
Großhadern
Marchioninistr. 15
81337 Munich
Germany

Marius Horger
Department of Diagnostic Radiology
Eberhard-Karls University
Hoppe-Seyler-Str. 3
72076 Tübingen
Germany

Tobias F. Jakobs
Institute of Clinical Radiology
Clinic of the University of Munich –
Großhadern
Marchioninistr. 15
81337 Munich
Germany

Marc Keberle
Department of Diagnostic Radiology
Medical High School Hanover
Carl-Neuberg-Str. 1
30625 Hanover
Germany

Andreas F. Kopp
Department for Diagnostic Radiology
University of Tübingen
Hoppe-Seyler-Str. 3
72076 Tübingen
Germany

Eva Coppenrath
Institute of Clinical Radiology
University of Munich – Innenstadt
Nussbaumstr. 20
80336 Munich
Germany

Raimund Kottke
Department of Diagnostic Radiology
Eberhard-Karls University
Hoppe-Seyler-Str. 3
72076 Tübingen
Germany

Axel Kuettner
Institute for Diagnostic Radiology (IDR)
Friedrich-Alexander University
Erlangen–Nürnberg
Maximiliansplatz 1
91054 Erlangen
Germany

Andreas H. Mahnken
Department of Diagnostic Radiology
University of Aachen
Pauwelsstr. 30
52074 Aachen
Germany

David Maintz
Department of Clinical Radiology
University of Muenster
Albert-Schweitzer-Str. 33
48149 Münster
Germany

Dominik Morhard
Institute of Clinical Radiology
Clinic of the University of Munich –
Großhadern
Marchioninistr. 15
81337 Munich
Germany

Ullrich G. Müller-Lisse
Institute of Clinical Radiology
Clinic of the University of Munich –
Innenstadt
Zremssenstr. 1
80336 Munich
Germany

Hans-Dieter Nagel
Philips Medical Systems
Clinical Science & Technology Group
Roentgenstr. 24
22335 Hamburg
Germany

Jean-François Paul
Radiology Unit
Marie Lannelongue Hospital
133 av. de la Résistance
92350 Plessis Robinson
France

Philippe L. Pereira
Department of Diagnostic Radiology
Eberhard-Karls University
Hoppe-Seyler-Str. 3
72076 Tübingen
Germany

Rainer Raupach
Siemens Medical Solutions
Computed Tomography
Siemensstr. 1
91301 Forchheim
Germany

Maximilian F. Reiser
Institute of Clinical Radiology
Clinic of the University of Munich –
Großhadern
Marchioninistr. 15
81337 Munich
Germany

Rupert A. Schmid
Clinic for Nuclear Medicine
Ludwig-Maximilians University
Marchioninistr. 15
81377 Munich
Germany

Astrid Wallnöfer
Institute of Clinical Radiology
Clinic of the University of Munich –
Großhadern
Marchioninistr. 15
81337 Munich
Germany

Martin Wiesmann
Department of Neuroradiology
Clinic of the University of Munich –
Großhadern
Marchioninistr. 15
81377 Munich
Germany

Contents

Abbreviations

CCT	cranial CT
CT	computed tomography
CTA	CT angiography
FOV	field of view
HR	high resolution
MDCT	multidetector CT
MIP	maximum intensity projections
MPR	multiplanar reformats
MRI	magnetic resonance imaging
MSCT	multislice CT
SSD	shaded surface display
STS	sliding thin slices
US	ultrasound
VRT	volume rendering techniques

How to Read the Tables

T. Flohr

In the following chapters, please find a selection of scan protocols for various categories of MDCT systems, ranging from 4 to 64 slices. These protocols are meant as suggestions; they can be modified and adapted to individual clinical needs or individual patient requirements.

There are some common rules that apply to the scan protocol definitions.

Pitch

- All authors use the standard IEC pitch definition, where pitch is defined as table feed per rotation divided by the total width of the collimated beam. The total width of the collimated beam is the number of active detector rows times the collimated width of one detector row. It must be kept in mind that the Siemens SOMATOM Sensation 64, although acquiring 64 overlapping 0.6-mm slices per rotation, has a total beam width of 32×0.6 mm.
- When pitch ranges are indicated for a scan protocol, they apply to scanner types with freely selectable pitch. For scanner types with fixed pitch values, the value closest to the indicated pitch range should be chosen.
- The pitch recommendations show whether an acquisition can be performed at high pitch to optimize volume coverage, such as in thorax or abdominal CTA examinations, or whether the pitch should be reduced to optimize image quality, such as in head or spine examinations.
- ECG-gated cardiac scanning is a special case that requires very low pitch (typically p = 0.2–0.35, depending on the number of rows, the gantry rotation time, and the number of data segments from different cardiac cycles used for image reconstruction) to ensure gapless coverage of the heart volume in all phases of the cardiac cycle.

Tube Current Time Product

All authors differentiate between mAs and effective mAs. Some manufacturers, such as Siemens, use the "effective" mAs concept for their scanners, which includes the pitch dependence into the mAs definition by multiplying mAs with 1/p. For spiral scans, $(mAs)_{eff}$ is indicated on the user interface for Siemens users. Some other manufacturers, such as Toshiba and GE, use the conventional mAs definition.

- When comparing the scan parameters for CT systems of different manufacturers, the underlying mAs definition has to be taken into account. The difference is most obvious for low pitch protocols, in particular for cardiac scanning. Consider the example of an ECG-gated cardiac CTA examination at 0.4-s rotation time and pitch 0.25, using 120 kV and a tube current of 500 mA. These parameters result in 500 mA×0.4 s = 200 mAs, but in 500 mA×0.4 s×1/0.25 = 800 eff. mAs. To reduce the confusion, the authors list both mAs and effective mAs for each protocol in the scan protocol tables of this book.
- When mAs ranges are indicated, they usually refer to different patient constitutions. Adaptation of the dose to patient size and weight is the most important

factor for reducing radiation exposure [1–3].

- As a general rule, the dose necessary to maintain constant image noise has to be doubled if the patient diameter is increased by 4 cm. This is of particular importance in pediatric imaging (see Chap. 5).

Tube Current Modulation Techniques

- With this technique the tube output is automatically adapted to the patient geometry during each rotation of the scanner to compensate for strongly varying X-ray attenuations in asymmetrical body regions, such as the shoulders and pelvis. The variation of the tube output is either predefined by an analysis of the localizer scan (topogram, scout view) or determined online by evaluating the detector signal. With use of this technique, dose can be reduced by 15–35% without degrading image quality depending on the body region [4,5]. In more sophisticated approaches, the tube output is modified according to the patient geometry not only during each rotation, but also in the longitudinal direction to maintain an adequate dose when moving to different body regions, for instance, from thorax to abdomen (automatic exposure control).
- Users of scanners equipped with CARE-Dose 4D software or other similar software should not adapt the mAs settings manually, as indicated in the scan protocol recommendations of this book. This will be done automatically by the CARE-Dose 4D software. Instead use a mean mAs value within the specified range as a "reference."

Contrast Material

- Contrast material recommendations are intended for 75-kg male patients;

otherwise the amount, injection speed, and density of contrast material must be adapted.

Reconstruction Kernels

- Each vendor of CT scanners provides different convolution kernels – also called "filters" – to trade off in-plane spatial resolution and image noise according to the underlying clinical application. Since there is no naming convention for these kernels, the authors in this volume use the terms soft, standard, bone, or high resolution to indicate the desired imaging characteristics independent of the individual scanner type.

References

1. Donelly LF, Emery KH, Brody AS et al. (2001) Minimizing radiation dose for pediatric body applications of single-detector helical CT: strategies at a large children's hospital. AJR 176:303–306
2. Frush DP, Soden B, Frush KS, Lowry C (2002) Improved pediatric multidetector body CT using a size-based color-coded format. AJR 178:721–726
3. Wildberger JE, Mahnken AH, Schmitz-Rode T, Flohr T, Stargardt A, Haage P, Schaller S, Guenther RW (2001) Individually adapted examination protocols for reduction of radiation exposure in chest CT. Investigative Radiology 36(10):604–611
4. Kalender WA, Wolf H, Suess C (1999) Dose reduction in CT by anatomically adapted tube current modulation. II. Phantom measurements. Med Phys 26:2248–2253
5. Greess H, Wolf H, Baum U et al. (2000) Dose reduction in computed tomography by attenuation-based on-line modulation of the tube current: evaluation of six anatomical regions. Eur Radiol 10:391–394

I Technical and Dose Considerations

1 Technical Principles and Applications of Multislice CT

T. Flohr

1.1 Introduction

The introduction of spiral computed tomography (CT) in the early 1990s constituted a fundamental evolutionary step in the development and ongoing refinement of CT-imaging techniques [1,2]. For the first time, volume data could be acquired without the danger of misregistration or double registration of anatomical details. Images could be reconstructed at any position along the patient axis (longitudinal axis, z-axis) and overlapping image reconstruction could be used to improve longitudinal resolution. Volume data became the very basis for applications such as CT angiography [3], which has revolutionized noninvasive assessment of vascular disease. The ability to acquire volume data also paved the way for the development of three-dimensional image processing techniques such as multiplanar reformations (MPR), maximum-intensity projections (MIP), surface-shaded displays (SSP), or volume-rendering techniques (VRT) [4], which have become a vital component of medical imaging today.

The main drawbacks of single-slice spiral CT are either insufficient volume coverage within one breath hold time of the patient or missing spatial resolution on the z-axis due to wide collimation. With single-slice spiral CT the ideal of isotropic resolution, i.e., of equal resolution in all three spatial axes, can only be achieved for very limited scan ranges [5].

Larger volume coverage and improved longitudinal resolution may be achieved by simultaneous acquisition of more than one slice and by faster gantry rotation. In 1998, all major CT manufacturers introduced multislice CT (MSCT) systems, which typically offered simultaneous acquisition of four slices at a rotation time of 0.5 s, thus providing considerable improvement of scan speed and longitudinal resolution and better utilization of the available X-ray power [6–9]. Simultaneous acquisition of M slices results in an M-fold increase in speed if all other parameters, such as slice thickness are unchanged. The increased performance allowed for the optimization of a variety of clinical protocols. The examination time for standard protocols could be significantly reduced, which proved to be of immediate clinical benefit for the quick and comprehensive assessment of trauma victims and of uncooperative patients. Alternatively, the scan range that could be covered within a certain scan time was extended by a factor of M, which is relevant for oncological staging or for CT angiography with extended coverage, for example of the lower extremities [10].

The most important clinical benefit, however, proved to be the ability to scan a given anatomic volume within a given scan time with substantially reduced slice width at M times increased longitudinal resolution. This way, for many clinical applications the goal of isotropic resolution was within reach with 4-slice CT systems. Examinations of the entire thorax [11] or abdomen could now routinely be performed with a 1-mm or 1.25-mm collimated slice width (Fig. 1.1). MSCT also dramatically expanded into areas previously considered beyond the scope of third-generation CT scanners based on the mechanical rotation of the X-ray tube and detector, such as cardiac imaging with the addition of ECG gating capability. With a gantry rotation time of 0.5 s and dedicated image reconstruction

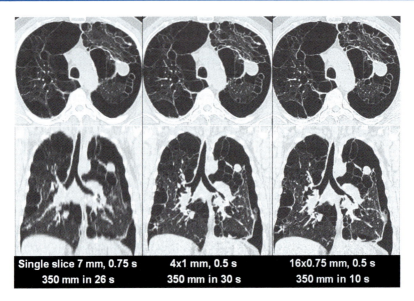

| Single slice 7 mm, 0.75 s | 4x1 mm, 0.5 s | 16x0.75 mm, 0.5 s |
| 350 mm in 26 s | 350 mm in 30 s | 350 mm in 10 s |

Fig. 1.1. Case study (axial slices and coronal MPRs) of a thorax examination illustrating the clinical performance of single-slice CT (7-mm slices, *left*), 4-slice CT (1-mm slices, *center*) and 16-slice CT (0.75-mm slices, *right*). The difference in diagnostic image quality is most obvious in the MPRs. The single-slice and 4-slice images were synthesized from the 16-slice CT data

approaches, the temporal resolution for the acquisition of an image was improved to 250 ms or less [12,13], which proved to be sufficient for motion-free imaging of the heart in the mid- to end-diastolic phase at slow to moderate heart rates (i.e., up to 65 bpm [14]).

Despite all these promising advances, clinical challenges and limitations remained for 4-slice CT systems. True isotropic resolution for routine applications had not yet been achieved, since the longitudinal resolution of about 1 mm does not fully match the in-plane resolution of about 0.5–0.7 mm in a routine scan of the chest or abdomen. For large volumes, such as CT angiography (CTA) of the lower extremity run-off [10], even thicker (i.e., 2.5-mm) collimated slices had to be chosen to complete the scan within a reasonable timeframe. For ECG-gated coronary CTA, stents or severely calcified arteries constituted a diagnostic dilemma, mainly due to partial volume artifacts as a consequence of insufficient longitudinal resolution [15], and reliable imaging of patients with higher heart rates was not possible due to limited temporal resolution.

As a next step, the introduction of an 8-slice CT-system in 2000 enabled shorter scan times, but did not yet provide improved longitudinal resolution (the thinnest collimation was 8×1.25 mm). The latter was achieved with the introduction of 16-slice CT [16,17], which made it possible to routinely acquire substantial anatomic volumes with isotropic submillimeter spatial resolution. Improved longitudinal resolution goes hand in hand with considerably reduced scan times that enable high-quality examinations in severely debilitated and severely dyspneic patients (Fig. 1.1). CTAs in particular benefit from the gain in spatial resolution, and clinical praxis suggests the potential of 16-slice CT to replace conventional catheter examinations for many indications. ECG-gated cardiac scanning is enhanced by both, improved temporal resolution achieved by gantry rotation times down to 0.375 s and improved spatial resolution [18,19]. As a consequence of the increased robustness of the technology, characterization and classification of coronary plaques is becoming feasible even in the presence of calcifications.

Currently, the race for more slices is ongoing. In 2004, all major CT manufacturers introduced MSCT-systems with 32, 40 or 64 simultaneously acquired slices, which brought about a further leap in volume coverage speed. Some of these scanners use double z-sampling, a refined z-sampling technique enabled by a periodic motion of the focal spot in the z-direction (z-flying focal spot), to further enhance longitudinal resolution and image quality in clinical routine [20]. With the most recent generation of CT systems, CT angiographic examinations with submillimeter resolution in the pure arterial phase become feasible even for extended anatomical ranges. The improved temporal resolution due to gantry rotation times down to 0.33 s has the potential to increase clinical robustness of ECG-gated scanning at higher heart rates, thereby significantly reducing the number of patients requiring heart rate control and facilitating the successful integration of CT coronary angiography into routine clinical algorithms.

Very useful up-to-date information regarding MSCT is readily available on the Internet, for example on the UK MDA CT Web site www.medical-devices.gov.uk or at www.ctisus.org.

1.2 Technical Principles of MSCT

In the following subsections we will discuss the relevant design features for volumetric scanning with MSCT-systems.

1.2.1 Detector Design

Modern CT systems generally use solid-state detectors. Each detector element consists of a radiation-sensitive solid-state material (such as cadmium tungstate, gadolinium-oxide or gadolinium oxi-sulfide with suitable dopings), which converts the absorbed X-rays into visible light. The light

is then detected by a Si photodiode. The resulting electrical current is amplified and converted into a digital signal. Key requirements for a suitable detector material are good detection efficiency, i.e., high atomic number, and very short afterglow time to enable the fast gantry rotation speeds that are essential for ECG-gated cardiac imaging.

A CT detector must provide different slice widths to adjust the optimum scan speed, longitudinal resolution and image noise for each application. For the 4-slice CT systems introduced in 1998, two detector types have been commonly used. The fixed array detector consists of detector elements with equal sizes in the longitudinal direction. A representative example of this scanner type, the GE Lightspeed scanner, has 16 detector rows, each of them defining a 1.25-mm collimated slice width in the center of rotation [7,9,21]. The total coverage in the longitudinal direction is 20 mm at the isocenter; due to geometrical magnification the actual detector is about twice as wide. In order to select different slice widths, several detector rows can be electronically combined to a smaller number of slices according to the selected beam collimation and the desired slice width. The following slice widths (measured at the isocenter) are thus realized: 4×1.25 mm, 4×2.5 mm,   4×3.75 mm,   4×5 mm   (see Fig. 1.2, top left). The same detector design is used for the 8-slice version of this system, providing 8×1.25-mm and 8×2.5-mm collimated slice width.

A different approach uses an adaptive array detector design, which comprises detector rows with different sizes in the longitudinal direction. Scanners of this type, the Philips Mx8000 4-slice scanner and the Siemens SOMATOM Sensation 4 scanner, for example, have eight detector rows [6]. Their widths in the longitudinal direction range from 1 to 5 mm (at the isocenter) and allow for the following collimated slice widths: 2×0.5 mm, 4×1 mm, 4×2.5 mm, 4×5 mm, 2×8 mm and 2×10 mm (see Fig. 1.2, top center).

The established 16-slice CT systems have adaptive array detectors in general. A rep-

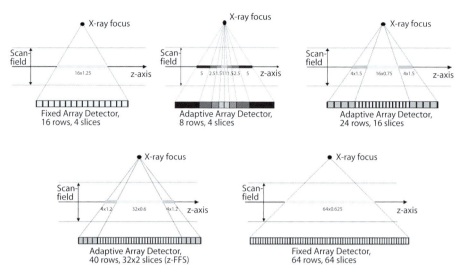

Fig. 1.2. Examples of fixed array detectors and adaptive array detectors used in commercially available 4-slice, 16-slice, and 64-slice CT systems

resentative example for this scanner type, the Siemens SOMATOM Sensation 16 scanner, uses 24 detector rows [16]. The 16 central rows define a 0.75-mm collimated slice width at the isocenter, the four outer rows on both sides define 1.5-mm collimated slice width (see Fig. 1.2, top right). The total coverage in the longitudinal direction is 24 mm at the isocenter. By appropriate combination of the signals of the individual detector rows, either 12 or 16 slices with 0.75- or 1.5-mm collimated slice widths can be acquired simultaneously. The GE Lightspeed 16 scanner uses a similar design, which provides 16 slices with either 0.625-mm or 1.25-mm collimated slice widths. The total coverage in the longitudinal direction is 20 mm at the isocenter. Yet another design, which is implemented in the Toshiba Aquilion scanner, allows the use of 16 slices with either 0.5-, 1- or 2-mm collimated slice widths, with a total coverage of 32 mm at the isocenter.

In 2004, MSCT systems providing more than 16 slices were introduced. The Siemens SOMATOM Sensation 64 scanner has an adaptive array detector with 40 detector rows [22]. The 32 central rows define 0.6-mm collimated slice widths at the isocenter and the four outer rows on both sides

define 1.2-mm collimated slice widths (see Fig. 1.2, bottom left). The total coverage at the isocenter in the longitudinal direction is 28.8 mm. Using a periodic motion of the focal spot in the z-direction (z-flying focal spot), two subsequent 32-slice readings with 0.6-mm collimated slice widths are slightly shifted in the z-direction and combined to one 64-slice projection with a sampling distance of 0.3 mm at the isocenter. With this technique, 64 overlapping 0.6-mm slices per rotation are acquired. Alternatively, 24 slices with 1.2-mm slice widths can be obtained. Toshiba, Philips and GE use fixed array detectors for their systems. The Toshiba Aquilion scanner has 64 detector rows with a collimated slice width of 0.5 mm. By appropriate combination of the signals of the individual detectors, 64 slices with 0.5-mm slice widths or 32 slices with 1-mm slice widths can be acquired simultaneously. The total z-coverage at the isocenter is 32 mm. Both the GE VCT scanner and the Philips Brilliance 64 have 64 detector rows with a collimated slice width of 0.625 mm, enabling the simultaneous read-out of 64 slices (see Fig. 1.2, bottom right) with a total coverage of 40 mm in the longitudinal direction. As a representative example, Fig. 1.3 shows a picture of a detector module of the SOMATOM Sensation 64. Each module consists of 40×16 detector pixels and the corresponding electronics. The antiscatter collimators are diagonally cut to open the view on the detector ceramics.

1.2.2 Multislice Spiral CT Scan and Image Reconstruction Techniques

With the advent of MSCT, axial "step-and-shoot" scanning has remained in use for only few clinical applications, such as head scanning, high-resolution lung scanning, perfusion CT and interventional applications. A detailed theoretical description to predict the performance of MSCT in sequential mode can be found in [23]. Spiral/helical scanning is the method of choice for the vast majority of all MSCT examinations.

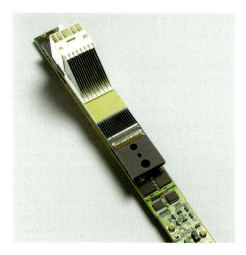

Fig. 1.3. Detector module of a commercially available MSCT scanner (SOMATOM Sensation 64, Siemens, Forchheim, Germany). Each module consists of 40×16 detector pixels with the corresponding electronics. The antiscatter collimators are diagonally cut to open the view on the detector ceramics (*yellow*)

Basic Parameters: Definition of Pitch and Dose

An important parameter to characterize a spiral/helical scan is the pitch. According to International Electrotechnical Commission (IEC) specifications [24], the pitch p is given by

$$p = \text{table feed per rotation/} \qquad (1.1)$$
$$\text{total width of the collimated beam.}$$

This definition holds for single-slice CT as well as for MSCT. It shows whether data acquisition occurs with gaps (p>1) or with overlap (p<1) in the longitudinal direction. With 4×1-mm collimation and a table feed of 6 mm/rotation, the pitch is p = 6/(4×1) = 6/4 = 1.5. With 16×0.75-mm collimation and a table feed of 18 mm/rotation, the pitch is also p = 18/(16×0.75) = 18/12 = 1.5. In the early days of 4-slice CT, the term volume pitch had been additionally introduced, which accounts for the width of one single slice in the denominator. For the sake of clarity and uniformity, the volume pitch should no longer be used.

In CT the average dose in the scan plane is best described by the weighted computerized tomographic dose index $CTDI_w$ [25,26], which is determined from $CTDI_{100}$ measurements both in the center and at the periphery of a 16-cm lucite phantom for head and a 32-cm lucite phantom for body. For the $CTDI_{100}$ measurements a 100-mm long ionization chamber is used. $CTDI_w$ is defined according to the following equation [25]:

$$CTDI_w = 1/3\ CTDI_{100}\ (\text{center}) + \qquad (1.2)$$
$$2/3\ CTDI_{100}\ (\text{periphery}).$$

$CTDI_w$, given in mGy, is always measured in an axial scan mode. It depends on scanner geometry, slice collimation and beam prefiltration as well as on X-ray tube voltage, tube current (mA) and gantry rotation time (t_{rot}). The product of mA and t_{rot} is the mAs-value of the scan. To obtain a parameter characteristic for the scanner used, it is helpful to eliminate the mAs-dependence and to introduce a normalized $(CTDI_w)_n$ given in mGy/mAs:

$$CTDI_w = mA \times t_{rot} \times (CTDI_w)_n = \qquad (1.3)$$
$$mAs \times (CTDI_w)_n.$$

$CTDI_w$ is a measure for the dose in a single axial scan. $(CTDI_w)_n$ still depends on X-ray tube voltage and on slice collimation. Scan protocols for different CT-scanners should always be compared on the basis of $CTDI_w$ and never on the basis of mAs, since different system geometries can lead to significant differences in the radiation dose that is applied at identical mAs.

To represent the dose in a spiral scan, it is essential to account for gaps or overlaps between the radiation dose profiles from consecutive rotations of the X-ray source [25]. For this purpose $CTDI_{vol}$, the volume $CTDI_w$, has been introduced:

$$CTDI_{vol} = 1/p \times CTDI_w = \qquad (1.4)$$
$$mAs \times 1/p \times (CTDI_w)_n =$$
$$mA \times t_{rot} \times 1/p \times (CTDI_w)_n.$$

The factor $1/p$ accounts for the increasing dose accumulation with decreasing spiral pitch due to the increasing spiral overlap. In principle, Eq. 1.4 holds for single-slice CT as well as for MSCT. Some manufacturers, such as Siemens, have introduced an "effective" mAs concept for spiral scanning, which includes the factor 1/p into the mAs definition:

$$(mAs)_{eff} = mA \times t_{rot} \times 1/p = \qquad (1.5)$$
$$mAs \times 1/p.$$

For spiral scans, $(mAs)_{eff}$ is indicated on the user interface. Inserting Eq. 1.5 into Eq. 1.4, the dose of a multislice spiral scan is simply given by

$$CTDI_{vol} = (mAs)_{eff} \times (CTDI_w)_n. \qquad (1.6)$$

Some other manufacturers, such as Toshiba and GE, stay with the conventional mAs definition, and the user must perform the 1/p correction himself. When comparing the scan parameters for CT systems of different manufacturers, the underlying mAs definition has to be considered.

$CTDI_w$ is a physical dose measure; it does not provide full information on the radiation risk associated with a CT examination. For this purpose the concept of "effective dose" has been introduced by the International Commission on Radiation Protection (ICRP). The effective dose is given in mSv. It is a weighted sum of the dose applied to all organs in a CT examination and includes both direct and scattered radiation. The weighting factors depend on the biological radiation sensitivities of the respective organs. The effective dose can be measured using whole body phantoms such as the Alderson phantom, or it is derived from computer simulations using Monte Carlo techniques to determine scattered radiation. The effective patient dose depends on the scanned range. For a comparison of effective dose values for different protocols, the scan ranges should be similar.

Short Review of Single-Slice Spiral CT

Spiral CT requires an interpolation of the acquired measurement data in the longitudinal direction to estimate a complete CT data set at the desired plane of reconstruction. The most commonly used single-slice spiral interpolation schemes are the 360° and 180° linear interpolations (360° LI and 180° LI). In spiral CT, z-axis resolution is not only determined by the collimated slice-width s_{coll} as in axial scanning, but by the effective slice width s, which is established in the spiral interpolation process. Usually, s is defined as the full width at half maximum (FWHM) of the slice sensitivity profile (SSP). For both 360° LI and 180° LI s increases with increasing pitch and longitudinal resolution degrades (Fig. 1.4). This is a consequence of the increasing longitudinal distance of the projections used for spiral interpolation. The image noise in single-slice spiral CT is independent of the pitch, if the tube current (mA) is kept constant and patient dose decreases with increasing pitch.

In clinical practice, single-slice spiral CT scanning is almost exclusively based on 180° LI due to the narrower SSP of this algorithm, despite its increased susceptibility to artifacts and increased image noise. For

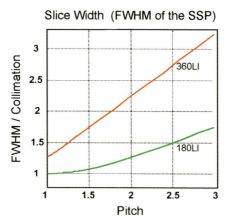

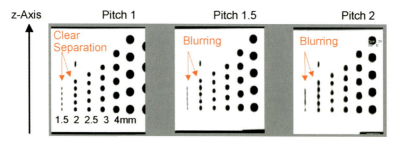

Fig. 1.4. FWHM of the spiral SSP as a function of the pitch for the two most commonly used single-slice spiral interpolation approaches, 180° LI and 360° LI. For both, the slice significantly broadens with increasing pitch. As a consequence, multiplanar reformats of a spiral z-resolution phantom scanned with 2-mm collimation (180° LI) show increased blurring of the 1.5-mm and 2-mm cylinders with increasing pitch

the same mAs, image noise is about 15% higher than in axial mode. With single-slice CT, scanning at higher pitch is often used to reduce patient dose at the expense of slice broadening – if the collimation is kept constant – and increased spiral artifacts. For CTA applications in particular it is more favorable to scan a given volume in a given time using narrow collimation at high pitch than using wider collimation at low pitch [27].

The Cone Angle Problem in MSCT

Two-dimensional image reconstruction approaches used in commercially available single-slice CT scanners require all measurement rays that contribute to an image to run in a plane perpendicular to the patient's longitudinal axis. In MSCT systems this requirement is violated; the measurement rays are tilted by the so-called cone angle with respect to the center plane. The cone angle is largest for the slices at the outer edges of the detector and it increases with an increasing number of detector rows if their width is kept constant. As a first approximation, the cone angle is neglected in MSCT reconstruction approaches and modified two-dimensional image reconstruction algorithms are used. The data, however, are then inconsistent, which produces cone–beam artifacts at high-contrast objects such as bones. It has been demonstrated that cone–beam artifacts can be tolerated if the maximum number M of simultaneously acquired slices does not

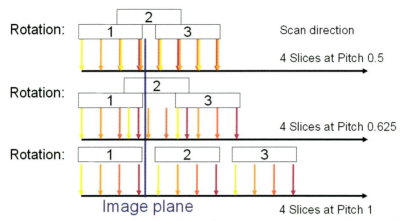

Fig. 1.5. Sampling scheme along the z-axis for a 4-slice CT-system at various pitch values. The sampling patterns are irregular and show a complicated dependence on the spiral pitch

significantly exceed M=4 [28]. As a consequence, the image reconstruction approaches of all commercially available CT systems with four slices and of some with even more slices neglect the cone angle of the measurement rays.

180° and 360° Multislice Linear Interpolation and z-Filtering

The 360° LI and 180° LI single-slice spiral reconstruction approaches can be extended to multislice spiral scanning in a straightforward way [21,29,30]. Both 360° MLI and 180° MLI are characterized by a projection-wise linear interpolation between two rays on either side of the image plane. The cone angle of the measurement rays is not taken into account. In general, scanners relying on 180° MLI or 360° MLI techniques and extensions thereof provide selected discrete pitch values to the user, such as 0.75 and 1.5 for 4-slice scanning [21] or 0.5625, 0.9375, 1.375 and 1.75 for 16-slice scanning [30]. This is a consequence of the complicated sampling patterns along the z-axis (see Fig. 1.5). The user has to be aware of pitch-dependent effective slice widths s. For low-pitch scanning (at p=0.75 using four slices and at p=0.5625 or 0.9375 using 16 slices), $s\sim s_{coll}$ and for a collimated 1.25-mm slice the resulting effective slice width stays at 1.25 mm. The narrow SSP, however, is achieved by a 180° MLI reconstruction using conjugate interpolation at the price of increased image noise [21,30]. For high-pitch scanning (at p=1.5 using four slices and at p=1.375 or 1.75 using 16 slices), $s\sim1.27s_{coll}$ and a collimated 1.25-mm slice results in an effective 1.5–1.6-mm slice. To obtain the same image noise as in an axial scan with the same collimated slice width, 0.73–1.68 times the dose, depending on the spiral pitch, is required, with the lowest dose at the highest pitch [30]. Scanners offering discrete optimized pitch values based on 180° MLI and 360° MLI techniques are comparable to single-slice CT systems in some core aspects: at high pitch the slice widens and longitudinal resolution degrades. At low pitch the narrowest possible SSP (comparable to 180° LI single-slice CT at pitch 1) can be obtained, but a higher dose is necessary to maintain the signal-to-noise ratio. Thus, when selecting the scan protocol for a particular application, scanning at low pitch optimizes image quality and longitudinal resolution at a given collimation, yet at the expense of increased patient dose. To reduce patient dose, either the mA settings should be reduced at low pitch or high pitch values should be chosen.

In a z-filter multislice spiral reconstruction [29,31] the spiral interpolation for each projection angle is no longer restricted to the two rays in closest proximity to the im-

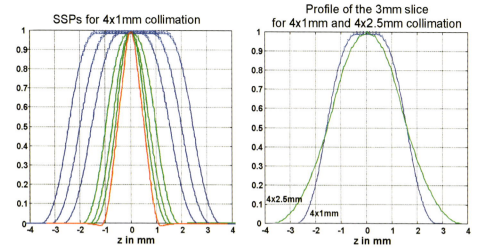

Fig. 1.6. Using *z*-filtering, images with different slice widths can be retrospectively reconstructed from the same CT raw-data. *Left*: SSPs for 4×1-mm collimation (SOMATOM Sensation 4, Siemens, Forchheim, Germany): 1-mm, 1.25-mm, 1.5-mm, 2-mm, 3-mm, 4-mm, and 5-mm slice width, not shown are the SSPs for 6-mm, 7-mm, 8-mm, and 10-mm slice width. *Right*: SSPs of the 3-mm slice for 4×1 mm and 4×2.5-mm collimation. The FWHM is equal, but the profile is more rectangular for the narrow collimation (4×1 mm)

age plane. Instead, all direct and complementary rays within a selectable distance from the image plane contribute to the image. Still, the cone angle is neglected. A representative example for a *z*-filter approach is the adaptive axial interpolation (AAI) [29] implemented in Siemens CT scanners. Another example is the MUS-COT algorithm [31] used by Toshiba. *z*-filtering allows the system to tradeoff z-axis resolution (SSP) with image noise (which directly correlates with required dose). From the same CT raw data, images with different slice widths can be retrospectively reconstructed (see Fig. 1.6). Only slice widths equal to or larger than the subbeam collimation can be obtained. With AAI, the spiral pitch is freely selectable in the range of 0.5 to 2 and the effective slice width is kept constant for all pitch values [6,29,32]. Therefore, longitudinal resolution is independent of the pitch, deviating from single-slice spiral CT and from MSCT relying on 180° MLI and 360° MLI [21,30]. Figure 1.7 shows SSPs of the SOMATOM Sensation 4 (2-mm slice for 4×1-mm col-

limation) and MPRs of a spiral *z*-resolution phantom for selected pitch values. As a consequence of the pitch-independent spiral slice width, the image noise for fixed effective mAs (see Basic Parameters above) is nearly independent of the spiral pitch – different from 180° MLI and 360° MLI. For a 1.25-mm spiral slice width reconstructed from 4×1-mm collimation, 0.61–0.69 times the dose is required to maintain the image noise of an axial scan at the same collimation [32]. Radiation dose, too, is independent of the spiral pitch and equals the dose of an axial scan with the same mAs. Thus, different from single-slice spiral CT, changing the pitch does not change the patient dose. Accordingly, using higher pitch does not result in dose saving, which is an important practical consideration with CT systems relying on AAI and the effective mAs concept.

With regard to image quality, narrow collimation is preferable to wide collimation, due to better suppression of partial volume artifacts and a more rectangular SSP (see Fig. 1.6), even if the pitch has to

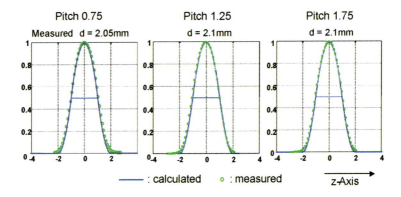

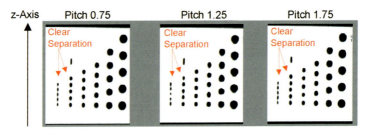

Fig. 1.7. Adaptive Axial Interpolation for a 4-slice CT-system (SOMATOM Sensation 4, Siemens, Forchheim, Germany): SSP of the 2-mm slice (for 4×1-mm collimation) at selected pitch values. The functional form of the SSP, and hence the slice width, is independent of the pitch. Consequently, multiplanar reformats of a spiral z-resolution phantom scanned with 2-mm slice width show clear separation of the 1.5-mm and 2-mm cylinders for all pitch values (compare with Fig. 1.4)

be increased for equivalent volume coverage. Similar to single-slice spiral CT, narrow collimation scanning is the key to reducing artifacts and improving image quality. Best suppression of spiral artifacts is achieved by using both narrow collimation relative to the desired slice width and reducing the spiral pitch. In general, challenging clinical protocols, such as examinations of the spine and skull base, rely on a combination of narrow collimation and low pitch.

Some manufacturers who use z-filter approaches do not provide completely free selection of the spiral pitch, but recommend a selection of fixed pitch values that are aimed at optimizing the z-sampling scheme and reducing spiral artifacts, such as 0.625, 0.75, 0.875, 1.125, 1.25, 1.375, and 1.5 for 4-slice scanning (MUSCOT algorithm [31]).

Cone–Beam Reconstruction:

3D Backprojection and Adaptive Multiple Plane Reconstruction

For CT scanners with 16 and more slices, modified reconstruction approaches accounting for the cone–beam geometry of the measurement rays have to be considered. Some manufacturers (Toshiba, Philips) use a 3D-filtered back-projection reconstruction [33–37]. With this approach, the measurement rays are back-projected into a 3D volume along the lines of measurement, this way accounting for their cone–beam geometry. Other manufacturers use variations and extensions of nutating slice algorithms [38–42], which split the 3D reconstruction task into a series of conventional 2D reconstructions on tilted intermediate image planes. Representative examples are the adaptive multiple plane

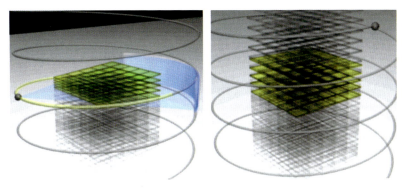

Fig. 1.8. Schematic diagram illustrating the adaptive multiple plane reconstruction. *Left*: depending on the spiral pitch the multislice raw data are divided into overlapping segments. As an intermediate step, a variety of partial images on double oblique image planes is calculated, which are individually adapted to the spiral path and to the multislice detector geometry and fan out like the pages of a book. *Right*: the final images are obtained by a longitudinal interpolation (*z*-interpolation) between the tilted partial image planes, similar to a multiplanar reformation.

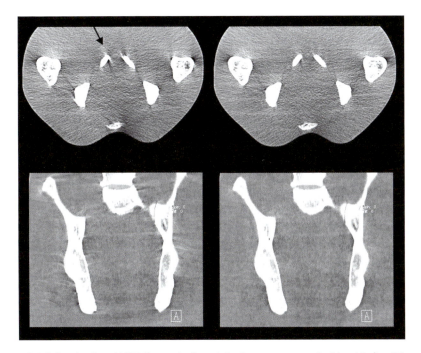

Fig. 1.9. Axial slice (*top*) and MPR (*bottom*) of a pelvis phantom scanned with a 16-slice CT-system, 16×1.5-mm collimation, 2-mm reconstructed slice width, 0.5-s rotation time, a pitch of 1.0, i.e., a table feed of 48 mm/s. *Left*: conventional multislice spiral reconstruction neglecting the cone angle of the measurement rays. Cone–beam artifacts are indicated by *arrows*. *Right*: AMPR. Cone–beam artifacts are effectively reduced

reconstruction (AMPR) used by Siemens [43,44] and the weighted hyperplane reconstruction (WHR) proposed by GE [45,46].

The AMPR approach delivers high quality images at optimum dose usage for a wide range of pitch values. As an inter-

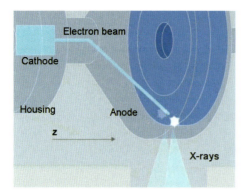

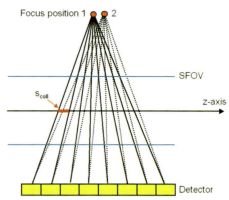

Fig. 1.10. Schematic drawing of a rotating envelope X-ray tube (Siemens STRATON, Forchheim, Germany) with z-flying focal spot technology. The entire tube housing rotates in an oil bath. The anode plate is in direct contact with the cooling oil to improve heat dissipation. The central cathode rotates as well, and continuous electromagnetic deflection of the electron beam is needed to control the position and the shape of the focal spot. The electromagnetic deflection unit is used to wobble the focal spot between two different positions on the anode plate (indicated by two asterisks). Due to the anode angle of typically 7–9° this translates into a motion both in the radial direction and in the z-direction

Fig. 1.11. Principle of improved z-sampling with the z-flying focal spot technique. Due to a periodic motion of the focal spot in the z-direction two subsequent M slice readings are shifted by half a collimated slice-width $s_{coll}/2$ at isocenter and can be interleaved to one $2M$ slice projection. Improved z-sampling is not only achieved at the isocenter, but maintained in a wide range of the SFOV. The simultaneous radial motion of the focal spot in an actual X-ray tube has been omitted to simplify the drawing

mediate step, partial images on double oblique image planes are calculated, which are individually adapted to the spiral path and to the multislice detector geometry and fan out like the pages of a book (see Fig. 1.8a). The final images with full-dose utilization are obtained by an appropriate longitudinal interpolation between the tilted partial image planes, similarly to a multiplanar reformation (Fig. 1.8b). The shape and the width of the interpolation function are freely selectable, different SSPs and hence different slice widths for retrospective reconstruction can therefore easily be adjusted similarly to z-filter approaches. Figure 1.9 shows images of a pelvis phantom scanned with 16×1.5-mm collimation, 0.5 s gantry rotation time, and a pitch p=1, corresponding to a table feed of 48 mm/s, on the left side for a reconstruction neglecting the cone angle of the measurement rays and on the right side for AMPR. The conventional approach leads

to severe artifacts and geometrical distortions of high-contrast objects (left). Cone artifacts are considerably reduced with the AMPR algorithm and the spatial integrity of the objects is restored (right).

Multislice spiral scanning using AMPR in combination with the effective mAs concept is characterized by the same key properties as AAI, which can be directly derived using the methods presented in the 180° and 360° Multislice Linear Interpolation and z-Filtering section above. Thus, all recommendations regarding the selection of collimation and pitch that have been discussed for AAI also apply to AMPR. In particular, changing the pitch does not change the radiation exposure to the patient, and using higher pitch does not result in dose saving. Narrow collimation scanning should be performed whenever possible. With 16×0.75-mm collimation, 1-mm slice width is recommended as the most suitable tradeoff between longitudinal resolution, image noise and artifacts when thin slices are reconstructed as an input for 3D postprocessing, such as MPR, MIP or VRT.

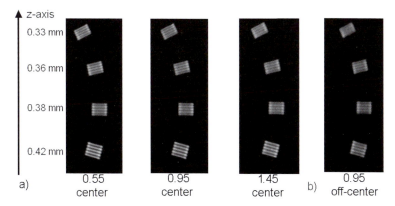

Fig. 1.12. MPRs of a z-resolution phantom (high-resolution insert of the CATPHAN, the Phantom Laboratories, Salem, NY, turned by 90°) for pitch 0.55, 0.95 and 1.45, scanned with a MSCT system with double z-sampling (SOMATOM Sensation 64, Siemens, Forchheim, Germany). Scan data has been acquired with 32×0.6-mm collimation in a 64-slice acquisition mode using the z-flying focal spot and reconstructed with the narrowest slice width (nominal 0.6 mm) and a sharp body kernel (B70). **a** z-resolution phantom positioned at the isocenter. Independent of the pitch all bar-patterns up to 15 lp/cm can be visualized, corresponding to 0.33 mm longitudinal resolution. **b** z-resolution phantom positioned 100 mm off-center (pitch 0.95). Longitudinal resolution is only slightly degraded (14 lp/cm, corresponding to 0.36 mm)

Double z-Sampling

The double z-sampling concept for multislice spiral scanning makes use of periodic motion of the focal spot in the longitudinal direction to improve data sampling along the z-axis [20,22]. By continuous electromagnetic deflection of the electron beam in a rotating envelope X-ray tube, the focal spot is wobbled between two different positions on the anode plate. Due to the anode angle of typically 7–9° this translates into a motion both in the radial direction and in the z-direction (Fig. 1.10). The radial motion is a side-effect that must be taken care of by the image reconstruction algorithms. The amplitude of the periodic z-motion is adjusted in a way that two subsequent readings are shifted by half a collimated slice width in the patient's longitudinal direction (Fig. 1.11). Therefore, the measurement rays of two subsequent readings with collimated slice-width s_{coll} interleave in the z-direction, and every two M-slice readings are combined into one 2M-slice projection with a sampling distance of $s_{coll}/2$.

The SOMATOM Sensation 64 (Siemens, Forchheim, Germany) as an example of a MSCT system relying on double z-sampling has a detector that provides 32 collimated 0.6-mm slices (see Sect. 1.2.1). Two subsequent 32-slice readings are combined into one 64-slice projection with a sampling distance of 0.3 mm at the isocenter. Thus, 64 overlapping 0.6-mm slices per rotation are acquired. The sampling scheme is similar to that of a 64×0.3-mm detector, and the AMPR algorithm is used for image reconstruction. Double z-sampling provides a sampling distance of $s_{coll}/2$ independent of the pitch. The improved sampling along the z-direction is not restricted to the isocenter, but is maintained in a wide range of the SFOV. As a consequence, spatial resolution in the logitudinal direction is increased, and objects <0.4 mm in diameter can be routinely resolved at any pitch (Fig. 1.12). Another benefit of double z-sampling is the suppression of spiral "windmill" artifacts at any pitch (Fig. 1.13). In contrast to conventional MSCT scan and reconstruction approaches, spiral image quality is largely independent of the pitch. Using conven-

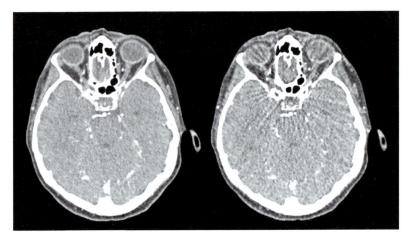

Fig. 1.13. Reduction of spiral artifacts with double *z*-sampling. *Left*: head scan acquired with 32×0.6 collimation in a 64-slice acquisition mode with *z*-flying focal spot at pitch 1.5. *Right*: same scan, using only one focus position of the *z*-flying focal spot for image reconstruction. Due to the improved longitudinal sampling with *z*-flying focal spot (*left*) spiral interpolation artifacts (windmill structures at high contrast objects) are suppressed without degradation of *z*-axis resolution

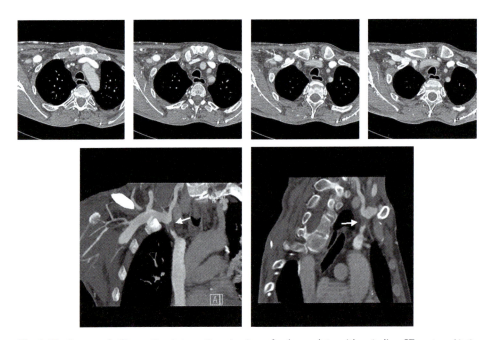

Fig. 1.14. Case study illustrating interactive viewing of volume data with a 4-slice CT system (4×1-mm collimation, pitch 2, reconstructed slice-width 1.25 mm). *Top*: axial images show the central thrombosis of the right subclavian vein. *Bottom*: MIP images show different views of the filiform stenosis of the right brachiocephalic vein proximal to the confluence of the superior cava vein (courtesy of M. Lell, University of Erlangen, Germany)

tional MSCT systems, demanding applications, such as neuroscanning, require low pitch protocols to reduce artifacts and to improve image quality. The z-flying focal spot technique maintains a low artifact level up to pitch 1.5, thus increasing the maximum volume coverage speed that can be used clinically.

1.3 Applications

1.3.1 Standard Applications

Clinical applications benefit from MSCT technology in several ways [6,9,16,32]:

- Shorter scan time (important for trauma victims, patients with limited ability to cooperate, pediatric cases, multiphase exams and CT angiography (CTA))
- Extended scan range (important for CTA or combined chest–abdomen–pelvis scans such as in oncological staging)
- Improved longitudinal resolution (beneficial for all reconstructions, in particular when 3D postprocessing is part of the clinical protocol)

Most protocols can benefit from a combination of these advantages. The wide availability of 4-slice CT systems started to change the way radiologists think about CT imaging and paved the way for CT from a cross-sectional slice modality to a volume imaging modality. In many applications, narrow collimation data is recommended independently from the desired slice width for primary viewing. In practice, two different slice widths are commonly reconstructed by default: thick slices for filming and thin slices for 3D postprocessing and evaluation (please also refer to the individual protocols). The image noise in close-to-isotropic high resolution volumes can be limited by making use of *thick* MPRs or *thick* MIPs. In this way, images with the desired slice-width can be obtained in arbitrary directions. As a consequence, the distinction between longitudinal and in-plane resolution is gradually becoming a historical remnant, and the traditional axial slice

is loosing its clinical predominance. It is replaced by interactive viewing and manipulation of volume images, with only the key slices or views in arbitrary directions used for filming or stored for a demonstration of the diagnosis. Figure 1.14 shows an example of a thorax study on a 4-slice CT-system that has been diagnosed interactively. Please note that MPRs and oblique MIPs are of similar resolution as the original axial images.

Meanwhile, 16-slice CT systems have been established in clinical practice, and isotropic submillimeter coverage of extended anatomical ranges has become the clinical standard for many applications. Clinical practice suggests the potential of 16-slice CTA to replace noninterventional catheter angiography in the evaluation of carotid artery stenosis [47]. For patients with suspicion of ischemic stroke both the status of the vessels supplying the brain and the location of the intracranial occlusion can be assessed in the same examination [48]. Additional brain perfusion CT permits differentiation of irreversibly damaged brain tissue from reversibly impaired tissue at risk [49]. Examining the entire thorax (350 mm) with submillimeter collimation requires a scan time of approximately 11 s. Due to the short breath hold time, central and peripheral pulmonary embolism can be reliably and accurately diagnosed [50,51]. Sixteen-slice CT enables whole body angiographic studies with submillimeter resolution in a single breath hold. Compared to invasive angiography, the same morphological information is revealed [52,53] (see Fig. 1.15 for an example of a patient with Leriche-syndrome).

Insufficient volume coverage speed, which was a serious problem in the days of single-slice CT [5], only rarely becomes a limiting factor with 16-slice CT. Clinical progress from further technical development of MSCT can more likely be expected from improvements in spatial and temporal resolution rather than from a mere increase in the volume-coverage speed. The new concept of double z-sampling implemented in some of the recently introduced 64-slice CT-systems allows for a pitch-independent

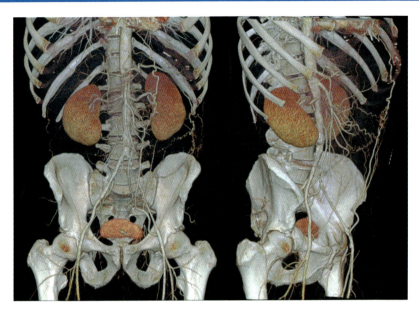

Fig. 1.15. Case study illustrating the clinical performance of 16-slice CT: patient with occlusion of the left common iliac artery. Scan parameters: 16×0.75-mm collimation, reconstructed slice-width 1 mm, 0.5 s gantry rotation time (courtesy of M. Heuschmid and A. Küttner, University of Tübingen, Germany)

increase of longitudinal resolution and suppression of spiral artifacts. Isotropic submillimeter CTAs of the carotid arteries and the circle of Willis with a scan range of 350 mm require 5–6 s scan time with these systems, hence they can be acquired in the purely arterial phase (see the example in Fig. 1.16). The entire thorax (350 mm) can be scanned in about 6 s, facilitating the examination of emergency patients, e.g., with suspicion of acute pulmonary embolism. Early experience in neuro-CT has already demonstrated a substantial improvement in spatial resolution and artifact level made possible by the double z-sampling concept for MSCT systems [54].

1.3.2 Special Applications

Cardiac CT

One of the most exciting new applications of multislice CT is the ability to image the heart. Increased rotation speed combined with dedicated ECG-synchronized recon-struction algorithms effectively allow one to freeze the heart motion [13,55,56]. The details of this new technique have been discussed extensively in several recent publications [57–59] so we restrict this section to a brief overview.

One important application of cardiac CT is the quantitative evaluation of coronary calcification as a risk indicator in non-symptomatic patients, which previously was a domain of electron beam CT (EBT) technology. Studies have shown that ECG-gated spiral imaging with reconstruction of overlapping images can significantly reduce inter-scan variability [60]. Good repeatability of the quantitative measurements is a prerequisite for longitudinal studies, such as controlling the same individual for effectiveness of medication. Advanced software platforms allow assessment of the established Agatston score as well as other score values, such as equivalent lesion volume and total calcified plaque burden in terms of absolute calcium mass, based on scanner-specific calibration [60, 61]. The mass score in particular has the potential

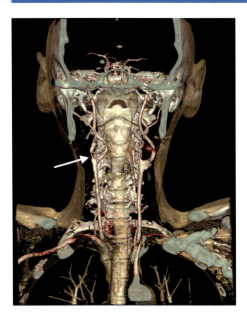

Fig. 1.16. Case study illustrating the clinical performance of 64-slice CT with *z*-flying focal spot: CTA of the carotid arteries and the circle of Willis. Scan parameters: 120 kV, 150 eff. mAs, 64×0.6-mm slice acquisition, reconstructed slice-width 0.6 mm, 0.375-s gantry rotation time, pitch 1.4, scan time 6 s for 350 mm. The *arrow* indicates a severe stenosis (courtesy of M. Lell and K. Anders, University of Erlangen, Germany)

to increase the accuracy, consistency, and reproducibility of coronary calcium assessment [61].

With four simultaneously acquired slices, coverage of the entire heart with thin slices (1 mm/1.25 mm) and ECG-gating within a single breath hold became feasible, enabling noninvasive visualization of the coronary arteries [15,56,62,63]. Due to the improved signal-to-noise ratio when compared to EBT and the better longitudinal resolution, the initial clinical studies demonstrated MSCT's potential to not only detect but to some degree characterize noncalcified plaques in the coronary arteries based on their CT attenuation [64,65]. Despite all promising advances, challenges and limitations with respect to motion artifacts in patients with higher heart rates, limited spatial resolution and long breath hold times remain for 4-slice cardiac CT.

Sixteen-slice MSCT systems with gantry rotation times down to 0.375 s have improved spatial and temporal resolution, while examination times have been considerably reduced: the entire heart volume can be covered with submillimeter slices in 15–20 s [17,44]. Sixteen-slice systems have been used to establish ECG-triggered or ECG-gated MSCT examinations of the heart and the coronary arteries in clinical practice. Detection and characterization of coronary plaques, even in the presence of severe calcifications benefit from the increased robustness of the technology. A study of coronary CTA with a 16-slice system in 59 patients demonstrated 86% specificity and 95% sensitivity for identifying significant coronary artery stenosis. None of the patients had to be excluded [18], as in previous studies based on less-advanced scanner technology. Meanwhile, other investigators report similar results [19].

The latest generation of 64-slice CT systems provides further increased spatial resolution (0.4-mm isotropic voxels) and improved temporal resolution due to gantry rotation times down to 0.33 s, and will be a further leap in integrating coronary CTA into routine clinical algorithms. Due to the fast volume coverage of these systems, ECG-gated examinations of the entire thorax for a comprehensive examination of patients with acute thorax pain are feasible, opening new perspectives for emergency care.

Figure 1.17 shows an example of a coronary CTA in a follow-up examination and demonstrates the improvement in image quality from 4 to 64 slices.

Lung Cancer Screening and CT Colonography

Early detection of lung cancer and CT colonography are promising applications in the field of preventive care.

Initial studies using CT to detect lung cancer at an early stage in a screening population were published in 1999 [66]. Basic system requirements are coverage of the entire lung in a single breath hold at sufficient

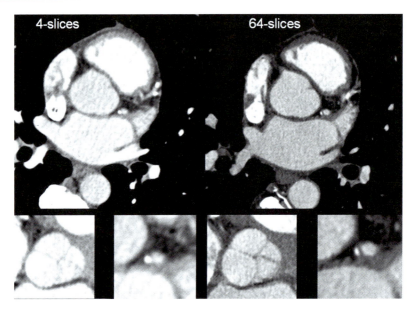

Fig. 1.17. Case study comparing ECG-gated cardiac CT with a 4-slice CT system and a 64-slice CT system with z-flying focal spot. The follow-up CTA examination demonstrates the improvement in spatial resolution with 64 slices (courtesy of C. Becker, Klinikum Großhadern, Ludwigs-Maximilians University Munich, Germany)

resolution to detect small, suspicious nodules while keeping the dose at an acceptable level. In principle, single-slice CT is able to meet these requirements, but clinical workflow improves substantially with MSCT. In the ELCAP study [66], which was performed using single-slice CT, suspicious nodules were found in about 25% of the screened population. These patients received further work-up, either monitoring and follow-up of small nodules or surgical removal, depending on various factors. Since accurate volume assessment of small nodules requires high spatial resolution, which was not available in the initial screening examination due to limited volume coverage, the respective patients had to be rescheduled. With MSCT the screening examination can be done at high resolution, obviating the need for rescheduling. With 4×1-mm collimation and 0.5 s gantry rotation time, the entire thorax (350 mm) can be covered in 25–30 s. With 16×0.75-mm collimation, the scan time is reduced to about 10 s. The use of CT as a screening tool in a healthy population at risk for lung cancer requires

reduction of the patient dose to the lowest clinically acceptable level. With 120 kV and 20 effective mAs, the effective patient dose is below 1 mSv, which is less than the natural background radiation exposure of half a year.

The ELCAP study has shown that CT screening can detect lung cancer significantly earlier than chest X-rays [66]. While it has not been proven that CT screening for lung cancer reduces mortality, earlier detection of lung cancer is commonly considered to have a favorable effect on the effectiveness of therapy.

Recently, new software tools have been developed that automatically detect suspicious nodules and can be used as a "second reader" to support the radiologist (nodule enhanced visualization NEV, Siemens Medical Solutions, Forchheim, Germany). Initial studies have demonstrated higher detection sensitivity of nodules smaller than 8 mm in diameter with the help of NEV.

CT colonography is used to detect suspicious polyps in the colon. Although controversially discussed, the method has been shown to compare well with conventional colonoscopy in detecting polyps with a diameter of at least 10 mm in a recent study [67]. Sixty-eight asymptomatic men at average risk underwent CT colonography followed by optical colonoscopy on the same day, and a per-patient specificity of 89.7% could be obtained for CT colonography [67]. A similar study on 1233 asymptomatic adults resulted in sensitivities of 93.8, 93.9, and 88.7% for the detection of adenomatous polyps at least 10, 8, and 6 mm in diameter, respectively. The specificity was 96.0, 92.2, and 79.6% for the three sizes of polyps, respectively. Two polyps in the screening population were malignant. Both were detected on virtual colonography, but one of them was missed on optical colonscopy [68].

Narrow-collimation scanning (4×1 mm/ 4×1.25 mm,   16×0.625 mm/16×0.75 mm) is the method of choice for CT colonography [69]. While no difference in sensitivity could be observed with thick-section reconstructions, specificity markedly improved with thin sections [70]. Again, the radiation dose should be kept as low as possible, e.g., by using 120 kV and 120 effective mAs or 40 effective mAs for the supine or prone scans, respectively. Similarly to the early detection of lung cancer, new software tools are being developed that automatically detect suspicious polyps and can be used as a second reader to support the radiologist (polyp enhanced viewing PEV, Siemens, Forchheim, Germany).

References

1. Kalender W, Seissler W, Klotz E, Vock P (1990) Spiral volumetric CT with single-breath-hold technique, continuous transport and continuous scanner rotation. Radiology 176:181–183
2. Crawford CR, King KF (1990) Computed tomography scanning with simultaneous patient translation. Med Phys 17:967–982
3. Rubin GD, Dake MD, Semba CP (1995) Current status of three-dimensional spiral CT scanning for imaging the vasculature. Radiol Clin North Am 33(1):51–70
4. Napel S, Rubin GD, Jeffrey RB (1993) STS-MIP: a new reconstruction technique for CT of the chest. JCAT 17(5):832–8
5. Kalender W (1995) Thin-section three-dimensional spiral CT: is isotropic imaging possible? Radiology 197:578–580
6. Klingenbeck-Regn K, Schaller S, Flohr T, Ohnesorge B, Kopp AF, Baum U (1999) Subsecond multislice computed tomography: basics and applications. EJR 31:110–124
7. McCollough CH, Zink FE (1999) Performance evaluation of a multislice CT system. Med Phys 26:2223–2230
8. Ohnesorge B, Flohr T, Schaller S, Klingenbeck-Regn K, Becker C, Schöpf U J, Brüning R, Reiser MF (1999) Technische Grundlagen und Anwendungen der Mehrschicht-CT. Radiologe 39:923–931
9. Hu H, He HD, Foley WD, Fox SH (2000) Four multidetector-row helical CT: image quality and volume coverage speed. Radiology 215:55–62
10. Rubin GD, Schmidt AJ, Logan LJ, Sofilos MC (2001) Multi-detector row CT angiography of lower extremity arterial inflow and runoff: initial experience. Radiology 221(1):146–58
11. Schöpf UJ, Bruening RD, Hong C, Eibel R, Aydemir S, Crispin A, Becker C, Reiser MF (2001) Multislice helical CT of focal and diffuse lung disease: comprehensive diagnosis with reconstruction of contiguous and high-resolution CT sections from a single thin-collimation scan. Am J Roentgenol 177(1):179–84
12. Kachelrieß M, Ulzheimer S, Kalender W (2000) ECG-correlated image reconstruction from subsecond multi-slice spiral CT scans of the heart. Med Phys 27:1881–1902
13. Ohnesorge B, Flohr T, Becker C, Knez A, Kopp A, Fukuda K, Reiser M (2000) Herzbildgebung mit schneller, retrospektiv EKG-synchronisierter Mehrschichtspiral CT. Radiologe 40:111–117
14. Hong C, Becker CR, Huber A, Schoepf UJ, Ohnesorge B, Knez A, Brüning R, Reiser MF (2001) ECG-gated reconstructed multi-detector row CT coronary angiography: effect of varying trigger delay on image quality. Radiology 220:712–717
15. Nieman K, Oudkerk M, Rensing B, van Oijen P, Munne A, van Geuns R, de Feyter P (2001) Coronary angiography with multi-slice computed tomography. Lancet 357:599–603
16. Flohr T, Stierstorfer K, Bruder H, Simon J, Schaller S (2002) New technical developments in multislice CT, part 1: approaching isotropic resolution with sub-mm 16-slice scanning. Röfo Fortschr Geb Rontgenstr Neuen Bildgeb Verfahr 174:839–845
17. Flohr T, Bruder H, Stierstorfer K, Simon J, Schaller S, Ohnesorge B (2002) New technical developments in multislice CT, part 2: sub-millimeter 16-slice scanning and increased gantry rotation speed for cardiac imaging. Röfo Fortschr Geb Rontgenstr Neuen Bildgeb Verfahr 174:1022–1027

18. Nieman K, Cademartiri F, Lemos PA, Raaijmakers R, Pattynama PMT, de Feyter PJ (2002) Reliable noninvasive coronary angiography with fast submillimeter multislice spiral computed tomography. Circulation 106:2051–2054

19. Ropers D, Baum U, Pohle K et al. (2003) Detection of coronary artery stenoses with thin-slice multi-detector row spiral computed tomography and multiplanar reconstruction. Circulation 107:664–666

20. Flohr T, Bruder H, Stierstorfer K, Schaller S (2003) Evaluation of approaches to reduce spiral artifacts in multi-slice spiral CT. Abstract Book of the 89th Scientific Assembly and Annual Meeting of the RSNA 2003, p 567

21. Hu H (1999) Multi-slice helical CT: scan and reconstruction. Med Phys 26(1):5–18

22. Flohr T, Stierstorfer K, Raupach R, Ulzheimer S, Bruder H (2004) Performance evaluation of a 64-slice CT-system with z-flying focal spot. Röfo Fortschr Geb Rontgenstr Neuen Bildgeb Verfahr 176:1803–1810

23. Hsieh J (2001) Investigation of the slice sensitivity profile for step-and-shoot mode multi-slice computed tomography. Med Phys 28:491–500

24. International Electrotechnical Commission (2002) 60601-2-44. Amendment 1: Medical electrical equipment, Part 2-44: Particular requirements for the safety of X-ray equipment for computed tomography. International Electrotechnical Commision, Geneva

25. Morin R, Gerber T, McCollough C (2003) Radiation dose in computed tomography of the heart. Circulation 107:917–922

26. McCollough C (2003) Patient dose in cardiac computed tomography. Herz 28:1–6

27. Rubin GD, Napel S (1995) Increased scan pitch for vascular and thoracic spiral CT. Radiology 197:316–317

28. Saito Y, Suzuki T (1998) Evaluation of the performance of multi-slice CT system in non-helical scanning. Abstract Book of the 84th Scientific Assembly and Annual Meeting of the RSNA 1998, p 578.

29. Schaller S, Flohr T, Klingenbeck K, Krause J, Fuchs T, Kalender WA (2000) Spiral interpolation algorithm for multi-slice spiral CT – part I: theory. IEEE Trans Med Imag 19(9):822–834

30. Hsieh J (2003) Analytical models for multi-slice helical CT performance parameters. Med Phys 30(2):169–178

31. Taguchi T, Aradate H (1998) Algorithm for image reconstruction in multi-slice helical CT. Med Phys 25(4):550–561

32. Fuchs T, Krause J, Schaller S, Flohr T, Kalender WA (2000) Spiral interpolation algorithms for multislice spiral CT – part 2: measurement and evaluation of slice sensitivity profiles and noise at a clinical multislice system. IEEE Trans Med Imag 19(9):835–847

33. Feldkamp LA, Davis LC, Kress JW (1984) Practical cone-beam algorithm. J Opt Soc Am A 1:612–619

34. Wang G, Lin T, Cheng P (1993) A general cone-beam reconstruction algorithm. IEEE Trans Med Imag 12:486–496

35. Schaller S (1998) Practical image reconstruction for cone-beam computed tomography. PhD thesis, University Erlangen, Nürnberg, Germany

36. Grass M, Köhler T, Proksa R (2000) 3D cone-beam CT reconstruction for circular trajectories. Phys Med Biol 45(2):329–347

37. Hein I, Taguchi K, Silver MD, Kazarna M, Mori I (2003) Feldkamp-based cone-beam reconstruction for gantry-tilted helical multislice CT. Med Phys 30(12):3233–3242

38. Larson G, Ruth C, Crawford C (1998) Nutating slice CT image reconstruction apparatus and method. US Patent 5802134

39. Turbell H, Danielsson PE (1999) An improved PI-method for reconstruction from helical cone beam projections. IEEE Medical Imaging Conference, Seattle

40. Proksa R, Koehler T, Grass M, Timmer J (2000) The n-PI method for helical cone-beam CT. IEEE Trans Med Imag 19:848–863

41. Kachelrieß M, Schaller S, Kalender WA (2000) Advanced single-slice rebinning in cone-beam spiral CT. Med Phys 27(4):754–772

42. Bruder H, Kachelrieß M, Schaller S, Stierstorfer K, Flohr T (2000) Single-slice rebinning reconstruction in spiral cone-beam computed tomography. IEEE Trans Med Imag 19(9):873–887

43. Schaller S, Stierstorfer K, Bruder H, Kachelrieß M, Flohr T (2001) Novel approximate approach for high-quality image reconstruction in helical cone beam CT at arbitrary pitch. Proc SPIE Int Symp Med Imag 4322:113–127

44. Flohr T, Stierstorfer K, Bruder H, Simon J, Polacin A, Schaller S (2003) Image reconstruction and image quality evaluation for a 16-slice CT scanner Med Phys 30(5):832–845

45. Hsieh J, Toth TL, Simoni P, Grekowicz B, Slack CC, Seidenschnur GE (2001) A generalized helical reconstruction algorithm for multi-slice CT. Abstract Book of the 87th Scientific Assembly and Annual Meeting of the RSNA 2001, p 271

46. Hsieh J, Grekowicz B, Simoni P, Thibault JB, Joshi MC, Dutta S, Williams EC, Shaughnessy C, Sainath P (2003) Convolution reconstruction algorithm for multi-slice helical CT. In: Proc. SPIE Int. Symp. Med. Imag. 2003

47. Lell M, Wildberger J, Heuschmid M, Flohr T, Stierstorfer K, Fellner F, Lang W, Bautz W, Baum U (2002) CT-Angiographie der A. carotis: Erste Erfahrungen mit einem 16-Schicht-Spiral-CT – CT-angiography of the carotid artery: First results with a novel 16-slice-spiral-CT scanner. Röfo Fortschr Geb Rontgenstr Neuen Bildgeb Verfahr 174:1165–1169

48. Ertl-Wagner B, Hoffmann RT, Brüning R, Dichgans M, Reiser MF (2002) Supraaortale Gefäßdiagnostik mit dem 16-Zeilen-Multidetektor-Spiral-CT. Untersuchungs-protokoll und erste Erfahrungen. Radiologe 42:728–732

49. Tomandl BF, Klotz E, Handschu R, Stemper B, Reinhardt F, Huk WJ, Eberhardt KE, Fateh-Moghadem S (2003) Comprehensive imaging of ischemic stroke with multisection CT. RadioGraphics 23(3):565–592

50. Remy-Jardin J, Tillie-Leblond I, Szapiro D et al. (2002) CT angiography of pulmonary embolism in patients with underlying respiratory disease: impact of multislice CT on image quality and negative predictive value. Eur Radiol 12:1971–1978

51. Schoepf UJ, Becker CR, Hofmann LK, Das M, Flohr T, Ohnesorge BM et al. (2003) Multislice CT angiography. Eur Radiol 13:1946–1961

52. Wintersperger B, Helmberger T, Herzog P, Jakobs T, Waggershauser T, Becker C, Reiser M (2002) Hochaufgelöste abdominelle Übersichtsangiographie mit einem 16-Detektorzeilen-CT-System – New abdominal CT angiography protocol on a 16 detector-row CT scanner. Radiologe 42:722–727

53. Wintersperger B, Herzog P, Jakobs T, Reiser M, Becker C (2002) Initial experience with the clinical use of a 16 detector row CT system. Crit Rev Comput Tomogr 43:283–316

54. McCollough CH, Lindell EP, Primak AN, Fletcher JG, Stierstorfer K, Flohr TG (2004) Early experience with 64-slice CT and z-axis oversampling: novel applications and the elimination of helical artifacts in neuro CT. On-line Abstract Book of the 90th Scientific Assembly and Annual Meeting of the RSNA

55. Ohnesorge B, Flohr T, Becker C, Kopp A, Schoepf U, Baum U, Knez A, Klingenbeck-Regn K, Reiser M (2000) Cardiac imaging by means of electro-cardiographically gated multisection spiral CT – initial experience. Radiology 217:564–571

56. Becker C, Knez A, Ohnesorge B, Schöpf U, Reiser M (2000) Imaging of non calcified coronary plaques using helical CT with retrospective EKG gating. AJR 175:423–424

57. Flohr T, Schoepf U, Kuettner A et al. (2003) Advances in cardiac imaging with 16-section CT systems. Acad Radiol 10:386–401

58. Schöpf UJ, Becker CR, Ohnesorge BM, Yucel EK (2004) CT of coronary artery disease. Radiology 232:18–37

59. Schönhagen P, Halliburton SS, Stillman AE, Kuzmiak SA, Nissen S E, Tuzcu EM, White RD (2004) Noninvasive imaging of coronary arteries: current and future role of multi-detector row CT. Radiology 232:7–17

60. Ohnesorge B, Flohr T, Fischbach R, et al. (2002) Reproducibility of coronary calcium quantification in repeat examinations with retrospectively ECG-gated multi- section spiral CT. Eur Radiol 12:1532–1540

61. Ulzheimer S, Kalender W (2003) Assessment of calcium scoring performance in cardiac computed tomography. Eur Radiol 13:484–497

62. Achenbach S, Ulzheimer S, Baum U et al. (2000) Noninvasive coronary angiography by retrospectively ECG-gated multi-slice spiral CT. Circulation 102:2823–2828

63. Knez A, Becker C, Leber A, Ohnesorge B, Reiser M, Haberl R (2000) Non-invasive assessment of coronary artery stenoses with multidetector helical computed tomography. Circulation 101: e221–e222

64. Schroeder S, Kopp A, Baumbach A, Meisner C, Kuettner A, Georg C, Ohnesorge B, Herdeg C, Claussen C, Karsch K (2001) Noninvasive detection and evaluation of atherosclerotic coronary plaques with multi-slice computed tomography. JACC 37(5):1430–1435

65. Schroeder S, Flohr T, Kopp AF, Meisner C, Kuettner A, Herdeg C, Baumbach A, Ohnesorge B. Accuracy of density measurements within plaques located in artificial coronary arteries by X-ray multislice CT: results of a phantom study. JCAT 25(6):900–906

66. Henschke CI, McCauley DI, Yankelevitz DF, Naidich DP, McGuinness G, Miettinnen OS, Libby DM, Pasmantier MW, Koizumi J, Altorki AK, Smith JP (1999) Early lung cancer action project: overall design and findings from baseline screening. Lancet 354:99–105

67. Macari M, Bini EJ, Jacobs SL, Naik S, Lui YW, Milano A, Rajapaksa R, Megibow AJ, Babb J (2004) Colorectal polyps and cancers in asymptomatic average-risk patents: evaluation with CT colonography. Radiology 230(3):629–36

68. Pickhardt PJ, Choi JR, Hwang I, Butler JA, Puckett ML, Hildebrandt H A, Wong RK, Nugent PA, Mysliwiec PA, Schindler WR (2003) Computed tomographic virtual colonoscopy to screen for colorectal neoplasia in asymptomatic adults. N Engl J Med 349(23):2191–200

69. Wessling J, Fischbach R, Meier N, Allkemper T, Klusmeier J, Ludwig K, Heindel W (2003) CT colonography: protocol optimization with multi-detector row CT – study in an anthropomorphic colon phantom. Radiology 228(3):753–9

70. Lui YW, Macari M, Israel G, Bini EJ, Wang H, Babb J (2003) CT colonography data interpretation: effect of different section thicknesses – preliminary observations. Radiology 229(3):791–7

2 Future Perspectives of Multislice CT

T. Flohr

Owing to its ease of use and its widespread availability, general purpose CT continues to evolve into the most widely used diagnostic modality for routine examinations, especially in emergency situations or for oncological staging. CT primarily provides morphological information. In combination with other modalities, however, functional and metabolic information can also be obtained [1]. Therefore, combined systems for obtaining comprehensive structural and functional diagnoses will gain increasing importance in the near future. Major clinical applications of PET/CT so far have been oncological staging and the search for inflammatory foci. CT can add sensitivity to PET, as certain small lesions (e.g., lung nodules) may not be visualized on PET alone, and PET adds specificity to CT because indeterminate lesions seen on CT can often be diagnosed unequivocally as benign or malignant using PET information [2]. Occult sites of cancer recurrence can be identified to guide subsequent treatment in many patients. If the respective CT system is a state-of-the-art MSCT providing submillimeter collimation and fast gantry rotation, the additional potential for comprehensive cardiac examinations is opened. While CT delivers morphological information about stenoses or plaques in the coronaries, PET can add the assessment of cardiac function, e.g., by determining the hemodynamic relevance of a stenosis. The diagnostic benefit of PET/CT for cardiac applications is currently being evaluated [3]. Other potential applications include PET/CT guided biopsy or the use of PET/CT in radiation therapy planning to reduce the irradiated volume.

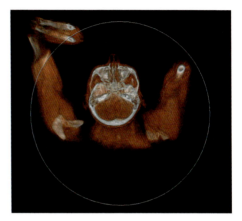

Fig. 2.1. Example of a CT scan with enlarged FOV of 70 cm achieved by an extrapolation of the original CT data. The original SFOV with 50-cm diameter is indicated by a circle

Reconstruction of the CT images in a sufficient field of view without truncation of anatomical structures (e.g., arms) is a prerequisite for adequate attenuation correction of the PET images. An enlarged FOV of up to 70 cm can be realized by extrapolation of the measured CT data. Pertinent algorithms can be found, e.g., in [4,5] (see Fig. 2.1).

Figure 2.2 shows sagittal and coronal MPRs with superimposed PET images of a 46-year-old patient with renal cancer, status post nephrectomy and chemotherapy (courtesy of Indiana University, Indianapolis, USA). The CT/PET examination identified a mediastinal lymph node metastasis by increased focal uptake of the FDG tracer (arrow), which supports the notion of PET scanning as adding a "new contrast agent" to CT.

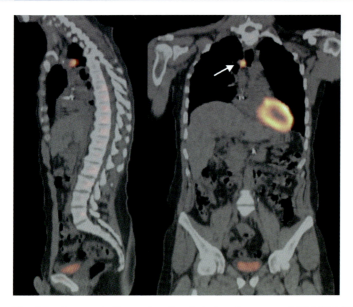

Fig. 2.2. Case study illustrating the clinical performance of PET-CT. MPR with superimposed PET images of a patient with renal cancer. A mediastinal lymph node metastasis (*arrow*) is identified by increased focal uptake of the FDG tracer (courtesy of Indiana University, Indianapolis, USA)

Combined CT/SPECT systems are another promising modality. Potential applications are currently being investigated and range from the localization of parathyroid lesions [6] and heterotopic splenic tissue [7] and the detection of recurrent nasopharyngeal carcinomas [8] to imaging of aortic prosthesis infection [9]. Again, the combination of state-of-the-art MSCT systems with SPECT scanners can open new potentials for cardiac diagnosis.

CT virtual simulation is gaining increasing importance with a more widespread adoption of three-dimensional conformal and intensity modulated radiation therapy. Using respiratory gating of the CT scan, i.e., the correlation of CT data acquisition with the breathing curve of the patient similar to ECG-gated cardiac scanning, 4D tumor motion can be evaluated to minimize the irradiated volume during radiation therapy, to concentrate the radiation dose in the tumor and to save healthy tissue. Figure 2.3 shows an example for a CT acquisition with respiratory gating on a patient with lung metastases. The VRTs have been obtained

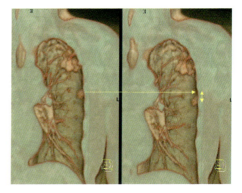

Fig 2.3. Case study illustrating CT data acquisition with respiratory gating. VRTs in end-inspiration and end-expiration for a patient with lung metastases. Metastases attached to the pleura (*arrow*) show significant movement during the breathing cycle (courtesy of J. Debus, University of Heidelberg, Germany)

for end-inspiration and end-expiration, metastases attached to the pleura (arrow) show significant movement during the breathing cycle.

Using general-purpose CT systems with gantry openings of typically 70-cm diameter, some patients, e.g., women with breast cancer, cannot always be scanned in the treatment position. These applications, along with interventional procedures and trauma protocols, will be facilitated by CT systems with larger bore [10]. Recently, concepts of 4-slice, 16-slice and 40-slice CT scanners with bore diameters of up to 85 cm and reconstruction fields of up to 82 cm were introduced, owing to image reconstruction based on data extrapolation. These systems will probably gain considerable importance in the near future, in radiation therapy, in emergency rooms and in particular with regard to the dramatically increasing number of severely obese patients in western societies.

For general purpose CT, we are currently witnessing a further increase in the number of simultaneously acquired slices. The latest generation of MSCT systems with up to 64 simultaneously acquired slices was introduced in 2004. In contrast to the transition from single-slice to 4-slice and 16-slice CT clinical performance will improve only incrementally with a further increase in the number of detector rows. Clinical progress can more likely be expected from further improved spatial resolution, enabled, e.g., by novel z-sampling schemes, such as double z-sampling, and improved temporal resolution, enabled by faster gantry rotation, rather than from an increase in the volume coverage speed. In clinical reality the latter only rarely becomes a limiting factor since the introduction of 16-slice CT. As soon as all relevant examinations can be performed in a comfortable breath hold of not more than 10 s, a further increase of the slice number will not provide significant clinical benefit.

The trend towards a larger number of slices in the future will therefore not be driven by the need to increase scan speed in spiral acquisition modes, but rather by the desire to increase volume coverage in non-spiral dynamic acquisitions, e.g., by the introduction of area detectors large enough to cover entire organs, such as the heart, the kidneys or the brain, in one axial scan (~120 mm scan range). With these systems, dynamic volume scanning will become feasible, opening up a whole spectrum of new applications, such as functional or volume perfusion studies. Area detector technology is currently under development, but no commercially available system so far fulfills the requirements of medical CT with regard to contrast resolution and fast data readout. A scanner with 256×0.5 mm detector elements has been proposed by one manufacturer and appears conceptually promising, but has not left the prototype stage so far. Prototype systems by other vendors use CsI-aSi flat panel detector technology, originally used for conventional catheter angiography, which is limited in low contrast resolution and scan speed. Due to the intrinsic slow signal decay of flat panel detectors rotation times of at least 20 s are needed to acquire a sufficient number of projections (≥ 600). Short gantry rotation times < 0.5 s, which are a prerequisite for successful examination of moving organs such as the heart, are therefore still beyond the scope of such systems. Spatial resolution is excellent, though, due to the small detector pixel size. Figure 2.4 shows a prototype setup, where a flat panel detector was incorporated into a standard CT gantry (SOMATOM Sensation 16, Forchheim, Germany). The detector covers a 25×25×18 cm^3 scan field of view and the spatial resolution is approximately 250×250×250 μm^3, both measured in the center of rotation. With a novel dynamic gain-switching mode, low-contrast detectability has been significantly enhanced. Small contrast differences down to 5 HU can be differentiated (see the image of a low contrast phantom in Fig. 2.5). This is an important step on the way towards expanding the application spectrum of such a system from mere high-contrast scanning to general radiology CT applications. Intracranial hemorrhage, for instance, can now be reliably detected.

In preclinical installations, potential clinical applications of flat-panel volume CT systems are currently being evaluated [11–13]. The application spectrum ranges from ultrahigh resolution bone imaging to dynamic CT angiographic studies and functional examinations. Inner ear imaging can substantially benefit from the in-

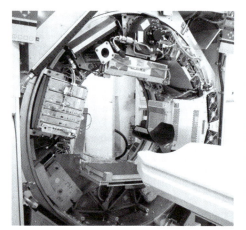

Fig. 2.4. Prototype setup incorporating a CsI-abi flat-panel detector in a standard CT gantry (SOMATOM Sensation 16, Siemens, Forchheim, Germany)

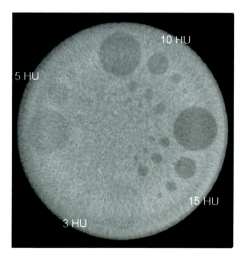

Fig. 2.5. Axial scan of a low-contrast phantom acquired with the flat-panel CT prototype shown in Fig. 2.4 demonstrating low contrast resolution down to 5 HU, enabled by a novel, dynamic gain-switching mode

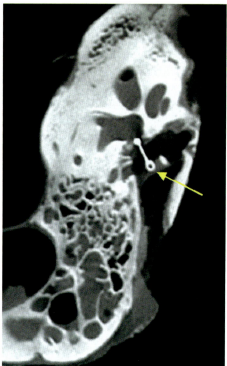

Fig. 2.6. Multiplanar reformation of an inner ear specimen with a stapes prosthesis scanned with the flat-panel CT prototype with CsI-aSi detector shown in Fig. 2.4. An isotropic resolution of 0.25 mm³ enables excellent detail visualization (courtesy of R. Gupta, MGH, Boston, USA)

creased spatial resolution (see Fig. 2.6 for the example of a scan of an inner ear specimen with a prosthesis of the stapes). Figure 2.7 shows VRTs of a contrast-filled heart specimen demonstrating excellent spatial resolution, which enables visualization of even very small side branches of the coronary artery tree. Potentially, the lumen of small stents in the coronary arteries can be evaluated, and in-stent restenosis can be reliably detected. Other interesting applications for volume CT include dynamic CTA examinations, e.g., of the carotids and the circle of Willis. Figure 2.8 shows an example of a CTA of the head and neck of a living rabbit.

The combination of area detectors that provide sufficient image quality with fast gantry rotation speeds will be a promising technical concept for medical CT systems. Yet, a potential increase in spatial resolution to the level of flat-panel CT will be associated with increased dose demands, and the clinical benefit has to be carefully considered in the light of the applied patient dose.

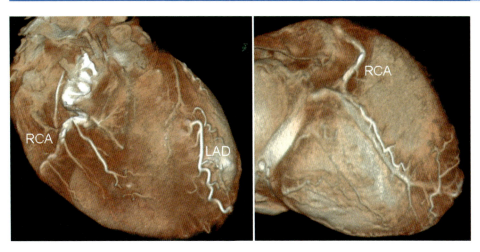

Fig. 2.7. Volume-rendered display of a stationary heart specimen scanned with the flat-panel CT prototype with CsI-aSi detector shown in Fig. 2.4. An isotropic resolution of 0.25 mm³ enables exquisite delineation of small side branches of the contrast filled coronary artery tree (courtesy of U. J. Schoepf, MUSC, Charleston, USA)

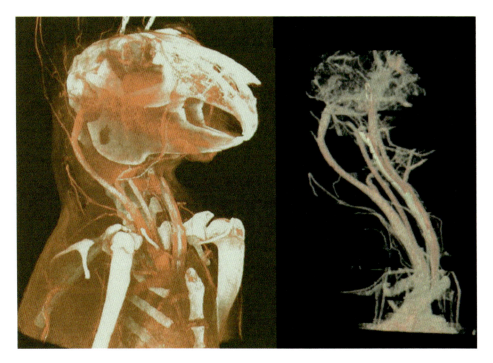

Fig. 2.8. CTA of the head and neck of a rabbit scanned with the flat-panel CT prototype with CsI-aSi detector shown in Fig. 2.4 (courtesy of R. Gupta, MGH, Boston, USA)

References

1. Townsend DW, Cherry SR (2001) Combining anatomy and function: the path of true image fusion. Eur Radiol 11(10):1968–1974
2. von Schulthess GK (2004) Positron emission tomography versus positron emission tomography/computed tomography: from "unclear" to "new-clear" medicine. Mol Imaging Biol 6(4):183–7
3. Namdar M, Kaufmann P, Hany T, von Schulthess G (2003) Combined CT-angiogram and PET perfusion imaging for assessment of CAD in a novel PET/CT: a pilot feasibility study. Eur Radiol 13(S):165
4. Ohnesorge B, Flohr T, Schwarz K, Heiken JP, Bae KT (2000) Efficient correction for CT image artifacts caused by objects extending outside the scan field of view. Med Phys 27(1):39–46
5. Hsieh J, Chao E H, Grekowicz B, Horst A, McOlash S, Myers T J. A Reconstruction Algorithm to Extend the Field-of-view Beyond the Scanner Limit, *Abstract Book of the 89th Scientific Assembly and Annual Meeting of the RSNA* 2003, 168
6. Kaczirek K, Prager G, Kienast O, Dobrozemsky G, Dudzak R, Niederle B, Kurtaran A (2003) Combined transmission and (99m)Tc-sestamibi emission tomography for localization of mediastinal parathyroid glands. Nuklearmedizin 42(5):220–3
7. Horger M, Eschmann SM, Lengerke C, Claussen CD, Pfannenberg C, Bares R (2003) Improved detection of splenosis in patients with haematological disorders: the role of combined transmission-emission tomography. Eur J Nucl Med Mol Imaging 30(2):316–9
8. Tai CJ, Shian YC, Wang IJ, Ho YJ, Ho ST, Kao CH (2003) Detection of recurrent or residual nasopharyngeal carcinomas after radiotherapy with technetium-99m tetrofosmin single photon emission computed tomography and comparison with computed tomography – a preliminary study. Cancer Invest 21(4):536–41
9. Hofmann A, Zetting G, Wachter S, Kurtaran A, Kainberger F, Dudzak R (2002) Imaging of aortic prosthesis infection with a combined SPECT-CT device. Eur J Nucl Med Mol Imaging 29(6):836
10. Garcia-Ramirez IJ, Mutic S, Dempsey JF, Low DA, Purdy JA (2002) Performance evaluation of an 85 cm bore X-ray computed tomography scanner designed for radiation oncology and comparison with current diagnostic CT scanners. Int J Radiat Oncol Biol Phys 52(4):1123–31
11. Enzweiler C, Chan P, Hoffmann U et al. (2003) In vitro coronary stent imaging: novel flat-panel volume CT versus multidetector CT. Eur Radiol 13(S):195
12. Knollmann F, Pfoh A (2003) Image in cardiovascular medicine. Coronary artery imaging with flat-panel computed tomography. Circulation 107(8):1209
13. Gupta R, Stierstorfer K, Popescu S, Flohr T, Schaller S, Curtin HD (2003) Temporal bone imaging using a large field-of-view rotating flat-panel CT scanner. Abstract Book of the 89th Scientific Assembly and Annual Meeting of the RSNA 2003, p 375

3 Dose Considerations and Radiation Protection Issues in Multislice CT

G. Brix and H.D. Nagel

3.1 Introduction

After the introduction of single-slice spiral CT (SSCT) scanners into clinical practice in 1989, the next considerable advance was the development of multislice spiral CT (MSCT) systems a few years ago. MSCT scanners are capable of simultaneously scanning a number of slices (N=2, 4, 8, 16,...) within a reduced scan time. As will be described in the subsequent chapters, the resulting improvement in scanner performance has increased the clinical efficacy of CT procedures and offered promising new applications in diagnostic imaging.

On the other hand, data from various national surveys have confirmed, as a general pattern, the growing impact of CT as a major source of patient and population exposure. In Germany, for example, it accounted for 6% of all X-ray examinations conducted in 2001, but for 47% of the resultant collective effective dose, with an increase of about 7% per year. Even higher numbers are reported for Japan and the USA. To limit patient exposure related to CT procedures, the following general principles of radiological protection have to be taken into account [1,2]:

- *Justification*: There must be sufficient net benefit for the individual patient, balancing the potential benefits of a CT examination against the individual detriment that may be caused by radiation exposure. In this context, the efficacy, benefits and risks of available alternative imaging techniques must be considered as having the same objective but either no or less exposure to ionizing radiation.

- *Optimization:* Radiation exposure of patients undergoing a CT procedure shall be kept "as low as reasonably achievable" (ALARA principle), which means that the scan protocols employed have to be optimized in order to define an acceptable balance between patient exposure and necessary diagnostic image quality.

It is the purpose of this chapter (1) to summarize the most relevant dosimetric quantities used for dose assessment in CT, (2) to give an overview on the specific factors determining radiation exposure of patients in MSCT, (3) to present the main results of the first dedicated survey on MSCT practice worldwide, and (4) to provide suggestions for the optimization of MSCT protocols to balance patient exposure against image quality.

3.2 Quantities for Dose Assessment in CT

3.2.1 Organ and Effective Dose

For the assessment of detrimental radiation effects, it is generally assumed that the probability of biological damage is directly proportional to the energy deposited by ionizing radiation in a specified organ or tissue. Therefore, the fundamental dosimetric quantity is the *absorbed dose*, which is defined as the radiation energy absorbed in a small volume element of matter divided by its mass. In the SI system the absorbed dose is given in the unit *Gray* (1 Gy = 1 J/kg). The absorbed dose averaged over the total mass of an organ or tissue T is denoted as organ dose, D_T. Whenever an organ

Table 3.1. Tissue weighting factors w_T given in [1] reflecting the relative susceptibility of various tissues and organs to ionizing radiation

Tissue or organ	w_T	$\sum w_T$
Gonads	0.20	0.20
Bone marrow, lungs, colon, stomach	0.12	0.48
Liver, thyroid, esophagus, breast, bladder	0.05	0.25
Bone surface, skin	0.01	0.02
Remaining organs*	-	0.05

* Remaining organs consist of a group of additional organs and tissues with a lower sensitivity to radiation-induced effects for which the average dose must be used: small intestine, brain, spleen, muscle tissue, adrenals, kidneys, pancreas, thymus and uterus. If a single one of the remaining organs receives a higher dose than any of the 12 organs with specific weighting factors, then the dose to that particular remaining organ is weighted by a factor of 0.025. In this case, the average dose to the other organs in the remainder group is weighted by a factor of only 0.025. This scenario is of particular importance for head examinations

is only partially irradiated, as in the case of an organ extending over the whole body (e.g., red bone marrow or skin) or an organ situated at the border of the irradiated body region, the organ dose may differ markedly from the absorbed dose at different positions within that organ.

Tissues and organs are not equally sensitive to the effects of ionizing radiation. For this reason, tissue weighting factors, w_T, were provided by the International Commission on Radiological Protection (ICRP) [1] for a reference population of equal numbers of both sexes and a wide range of ages (Table 3.1). These factors indicate the relative proportion of each organ or tissue to the total health detriment – in terms of the risk of fatal cancers and hereditary defects – resulting from uniform irradiation of the whole body. If the body is exposed in a nonuniform manner as, for example, in a patient undergoing a CT examination, the sum of the products of the organ dose and the corresponding tissue weighting factor determined for each of the various organs or tissues exposed must be computed:

$$E = \sum_T w_T \cdot D_T \quad \text{with} \quad \sum_T w_T = 1. \quad (3.1)$$

The resulting quantity is denoted as effective dose E and expressed in the SI unit *Sievert* (Sv). On the basis of the effective dose, it is possible to assess and to compare the probability of stochastic radiation effects resulting from different radiation exposures as, for example, diverse X-ray or nuclear medicine procedures yielding a different pattern of dose distribution in the body. It should be mentioned, however, that the weighting factors provided by the ICRP are generic, rather than patient-specific, because the age and gender of patients are not taken into account. In fact, the radiation risk is somewhat higher for females and for younger patients when compared to males and older patients.

3.2.2 Operational Dose Quantities

In practice, neither organ nor effective doses can be measured directly. In order to overcome this difficulty, operational dose quantities are frequently used, which can easily be measured with an appropriate phantom. These quantities can be used for comparison of different devices and parameter settings within a particular diagnostic modality (e.g., CT). Moreover, they form

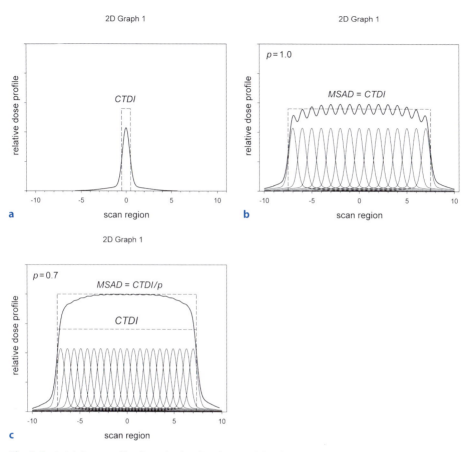

Fig. 3.1. Axial dose profiles for a single-slice CT scan (**a**), a CT scan series with 15 slices acquired with p = 1.0 (**b**), and a CT scan series with 21 slices acquired with p = 0.7 (**c**). The slice thickness is 10 mm in each case. Indicated are the *CTDI* and the *MSAD*

the basis for the estimation of organ and effective doses by means of complex Monte Carlo calculations performed for anthropomorphic mathematical models [3,4].

The most relevant dose descriptor for CT is the computed tomography dose index (*CTDI*) (given in mGy). As illustrated in Fig. 3.1a, the *CTDI* indicates the dose value inside an irradiated slice that would result if the dose profile were entirely concentrated in a rectangular profile of width equal to the nominal slice thickness. Accordingly, all dose contributions from outside the nominal slice width, such as the areas under the tails of the real dose profile, are added to the area inside the slice.

Whenever several adjacent slices are scanned instead of a single slice – as is usu-

ally the case in CT practice – the dose for a particular slice is increased due to the contributions from slices in its neighborhood (see Fig. 3.1b,c). For this reason, the dose in the central portion of the superimposed dose profile – the multiple scan average dose (*MSAD*) – is markedly larger than the peak value for a single slice. The degree of overlap of slice profiles is characterized by the pitch factor, *p*. In MSCT this factor is defined as

$$p = \frac{TF}{s_{coll}\,M} \qquad (3.2)$$

where TF is the table feed, s_{coll} is the slice (or detector) collimation, and M the number of simultaneously acquired slices. Using this definition, the MSAD is given by

$$\text{MSAD} = \frac{\text{CTDI}}{p} \qquad (3.3)$$

To obtain the average dose for a multiple-slice CT scan performed over a larger body region, it is thus sufficient to measure the CTDI from a single rotation by acquiring the dose over the entire dose profile. The situation is illustrated in Figs. 3.1b,c for two CT series carried out over the same scan length with $p = 1$ (MASD = CTDI) and $p < 1$ (MASD = CTDI), respectively.

In practice, CTDI measurements are usually performed with a pencil ionization chamber with an active length of 100 mm, which is positioned at the center ($\text{CTDI}_{100,c}$) and at the periphery ($\text{CTDI}_{100,p}$) of either a standard head or body CT dosimetry phantom (Fig. 3.2). On the assumption that the dose decreases linearly with the radial position from the surface to the center of the phantom, the average dose is given by the weighted CTDI:

$$\text{CTDI}_w = \frac{1}{3}\text{CTDI}_{100,c} + \frac{2}{3}\text{CTDI}_{100,p} \qquad (3.4)$$

Because the CTDI_w is directly proportional to the electrical current–time product (Q_{el} in mAs) chosen for the scan, it has to be measured for all combinations of tube potentials (U in kV) and slice collimations that can be realized at the specific type of scanner but only for a fixed Q_{el} value.

According to the revised IEC-standard 60601-2-44, the dose quantity displayed at the operator's console of a CT system is the effective or volume CTDI:

$$\text{CTDI}_{vol} = \frac{\text{CTDI}_w}{p} \qquad (3.5)$$

that takes the effect of overlap of slice profiles at the level of local dose into account. The CTDI_{vol} is the principal dose descriptor in CT, reflecting not only the combined effect of the scan parameters Q_{el}, U, p, and s_{coll} on the local dose level, but also of scanner specific factors such as beam filtration, beam shaping filter, geometry, and over-beaming (see below).

Besides the CTDI_{vol}, the length L of the scan region is the second important parameter that determines radiation exposure of

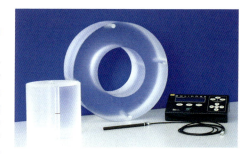

Fig. 3.2. Cylindrical standard CT dosimetry phantoms made from Perspex. The phantoms with a diameter of 16 cm and 32 cm are used for representative *CTDI* measurements of the head and trunk, respectively. For dose measurement the pencil ionization chamber with an active length of 100 mm is inserted into the five holes

patients undergoing a CT procedure. Therefore, the dose–length product (DLP)

$$\text{DLP} = \text{CTDI}_{vol}\, L \qquad (3.6)$$

(given in mGy·cm), is used as a further operational dose quantity.

Nevertheless, the relevant quantity for risk assessment is the effective dose, which takes not only the organ doses into account but also the relative radiation susceptibility of the various organs and tissues within the scanned body region (see Sect 3.2.1). According to the generic method presented in the *European Guidelines on Quality Criteria for CT* [5], coarse estimates of E can be derived from the *DLP* by using appropriate conversion factors given in that report for different body regions (head, neck, chest, abdomen, and pelvis).

3.2.3 Diagnostic Reference Levels

In its publication on *Radiological Protection and Safety in Medicine* [6] the ICRP recommends the use of diagnostic reference levels (DRLs) for patient examinations as a measure of optimization of protection. The DRLs apply to an easily measurable operational dose quantity and are intended for use as a simple test for identifying situations where the levels of

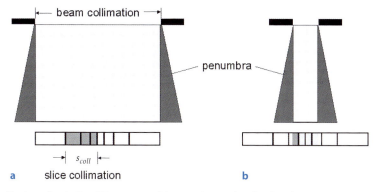

Fig. 3.3. Design of a 4-slice CT scanner with a nonisotropic adaptive detector array. By changing beam collimation and electronically binning different numbers of adjacent detector elements together, images from four slices with variable thickness can be acquired simultaneously. **a** Four thick slices. **b** Four thin slices. The figure reveals that the relative contribution of overbeaming (*dark grey* penumbra) to total patient exposure becomes more relevant with decreasing slice thickness

patient dose are unusually high. If patient doses related to a specific procedure consistently exceed the corresponding DRL, there should be a local review of the procedures and equipment. Measures aimed at the reduction of dose levels should be taken, if necessary.

The council of the European Union has adopted this concept in the Council Directive 97/43/EURATOM [2]. By this means, the member states of the EU are obliged to adopt the DRLs into national legislation and regulations concerning radiation protection. Additionally, DRLs for various CT examinations have been published – in terms of the operational dose quantities $CTDI_w$ and DLP – by the European Commission [5]. According to Eq. 3.5, the $CTDI_w$ can easily be determined from the $CTDI_{vol}$ displayed on the operator's console.

3.3 MSCT-Specific Features Influencing Radiation Exposure

There are a number of features specific to MSCT systems that systematically influence patient exposure compared to SSCT scanners. These are either inherent to the principle of MSCT scanning or a conse-

quence of the improved imaging capabilities provided by modern MSCT systems.

3.3.1 Detector Efficiency

Individual detectors in a multirow, solid-state detector array are separated by narrow strips (septa), which are not sensitive to radiation and thus do not contribute to the detector signal. Due to the large number of strips, these inactive zones result in geometrical losses, the degree of which depends on the design of the detector array. In addition, further losses occur due to a decrease in sensitivity at the edges of each row that results from cutting the scintillator crystal. In contrast to a single-row detector array whose width can be larger than the maximum slice thickness, the edges of the rows in a multirow detector array are located inside the beam (Fig. 3.3). Both effects result in a decrease of the net efficiency of a solid-state detector array.

3.3.2 Beam Geometry

By using cone beams instead of fan beams, the incidence of scatter is increased, which requires the use of either more dose to preserve the contrast-to-noise ratio or technical means associated with a decrease in geometric efficiency.

3.3.3 Overbeaming

In MSCT, data from each detector contribute to every reconstructed image. Therefore, the image noise and the slice sensitivity profile for each slice need to be similar to reduce image artifacts. To accommodate this condition for MSCT systems with more than two detector rows, beam collimation is usually adjusted in such a way that the focal spot-collimator blade penumbra falls outside the edge detectors (see Fig. 3.3). The resulting overbeaming causes an increased radiation dose compared to single-slice and (most) dual-slice scanners, where the collimator width is in general smaller than the maximum detector width. As shown in Fig. 3.3, this effect becomes more relevant for thinner slices, which are preferred for MSCT scanners with $N \geq 4$ in contrast to single- and dual-slice systems. However, with the availability of MSCT systems capable of scanning more than four slices simultaneously ($N = 8, 16,...$), overbeaming will become less significant in future.

3.3.4 Overranging

In spiral CT, the actual scan range is larger than the range defined on the operator's console, because additional data are required for interpolation at the beginning and the end of the body region to be scanned. At present, with a maximum total width of the detector arrays of typically 20 mm, overranging is still not a major issue. This will change in the future, however, as soon as much wider arrays become available.

3.3.5 Tube Output and Rotation Time

The improved utilization of tube output in combination with a reduced rotation time allow for significant changes in scan protocol settings. The ability to scan a given volume in the same time with reduced slice thickness, thus enabling the production of *isotropic voxels* is the most prominent implication. By using this approach, an increase in patient dose seems to be necessary, at least in clinical indications limited by noise, when thinner slices are used in order to improve spatial resolution in the z-direction.

3.3.6 ECG Gating

There are new applications, such as CT angiography (CTA) of the coronary arteries, that are preferentially performed with retrospective ECG gating, thereby making use of selected intervals during the cardiac cycle only while exposing the patient during the entire cycle.

3.4 Current MSCT Practice

3.4.1 German MSCT Survey 2002

At the beginning of 2002, a nationwide survey on MSCT practice was conducted in Germany. Similar to a previous nationwide survey on SSCT practice in 1999 [7], the recent survey was based on questionnaires sent to 207 hospitals and private practices operating an MSCT scanner at the end of 2001. The examinations considered are defined in Table 3.2 and details of the study design and methodology used for dose assessment can be found in [8]. The results summarized in Table 3.2 are based on data reported for 113 scanners: 39 2-slice scanners (most of them former Elscint CT Twin), 73 4-slice scanners (predominantly Siemens Volume Zoom), and one 8-slice scanner (GE LightSpeed Ultra).

In Fig. 3.4, average values of the scan length L, the number of scan series n_{ser}, the operational dose quantities $CTDI_{vol}$ and DLP per scan, as well as the effective dose E per examination (including precontrast and postcontrast scans) for 2- and 4-slice CT scanners are plotted for the 14 standard examinations considered relative to the corresponding mean values established for

Table 3.2. Definition of 14 standard and four special examinations frequently carried out on MSCT scanners along with the corresponding average scan parameters and dose values, as determined in a nationwide survey performed in Germany in 2002 [4][a]

Examinations		Scan parameters						Dose values per scan			Scan series
Type	Abbreviation	U (kV)	Q_{el} (mAs)	s_{coll} (mm)	p	s (mm)	L (cm)	$CTDI_{vol}$ (mGy)	DLP (mGy cm)	E (mSv)	n_{ser}
Brain	BR	122	317	5.7	1.0	7.3	13.2	60.6	813	2.2	1.3
Face and sinuses	FS	123	123	1.7	1.1	2.4	10.2	26.7	272	0.8	1.0
Face and neck	FA / NE[b]	122	202	3.0	1.1	4.2	19.5	14.4	288	1.9	1.1
Chest	CH	128	163	4.0	1.4	6.3	31.0	10.9	339	5.5	1.0
Abdomen & pelvis	AB / PE	121	200	4.3	1.3	6.6	41.9	12.6	529	9.7	1.5
Pelvis	PE	123	203	4.0	1.2	6.0	23.6	14.8	349	6.3	1.2
Liver / kidney	LI / KI	121	191	3.8	1.2	5.8	22.7	12.8	292	5.5	2.1
Whole trunk	WT	124	194	4.0	1.3	6.6	65.4	12.8	836	14.5	1.2
Aorta, thoratic	AT	123	176	2.7	1.4	4.1	28.5	12.6	361	6.1	1.1
Aorta, abdominal	AA	122	197	2.8	1.4	4.2	37.5	12.8	484	9.0	1.2
Pulmonary vessels	PV	124	179	1.9	1.4	3.2	23.5	12.8	300	5.2	1.0
Pelvis, skeleton	PS	129	204	2.3	1.2	3.4	22.3	19.4	438	8.2	1.0
Cervical spine	CS[b]	128	243	1.7	1.0	2.1	10.0	27.0	275	2.9	1.0
Lumbar spine	LS	130	285	2.3	1.0	2.8	13.5	32.4	441	8.1	1.0
Extremities	EX	122	120	1.1	1.1	1.7	12.6	14.4	169	--	1.0
Coronary CTA	COAN	121	133	1.2	0.4	1.7	13.1	43.1	564	10.2	1.1
Calcium scoring	CASO	121	88	2.4	0.7	2.7	13.8	12.4	171	3.1	1.0
Virtual colonoscopy	VICO	120	138	1.2	1.5	2.5	37.7	11.4	440	8.0	1.2

[a] U: tube potential, Q_{el}: electrical current–time product, s_{coll}: slice collimation, p: pitch factor, s: reconstructed slice thickness, L: scan length, $CTDI_{vol}$: volume CT dose index, DLP: dose–length product, E: effective dose

[b] Body mode

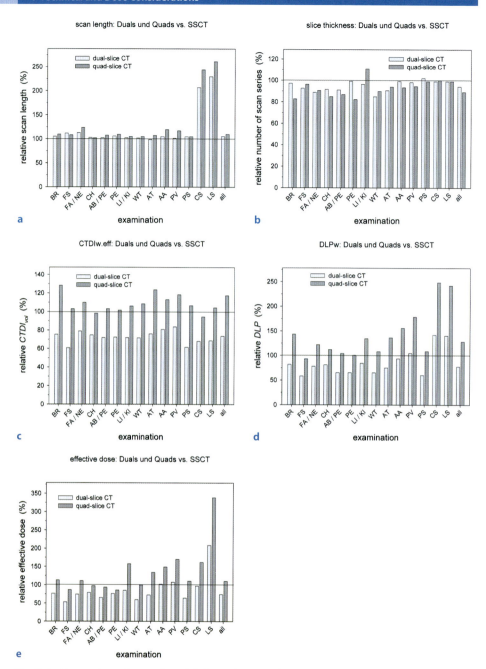

Fig. 3.4. Mean values of **a** scan length L, **b** number n_{ser} of scan series, **c** CTDI$_{vol}$ per scan series **d** DLP per scan series, and **e** effective dose E per examination determined for 2-slice and 4-slice scanners in a nationwide survey in Germany [8] for the 14 standard CT examinations defined in Table 3.2 along with the corresponding mean values averaged by weight over all CT examinations. Data are presented relative to the corresponding mean values determined in a previous survey [7] for modern SSCT scanners

conventional spiral CT examinations [7]. The reference group comprises 398 modern SSCT systems installed before June 1999. As an overall trend, the average effective dose to patients from CT examinations has changed from 7.4 mSv at single-slice to 5.5 mSv and 8.1 mSv for 2-slice and 4-slice scanners, respectively. The most relevant differences in the effective dose were found for standard brain, liver/kidneys, CTA, and spine examinations (see Fig. 3.4e). This increase is mainly explained by the following facts:

- For the majority of scanners, reduced beam filtration is used in the head scanning mode, resulting in an increased tube output per mAs. This does not hold for most single-slice scanners.
- In examinations of the liver or kidneys, the average number of scan series is somewhat increased.
- In CTA, the average scan length is somewhat increased. The main reason, however, is the increase in local dose to compensate for the increased noise owing to the selection of much narrower slices.
- For the spine, the average scan length is increased considerably, as there is now a clear preference to scan the entire spine section (cervical spine, lumbar spine) in the spiral mode instead of only selected segments.

3.5   Suggestions on How to Optimize MSCT Practice

The increased noise and the extended overbeaming associated with the preferred use of narrow slice collimations is the most important implication of MSCT scanning. The key factor towards optimization of current MSCT practice is how to handle this issue.

3.5.1   How to Avoid Overbeaming

As overbeaming is most pronounced on 4-slice scanners, data acquisition with very narrow slice collimation should be avoided for these systems unless there is a real diagnostic need to do so (e.g., for multiplanar reformatting (MPR) or if improved spatial z-resolution is mandatory). Otherwise, scans should be carried out with medium or wide collimation. This particularly holds for scanners with comparatively high overbeaming. For MSCT scanners with $N \geq 16$, there is less overbeaming and therefore no special attention is required.

3.5.2   How to Face Increased Noise

In order to reduce image noise, reconstructing thicker slices is recommended (multiplanar volume reconstruction, MPVR). This is already practiced by the majority of MSCT users, although the average (reconstructed) slice thickness still remains significantly smaller than for SSCT scanners. Another fact, however, deserves much more attention: the reduction of partial volume effects. Lesion contrast is enhanced with narrow slice collimation due to the reduction of partial volume effects, and thus the contrast-to-noise ratio is improved even in the presence of increased noise. Therefore, if a narrow slice thickness is used, the visibility of small details improves despite increased noise. There is thus no need to increase radiation dose when making use of thinner slices.

3.5.3   Technical Means

Dose reduction can be further facilitated by a variety of technical measures. Meanwhile, all CT manufacturers have developed systems for automatic dose control. These adjust the electrical current–time product to individual patient size and shape and are currently employed in the latest generation of MSCT scanners [3]. Dedicated smoothing filters that preserve spatial resolution are another approach. Even more sophisticated solutions can be expected in the next years.

3.6 Summary

Results from a recent survey on MSCT practice in Germany indicate that 2-slice scanners (which are mainly former Elscint Twin scanners) are used at dose levels comparable with modern SSCT scanners, while dose values related with 4-slice scanner protocols are currently significantly, but not alarmingly, higher. The main reasons are: (1) reduced slice thickness, which tempts the users to increase the electrical current–time product in order to compensate for increased noise, (2) overbeaming due to penumbral effects, which are most pronounced at narrow slice collimation, and (3) reduced transparency of the implications of parameter settings on dose.

The key factor to reduce dose at MSCT systems with N ≥ 4 to a level comparable to modern single-slice and dual-slice scanners is to appreciate the improved detail contrast achieved with thin slices due to reduced partial volume effect. This overcompensates for the drawback of increased noise. Thus, at least the same dose level as for modern SSCT scanners should be attainable. Furthermore, new technical means have the potential for dose reduction. It should be emphasized, however, that technical means are only a prerequisite, but no guarantee for dose reduction. Of greatest importance is appropriate training and guidance of the medical and technical staff operating the MSCT scanner with respect to the specific factors determining patient exposure and its reduction.

References

1. ICRP (1991) Publication 60: 1990 Recommendations of the International Commission on Radiological Protection. Ann ICRP 21(1–3)
2. Council of the European Union (1997) Council directive 97/43/Euratom of 30 June 1997 on health protection against the dangers of ionizing radiation in relation to medical exposure, and repealing directive 84/466/Euratom. Document 397L0043. Official journal no. L 180, 09/07/1997, p 0022–0027
3. Nagel HD, Galanski M, Hidajat N, Maier W, Schmidt T (2002) Radiation exposure in computed tomography – fundamentals, influencing parameters, dose assessment, optimisation, scanner data, terminology. CTB Publications, Hamburg, ctb-publications@gmx.de
4. Brix G, Lechel U, Veit R, Truckenbrodt R, Stamm G, Coppenrath EM, Griebel J, Nagel HD (2004) Assessment of a theoretical formalism for dose estimation in CT: an anthropomorphic phantom study. Eur Radiol 14:1275–1284
5. European Commission (1999) Report EUR 16262 EN – European guidelines on quality criteria for computed tomography
6. ICRP (1996) Publication 73: Radiological protection and safety in medicine. Ann ICRP 26(2)
7. Galanski M, Nagel HD, Stamm G (2001) CT-Expositionspraxis in der Bundesrepublik Deutschland – Ergebnisse einer bundesweiten Umfrage im Jahre 1999. Fortschr Röntgenstr 173:R1–R66
8. Brix G, Nagel HD, Stamm G, Veit R, Lechel G, Griebel J, Galanski M (2003) Radiation exposure in multi-slice versus single-slice spiral CT: results of a nationwide survey. Eur Radiol 13:1979–1991

4 Artifacts in MSCT

R. Raupach and T. Flohr

4.1 Introduction

Artifacts in CT are usually based on the misinterpretation of raw data due to various physical phenomena. As CT images are generally derived by means of a filtered back-projection [1], artifacts, i.e., image disturbances, do not occur only at the originating location, as known from conventional radiography, but may also affect the entire image. For example, a thin metallic wire causes streak artifacts emanating from its origin, but deteriorates the environmental region up to a greater distance as well. Artifacts can also occur if the source is located outside the reconstructed field of view or even out of the field of measurement (the maximum field of view, which is completely covered by the acquired raw data).

The challenge is to decide whether details in the CT image represent the reality or are produced artificially. Therefore, considerable experience as well as a profound knowledge of the technology behind a CT system are essential to be able to interpret images correctly. Although artifacts are commonly caused by a combination of different physical effects the diagnostic quality of CT images can be optimized by choosing appropriate scan parameters.

The most common sources for artifacts and their appearance are described in the following. General hints are given to minimize artifacts.

Therefore, this article aims to help optimize the MSCT protocols by describing both the appearance of artifacts and their origins.

4.2 Beam-Hardening Artifacts

The most prominent beam-hardening artifact is known as the *Hounsfield bar*, a dark band between the petrous bones in the base of the skull obliterating the mid-portion of the brain stem (Fig. 4.1a). The radiation generated by the tube shows a polychromatic spectrum, i.e., contains photons with different energies. This can be compared to a continuous mixture of colors in the case of visible light.

Attenuation of X-rays depends on the energy, but this attenuation decreases with higher photon energy. Therefore, the spectral composite of the X-rays changes when passing an object: radiation behind the object contains a higher ratio of high-energy photons than the primary beam, but a lower ratio of low-energy photons. Hence, the effect is commonly referred to as the *beam-hardening effect*. The measured signals at the detector, however, represent an averaged attenuation over all energies resulting in averaged data. As a result, reconstructed images show dark areas or streaks between, for example, thick bones.

Its strength depends significantly on the atomic composite, the size of the object and the voltage used. Heavy atoms like calcium in bones cause a more distinct effect than soft tissue. A lower voltage, corresponding to a lower peak energy of the X-ray photons, will intensify the artifacts.

Beam-hardening artifacts typically appear in the vicinity of dense bones, like in the base of the skull. Also, very concentrated iodine contrast media, or implanted metals may show significant artifacts due to the discussed phenomenon.

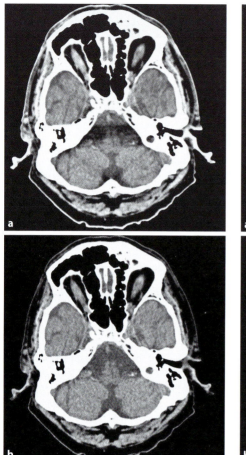

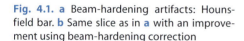

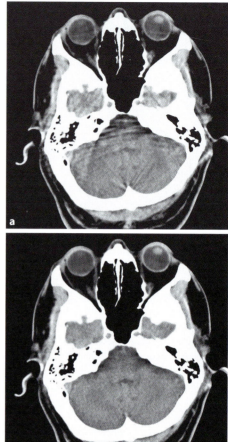

Fig. 4.1. a Beam-hardening artifacts: Hounsfield bar. **b** Same slice as in **a** with an improvement using beam-hardening correction

Fig. 4.2. a Partial volume artifacts in the base of the skull. **b** Same slice as in **a**, but scanned with thin-collimated slices

Correction of this effect for soft tissue is routinely performed during data processing to ensure a homogeneous soft tissue level over the entire object. Whereas, the simultaneous beam-hardening correction for a combination of soft tissue, bone, etc., requires more sophisticated algorithms, such as iterative reconstruction approaches.

As beam-hardening artifacts particularly deteriorate the diagnostic properties of head images, most CT systems provide dedicated soft tissue reconstruction algorithms for brain scans considering the two-component system soft tissue and bone [2], where artifacts are removed almost completely (Fig. 4.1b). Therefore, it is highly

recommended to use the dedicated scan protocols for brain examinations.

4.3   Partial-Volume Artifacts

Partial-volume artifacts occur if the edge of a structure with high contrast, e.g., bone or metal, partly shadows a particular channel when projected onto the detector. In this case, the measured signal is the cumulated intensity of rays passing through the object and the environmental tissue exclusively. This applies to the image plane as well as to the z-direction. Incorrect data then arise from the fact that signal attenuation is mea-

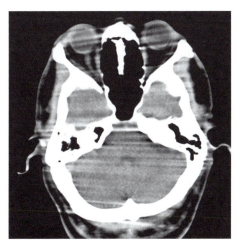

Fig. 4.3. Motion artifacts in a head scan

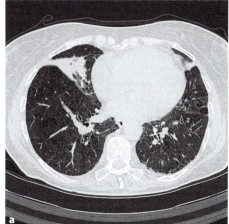

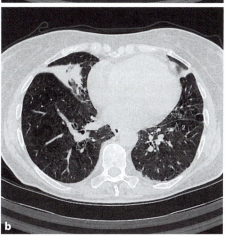

Fig. 4.4. a Artifacts in a thorax scan by breathing and movement of the heart. **b** Improvement by a motion artifact correction algorithm

sured but CT images are reconstructed by means of a filtered back-projection of attenuation integrals, i.e., the logarithm of the measured intensities [1]. Arising artifacts are typically streak-shaped and look very similar to beam-hardening artifacts (Fig. 4.2a).

In the case of partly in-plane coverage of a detector channel, artifacts are usually denoted as sampling errors. As the width of detector channels in MSCT is small, sampling artifacts occur only at edges of objects with very high attenuation coefficients like metallic objects.

The geometrical width of detector channels is fixed and cannot be changed, whereas the strength of partial volume artifacts due to finite size of the channels in the z-direction can be influenced by the collimation. As a rule, a thinner collimation reduces the level of partial volume artifacts because contours are sampled more precisely. Modern MSCT systems always provide scan modes with submillimeter collimation, which should be used if high-contrast structures are present. Figure 4.2b shows the same slice position and thickness as Fig 4.2a, but has been acquired with narrower (1 mm) collimation and subsequent fusing of the thin collimated slices. Obviously, partial volume artifacts are eliminated.

4.4   Motion Artifacts

CT images are reconstructed from a certain angular segment of projections. Movement of an object or patient during this time leads to inconsistent data. Artifacts typically occur as streaks (Fig. 4.3) or blurred or double contours (Fig. 4.4a). Protocols for critical examinations, may include special approaches to suppress those artifacts (Fig. 4.4b), known as motion correction algorithms.

Especially if a slow gantry rotation is selected for high resolution scans patients should be fixed properly using the assigned

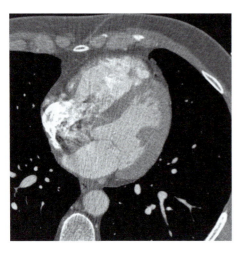

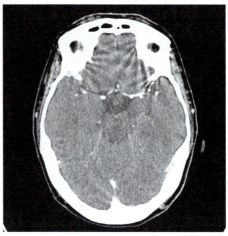

Fig. 4.5. Artifacts caused by dense contrast bolus

Fig. 4.6. Spiral or windmill artifacts

equipment like, e.g., head holders or restraining straps. Disturbances can also be introduced by a dense contrast bolus (Fig. 4.5).

Generally, a fast rotation speed of the gantry is recommended to minimize motion artifacts. State-of-the-art CT systems offer rotation times down to 0.33 s per 360°, fast enough to freeze most of the physiological processes. If submillimeter structures have to be displayed close to the heart, e.g., coronary arteries, retrospectively gated reconstruction algorithms are provided that use information from the parallel recorded ECG to determine optimized temporal windows. Temporal resolution can be much less than the full rotation time by employing so-called multisegment reconstruction techniques. However, they reduce motion artifacts efficiently only if the movement is exactly reproducible.

4.5 Spiral Artifacts (Windmill Artifacts)

CT scanners acquire raw data by using finite detector channels. For all spiral reconstruction algorithms, an interpolation in the z-direction of those data to axially aligned projections has to be performed. This induces errors for structured high-contrast objects, like bones or metals, compared to the idealized situation of an arbitrarily fine grid of sampled data points. Resulting artifacts are propeller-like, dark/bright structures in the vicinity of their sources (Fig. 4.6) that seem to rotate around their center when scrolling through the stack of axial images. For this reason, they are sometimes denoted as "windmill" artifacts.

Spiral artifacts can be reduced effectively by an improvement of the sampling pattern in the z-direction. The recently introduced z-sharp or double z-sampling technology [3] represents an advanced technological approach to overcome this well-known phenomenon of MSCT systems completely. This technical solution is superior to other measures trying to reduce spiral artifacts by scan and reconstruction parameters as discussed in the following.

The appropriate spiral feed or pitch may reduce the level of spiral artifacts by optimizing the data sampling. Some vendors offer fixed pitch values with improved sampling, while other scanners allow for adjusting the pitch over a range in order to continuously adapt scanning speed. However, default protocols usually provide the optimum settings and should not be changed freely with respect to pitch or table feed.

Disturbances by spiral artifacts also depend on the ratio between reconstructed slice width and collimation. Thin reconstructed slices close to the collimated slice width are more susceptible to such artifacts than thick reconstructed slices. By choosing thicker reconstructed slices, spiral artifacts can be reduced, however, at the cost of longitudinal resolution.

The effect of spiral artifacts should also be considered for reconstruction of thin images as a basis for multiplanar reformation (MPR), and for maximum or minimum intensity projections (MIP) as well. Windmills in axial images may lead to streak artifacts in secondary reconstructions, e.g., horizontal streaks in coronal or sagittal MPRs. Besides the slice thickness, the distance of two adjacent slices (slice increment) represents an essential parameter. Since the wing pattern of the windmills shows identical alignment after a shift of one collimation (not reconstructed slice!), a slice increment of half a collimation must be regarded as the worst case because a dark/bright streak pattern will be produced in MPRs consequently. Choice of the reconstruction increment is therefore a compromise between resolution and the level of artifacts. With regard to the first property, a smaller increment is preferred while the consideration of artifacts rather leads to an increment of a full collimation. Generally, the optimum can be found in between. For example, a spiral scan using the collimation 6×1 mm with reconstructed slices of 1.25 mm shall be considered. Then, an increment of 0.5 mm (1.0 mm) will show maximized (minimized) artifacts in MPRs based on windmills in axial images. Increments of 0.9 down to 0.8 mm improve the resolution by overlapping without significantly enhancing the visibility of streaks. Please remember that the slice increment has to be compared with collimation, not with reconstructed slice width.

4.6 Cone Artifacts

Cone artifacts arise due to an approximation of the measured slices of MSCT systems to truly parallel planes. If the

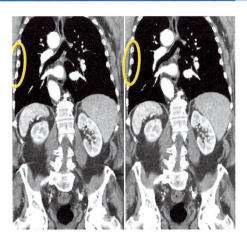

Fig. 4.7. a Cone beam artifacts. **b** Reduction of cone artifacts by a cone beam reconstruction

number of slices increases, deviations from this simplified description start to grow and result in characteristic artifacts (Fig. 4.7a). As the misfit increases away from the center of rotation, cone artifacts typically appear in the periphery, e.g., in the ribs.

However, most of the present MSCT scanners provide an effective cone correction or cone beam reconstruction, depending on the number of detector rows, if necessary (Fig. 4.7b). Users do not have the possibility to influence the reconstruction in this sense.

4.7 Metallic Objects

The term metal artifact includes almost all of the phenomena described above. Depending on the alloy, shape, size and position, one particular effect may dominate. Generally, the transition from environmental tissue to the metal is very sharp compared to the size of the detector channels that the partial volume effect or sampling errors, respectively, contribute to metal-induced artifacts, appearing as thin streaks emanating from the edges.

As discussed above, using the thinnest possible collimation will minimize partial volume artifacts. The conspicuousness can also be influenced by the convolution kernel. A smooth convolution kernel or smooth reconstruction algorithm can help to reduce thin streaks.

The most effective measure to avoid metal-induced artifacts is to exclude the metallic object from the scanned range. This can sometimes be realized by a careful patient positioning or using gantry tilt in special examinations, e.g., for excluding dental inlays from the scanned volume.

If the metallic object inevitably belongs to the range of interest or diagnostic information has to be gained close to implants, orientation of the scan plane is essential for optimal image quality. As a rule of thumb, the more metal being passed by the X-rays, the more severe artifacts appear. For example, a screw of a spine fixation causes more distinct disturbances if it is aligned in-plane. When cut perpendicular to the screw axis the artifact level will be reduced, which allows the evaluation of the area closer to the implant. Of course, a larger volume, i.e., more axial slices, might be influenced by long-range artifacts in the latter situation. Because of the sharp transitions of metallic objects, typical spiral artifacts may also occur of their edges (see previous section for details and hints).

Metal artifacts can also occur as a consequence of motion, e.g., in the case of electrodes, stents or clips close to the heart. Measures have already been discussed in the dedicated section.

If the size of metallic objects increases, the attenuation of X-rays grows significantly and beam hardening becomes relevant. On the other hand, the absolute signal measured in detector elements behind the implant becomes so low that the reading is not reliable due to a high level of noise. Both effects may completely destroy the image content on lines passing a large amount of metal. Artifacts are particularly visible between two metallic objects, e.g., hip implants. Using a higher voltage reduces beam hardening as well as a lack of detector signal due to smaller attenua-

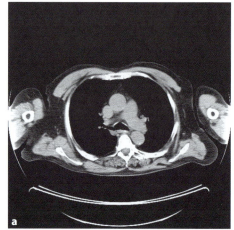

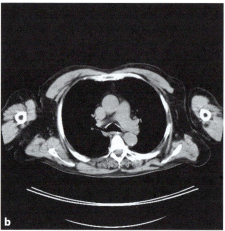

Fig. 4.8. a Patient exceeding the field of measurement without correction. **b** Same slice as in **a**, but including an extrapolation-type correction

tion at higher photon energies. Whereas, selecting higher mAs does not improve the situation significantly but will increase radiation dose. Please note that intelligent automatic exposure controls exclude metallic objects from calculating optimal mAs settings because no benefit with regard to image quality can be observed opposed to the higher dose. Furthermore, most state-of-the-art CT scanners employ advanced filters on the raw data to reduce disturbing noise structures.

4.8   Objects Outside the Field of Measurement (Shoulder Artifacts)

The relation between CT raw data and reconstructed images causes artifacts if objects are inside the gantry but exceed the field of measurement. For example, patients larger than the maximal scanning field or arms lateral to the body likewise produce artificial hyperdense edges (Fig. 4.8a) when not accounted for in the reconstruction. Some recent scanners automatically apply extrapolation-type algorithms in order to reduce those artifacts considerably (Fig. 4.8b) and, moreover, offer special reconstruction techniques to display objects located outside the field of measurement almost correctly.

ECG cables running through the gantry opening and contrast media on the gantry surface or in flexible tubes may also result in streak artifacts and sometimes are difficult to attribute to their origin.

References

1. Kalender WA (2000) Computed tomography. Publicis MCD, p 22ff
2. Herman GT, Trivedi SS (1983) A comparative study of two postreconstruction beam hardening correction methods. IEEE Trans Med Imaging 2(3):128–135
3. Flohr T, Stierstorfer K, Raupach R, Ulzheimer S, Bruder H (2004) Performance evaluation of a 64-slice CT-system with z-flying focal spot. *Röfo Fortschr Geb Rontgenstr Neuen Bildgeb Verfahr* 176:1803–1810

5 CT of the Heart and Great Vessels: Protocols in Congenital Heart Disease Patients

J.-F. Paul

5.1 Indications for MSCT

- Pulmonary atresia with ventricular septal defect
- Tetralogy of Fallot and other cyanotic cardiac disease
- Transposition of great arteries
- Double aortic arch
- Aortic coarctation
- Anomalous pulmonary venous return

5.2 Patient Preparation

In general, neonates are not necessarily sedated. The sedation protocol for infants includes the intrarectal administration of Midazomal at a dose of 0.3 mg/kg, given approximately 15 min before examination. Additional sedative drugs may be useful (Hydroxyzine at a dose of 1 mg/kg, per os, 1 h before examination).

5.3 Scan Parameters

See Table 5.1.

5.4 Tips and Tricks

5.4.1 Neonates and Babies

- Appropriate centric positioning of the baby is best facilitated with the assistance of the laser beam.
- In our institution, no preview scan is performed, as it constitutes an unnecessary additional radiation dose.
- Systematic use of 80 kV settings.

- Adaptation of the mAs to typical neonate/baby weights (e.g., 25 mAs for 3 kg, see Table 5.2).
- Only one phase acquisition when possible.
- Systematic protection of nonscanned organs.

5.4.2 Infants over Seven Years of Age

- Breath hold angio-CT acquisition or ECG-gated acquisition (for coronaries).
- Adaptation of the mAs to typical child weights.

5.4.3 Comments

Congenital heart disease (CHD) arises due to abnormal development of the cardiac structures during intrafetal life and consists of more or less complex malformations of the heart and great vessels. Most of the patients may benefit from surgical intervention to partially or totally correct the anatomical anomalies or percutaneous interventional radiologic procedures. For the clinical management of patients with complex congenital heart disease, three-dimensional accurate evaluation of their morphologic conditions is critical. 3D reconstructions should be routinely used and demonstrate the shape and spatial relation of the great arteries, proximal branch pulmonary arteries and anomalous pulmonary venous or systemic connections. The 3D information of extra cardiac morphologic characteristics may determine the choice and method of surgical intervention.

Table 5.1. Examples of kV and mAs settings in pediatric protocols depending on the infant weight

Parameters	4–8 slice scanners	10–16 slice scanners	32–64 slice scanners
Scanner settings			
Tube voltage (kV)	80 (see Table 5.2)	80 (see Table 5.2)	80 (see Table 5.2)
Rotation time (s)	0.5	0.37	0.33–0.42
Tube current time product (mAs)	See Table 5.2	See Table 5.2	See Table 5.2
Pitch corrected tube current time product (eff. mAs)	See Table 5.2	See Table 5.2	See Table 5.2
Collimation (mm)	2.5*	0.75	0.6/0.625
Norm. pitch	1.5	1.5	1.5
Reconstruction increment (mm)	1.5	0.8	0.4
Reconstr. slice thickness (mm)	3	1.25	1
Convolution kernel	Soft	Soft	Soft
Specials			
Scan range	Upper aperture/diaphram	Upper aperture/diaphram	Upper aperture/diaphram
Scan direction	Caudocranial	Caudocranial	Caudocranial
Contrast media application			
Concentration (mg iodine/ml)	300	300	300
Mono/Biphasic	Monophasic	Monophasic	Monophasic
Volume (mL)	2 cc/kg	2 cc/kg	2 cc/kg
Injection rate (mL/s)	0.5–1	0.5–1	0.5–1
Saline chaser (mL, mL/s)	No	No	No
Delay (s)	10 (central) or 15 (peripheral) access	10 (central) or 15 (peripheral) access	10 (central) or 15 (peripheral) access

* Limited use for pediatric CHD cases.

In pulmonary atresia with ventricular septal defect (absence of development of the right outflow tract and pulmonary valve) the pulmonary blood supply is provided by aorticopulmonary arteries (MAPCAs) or a patent ductus arteriosus. Several important aspects can be assessed using MSCT, such as the status of pulmonary arteries including size, exclusion of pulmonary artery stenosis [1, 2]. Evaluation of MAPCA should include their number and location, the assessment of a patent ductus arteriosus, and exclusion of usually proximal stenosis. Also, their position in relation to the central airways (in front of or behind) should be assessed and is essential for surgical planning. Coronary artery abnormalities can be detected noninvasively using thin collimation MSCT

Table 5.2. Examples of kV and mAs settings in pediatric protocols depending on the infant weight

Patient's weight	Tube kilovoltage (kV)	Tube current time product (mAs)	Pitch corrected tube current time product (eff. mAs)
Newborn–3 kg	80	25	37.5 (at pitch of 1.5)
20 kg	80	65	100 (at pitch of 1.5)
40 kg	80	100	150 (at pitch of 1.5)

(please see the chapters on coronary imaging in this book) and may include variations such as a left anterior descending artery originating from right coronary artery, a doubled left anterior descending (LAD) (anterior and posterior), or others.

Fallot's tetralogy (right ventricular outflow tract stenosis associated with ventricular septal defect, overriding aorta, and right ventricle hypertrophy) is the most common cyanotic cardiac disease. Various aspects such as the right ventricular enlargement can be followed using Doppler, echocardiography, or MSCT. Pulmonary insufficiency must therefore be excluded. In Fallot's tetralogy the status of pulmonary arteries (including size, especially regarding dilatation caused by pulmonary artery stenosis and ventricular size, if not determined by ultrasound) must be assessed.

If a transposition of great arteries (aorta arises from right ventricle and pulmonary artery arises from left ventricle) is present, MSCT may play a role in follow-up. The transposition of great arteries is generally treated surgically by the switch intervention, with reimplantation of the coronary arteries.

A double aortic arch (Fig. 5.1) is the persistence of both left and right aortic arch, responsible for an aortic ring. The ascending aorta lies in front of the trachea, passes the trachea on either side and then fuses again the posterior to the esophagus. CT can help evaluate the size of both arches, and the anatomic relationship of each arch to trachea and esophagus.

An aortic coarctation (Fig. 5.2) is a relatively common anomaly and can be de-

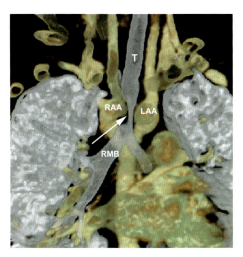

Fig. 5.1. Severe respiratory distress in a newborn. MSCT using VRT shows clearly a complete double aortic arch responsible for tracheal compression (5-month-old patient, 5 kg). VRT displaying both airways and vascular structures show clearly the compression of the trachea (arrow) by the right aortic arch. RAA: right aortic arch, LAA: left aortic arch, T: Trachea, RMB: right main bronchus

scribed as a narrowing of the aortic lumen at the level of the aortic arch. The term coarctation refers to an infolding of the posterolateral wall in the region of the ductus arteriosus insertion (adult form), or proximal to the insertion in which case it is then usually named infantile coarctation. CT helps to determine the degree of stenosis as well as the collateral flow patterns, presence of thrombus, or associated anomalies.

Variations of anomalous pulmonary venous return (Fig. 5.3) are seen if an absence of connection of at least one of the pulmo-

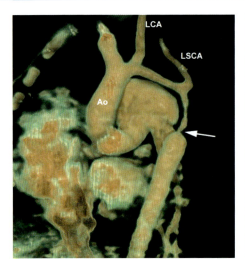

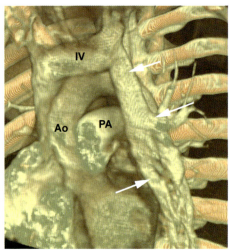

Fig. 5.2. Aortic coarctation in a 1-month-old baby. Total interruption of the aortic arch was suspected after echocardiography. MSCT showed long stenosis of aorta with postductal severe narrowing (*arrow*). Ao: Aorta, LCA: left carotid artery, LSCA: left subclavian artery

Fig. 5.3. MSCT image of a total abnormal left venous return in a 25-year-old man with dyspnea. All left pulmonary veins (*arrows*) are connected to the innominate vein. Ao: Aorta, PA: pulmonary artery, IV: innominate vein

nary vein to the left atrium occurs. 3D visualization of anomalous venous return should be performed, and the distance of the vein from left atrium needs to be evaluated before surgical treatment decision making.

5.5   Dose Issues

In general, we use 80 kV for thorax imaging of all children [3, 4]. We use 80 kV for thorax imaging of children weighing less than 60 kg [5]. Only if the weight of the child exceeds 60 kg, is the KV switched from 80 to 100 kV. Regarding the optimized rotation time, we always use the fastest possible speed in nongated acquisition, for example, in the 16-slice case: 0.42 s (0.37 s if applicable), and 0.33 s for the 64-slice CT. For the different weight groups of the pediatric population sample values of tube voltage and tube current time product, examples of our actual values are given in Table 5.2.

References

1. Paul JF, Lambert V, Losay J, Petit J, Mace L, Belli E, Serraf A, Planche C, Angel C (2002) Three-dimensional multislice CT : value in patients with pulmonary atresia with septal defect. Arch Mal Coeur Vaiss. 95(5):427–432

2. Westra SJ, Hurteau J, Galindo A, McNitt-Gray MF, Boechat MI, Laks H (1999) Cardiac electron-beam CT in children undergoing surgical repair for pulmonary atresia. Radiology 213(2):502–512

3. Paul JF, Abada HT, Sigal-Cinqualbre A (2004) Should low-kilovoltage chest CT protocols be the rule for pediatric patients? AJR Am J Roentgenol 183(4):1172

4. Honnef D, Wildberger JE, Stargardt A, Hohl C, Barker M, Gunther RW, Staatz G (2004) Multislice spiral CT (MSCT) in pediatric radiology: dose reduction for chest and abdomen examinations. Röfo 176(7):1021–1030

5. Sigal-Cinqualbre AB, Hennequin R, Abada HT, Chen X, Paul JF (2004) Low-kilovoltage multidetector row chest CT in adults: feasibility and effect on image quality and iodine dose. Radiology 231(1):169–174

6 Contrast Medium Applications for Multislice CT

D. Fleischmann

6.1 Introduction

Multislice or multiple detector-row CT (MDCT) technology continues to rapidly evolve; acquisition times have become substantially faster when 4-, 8-, 16-, and now 64-channel systems are compared. While fast acquisitions at unprecedented spatial resolution offer new opportunities in cardiovascular CT and body imaging, contrast material (CM) delivery becomes more difficult and less forgiving at the same time.

Several traditional concepts of CM injection for CTA that were conceived empirically in the single-detector row CT era do not hold true for faster scan times. For example, the assumption that a constant-rate intravenous injection of CM leads to an arterial enhancement plateau is simply not (and never was) true. Second, the ballpark rule to chose an injection duration equal to the scanning time works well for long scan times (>20 s or so), but obviously cannot be used for a 4 s or shorter acquisition time. Finally, the appealing idea that faster scans will naturally result in better arterial enhancement is not true either – the opposite is actually the case: faster scanners tend to result in lower arterial opacification if one applies traditional injection concepts. On the other hand, some well-established concepts with respect to parenchymal organ enhancement – such as the relationship of normal liver parenchymal enhancement being proportional to the total contrast medium volume administered – have not changed recently and will not change in the foreseeable future, even with the fastest of scanners.

The main purpose of this chapter is thus to explain the fundamentals of arterial and parenchymal enhancement in order to allow the reader to design his or her own strategy of contrast medium delivery. Such strategies are primarily tailored to the scan time, not specifically to a scanner generation, and require knowledge of the physiologic and pharmacokinetic principles of arterial and/or parenchymal enhancement, and knowledge of the effects of user-selectable injection parameters.

6.2 Principles of Arterial and Parenchymal Enhancement

6.2.1 Early Arterial Contrast Medium Dynamics

For a given individual, arterial enhancement is determined by the iodine administration rate (iodine flux) and the injection duration (Fig. 6.1). The iodine administration rate is directly proportional to arterial enhancement. Thus, an increase in the injection rate and/or a higher iodine concentration of the contrast medium directly translates into increased vascular enhancement. Furthermore, arterial enhancement continuously increases over time with longer injection durations. It follows that shorter injection durations lead to lower arterial enhancement [1]. The basic rules of early arterial contrast medium dynamics can be summarized as follows:

1. Arterial enhancement is directly proportional to the iodine administration rate (iodine flux), and can be controlled by the injection flow rate (mL/s) and the

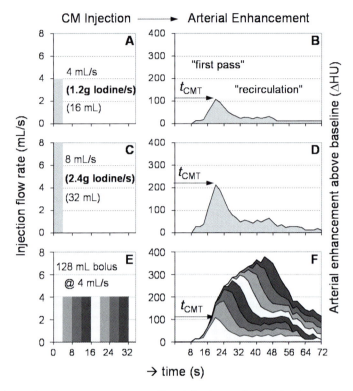

Fig. 6.1. Relationship between contrast medium injection and arterial enhancement. The simple additive model illustrates the effects of the injection flow rate (iodine flux) and injection duration on arterial enhancement. **a** Intravenous contrast medium injection causes **b** an arterial enhancement response, which consists of an early first pass peak and a lower recirculation effect. **c** Doubling the injection flow rate (doubling the iodine administration rate) results in **d** approximately twice the arterial enhancement. **e** The effect of the injection duration can be regarded as **f** the sum (time integral) of several enhancement responses. Note that due to the asymmetric shape of the test enhancement curve and due to recirculation effects, arterial enhancement following an injection of 128 mL (the time integral of eight consecutive injections of 16 mL) increases continuously over time

iodine concentration of the contrast medium (mg I/mL).

2. Arterial enhancement continuously increases over time with longer injection durations, due to the cumulative effects of bolus broadening and recirculation. Thus, increasing the injection duration also improves vascular opacification.

3. The strength of an individual's enhancement response to intravenously administrated CM is controlled by and inversely related to cardiac output and central blood volume, and correlates inversely with bodyweight.

6.2.2 Enhancement of Normal Liver Parenchyma

Parenchymal enhancement results not only from opacification of blood vessels, but also from CM distribution into the extravascular, extracellular interstitial space [2]. The dynamics of hepatic CM enhancement is also influenced by the dual blood supply of the liver, with the majority of hepatic blood flow (approximately 80%) derived from the portal venous system, where any CM bolus is substantially broadened (and delayed) within the splanchnic vasculature.

Hence, the enhancement of normal liver parenchyma is much lower than vascular enhancement and also peaks much later than arterial enhancement (approximately 40 or 50 s). Enhancement of normal liver parenchyma – and thus the contrast to low-attenuation liver lesions – is rather independent of the injection flow rate, but it is directly proportional to the total amount of CM. As a rule of thumb, 600 mg of iodine per kilogram of bodyweight achieves adequate hepatic parenchymal enhancement.

With faster scanners, correct timing is becoming increasingly important for phase-selective imaging, but the total amount of CM must not be changed.

6.2.3 Enhancement of Hypervascular Liver Lesions and Well-Perfused Organs

The enhancement dynamics of so-called *hypervascular* liver lesions is fundamentally different when compared to normal liver parenchyma (Fig. 6.2). Such lesions are characterized (among others) by their systemic arterial blood supply and their enhancement dynamics are comparable to splenic rather than normal liver parenchymal enhancement. Because of their intimate relationship to arterial contrast dynamics, the enhancement of hypervascular liver lesions can be controlled by the same parameters that affect arterial enhancement.

Hence, maximum lesion-to-background contrast in the setting of hypervascular liver lesions, can be achieved by maximizing the iodine flux (by using high injection flow rates and/or high iodine concentration of the CM), and selecting an appropriately long scanning delay (relative to the contrast medium transit time t_{CMT}, see below). The goal is to ensure strong lesion opacification before the onset of normal parenchymal enhancement. This particular phase of enhancement is commonly referred to as the late arterial phase, and occurs approximately 10 to 15 s after CM arrival in the aorta [3]. Note that at that time the portal vein branches will be slightly opacified – hence

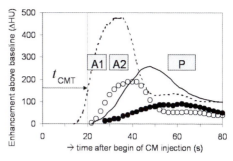

Fig. 6.2. Early contrast medium dynamics of the liver. Hepatic vascular and parenchymal time-attenuation curves modeled for an injection duration of 20 s. Normal hepatic parenchymal enhancement (●) is comparably low and delayed relative to enhancement of the portal vein (––). The enhancement of a hypervascular liver lesion (○) follows arterial enhancement (- - -), and thus slightly precedes portal venous and hepatic parenchymal enhancement. The early arterial phase (A1) begins immediately after the contrast medium transit time (t_{CMT}). The late arterial phase (A2) begins 10–15 s after the t_{CMT} and provides the best contrast between hypervascular liver lesion and normal liver parenchyma. The parenchymal phase occurs approximately 40 s after the t_{CMT}

the alternative term portal venous inflow phase (Fig. 6.2).

The enhancement kinetics of other solid organs, such as the pancreas, also follow arterial dynamics, with an additional delay necessary to opacify the interstitial spaces of the organ of interest. Pancreatic imaging thus also benefits from high iodine-flux and accurate timing relative to t_{CMT}, but also improves with larger CM volumes.

6.3 Contrast Medium Transit Time (t_{CMT}) and Individual Scan Timing

The time interval for an intravenously injected bolus of CM to appear in the arterial territory of interest is generally referred to as the contrast medium transit time (t_{CMT}). In patients with cardiocirculatory disease, the scanning delay needs to be individualized relative to the patient's t_{CMT}. The t_{CMT} can be determined either by using a test bolus injection or by using automated bolus triggering techniques.

Traditionally, the scanning delay in CTA studies has been chosen to equal a patient's t_{CMT}. However, with faster scan times and shorter injection durations, this is not necessarily the best strategy. Instead, a patient's t_{CMT} may be used as an individual landmark, with an additional time delay (diagnostic delay) before initiation of CT data acquisition. For example, a scanning delay of $t_{CMT}+8$ s means that scanning begins 8 s after arrival of the bolus in, e.g., a patient's aorta.

The same also applies to phase-selective abdominal imaging protocols: The t_{CMT} (as determined by a test-bolus or bolus triggering technique) serves as an individual landmark for optimized timing of, e.g., an early arterial ($t_{CMT}+2$ s), late arterial ($t_{CMT}+15$ s), or a pancreatic ($t_{CMT}+20$ s) CT acquisition.

6.4 Caveats of Automated Bolus Triggering

Automated bolus triggering has the advantage that it does not require a separate test-bolus injection for individualizing the scanning delay. It is important to be aware of the fact, however, that the use of automated bolus triggering inherently increases the scanning delay relative to the t_{CMT} obtained with the test-bolus technique. This is due to technical factors, such as the sampling interval for the monitoring slices, image reconstruction time, and a minimal delay required for changing the collimation and table repositioning after reaching the predefined threshold of opacification within the target vessel. Furthermore, when a prerecorded breath-hold command is used in conjunction with bolus triggering, this may further delay the initiation of CT data acquisition.

While an increase of the scanning delay for a few seconds improves rather than deteriorates arterial enhancement, the main problem with bolus triggering is that its inherent delay is not necessarily obvious to the user – and that it may dif-

fer substantially between scanner models and manufacturers. The obvious solution is to identify the inherent delay associated with bolus triggering for a given scanner model and factor this slight delay into the injection duration. So, for example, if bolus triggering results in an 8-s increase in the scanning delay relative to the true t_{CMT}, the injection duration needs to be 8 s longer than the scan time.

6.5 Double-Barrel Power Injectors and Saline-Flushing

The latest models of power injectors are equipped with two syringes, which can be filled with CM and normal saline, respectively. Routine flushing of the arm veins after CM injection improves CM utilization and slightly prolongs and increases arterial enhancement. Furthermore, saline-flushing may reduce perivenous streak artifacts in cardio-thoracic CT. Saline flushing is relatively more important when small amounts of contrast or high-concentration agents are being used.

Some injector models allow the simultaneous injection of saline and CM, which can be used to chase a full bolus with diluted CM. This may be useful for cardiac imaging because it maintains a minimum opacification for delineating the right ventricular cavity.

6.6 Avoiding the Valsalva Maneuver

Central venous blood flow is subject to intrathoracic pressure changes due to respiration [4]. In the setting of CM-enhanced CT this may be particularly harmful if a patient performs an ambitious Valsalva maneuver during breath holding. During a Valsalva maneuver, the intrathoracic and intraabdominal pressures increase, which causes a temporary interruption of venous return from the head and upper extremity veins (where CM is usually injected), and a

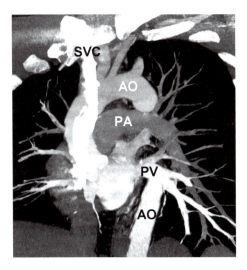

Fig. 6.3. Detrimental effect of Valsalva maneuver on pulmonary arterial enhancement. Oblique thin-slab MIP image of pulmonary CT angiogram of a 49-year-old man with suspected pulmonary embolism. The patient performed a strong Valsalva maneuver during breath holding for the CT acquisition, which was obtained in the caudocranial direction. Note that while CM is still being injected at the end of the study, as seen in the superior vena cava (SVC), and while there is good opacification of the aorta (AO) and pulmonary veins (PV), the opacification of the pulmonary arterial (PA) tree is nondiagnostic to rule out pulmonary embolism

temporary increase of (unopacified) venous blood flow from the inferior vena cava. The effect of this flow alteration is a temporary decrease of vascular opacification in the dependent territories, such as the pulmonary arterial tree, but also in the arterial system. In some cases (and notably with fast scanners) this may cause nondiagnostic opacification of the entire pulmonary arterial tree (Fig. 6.3).

It is thus important that the technologist explains to the patient not to "bear down" during breath holding, and/or advise him or her to keep the mouth open during breath holding. Minor respiratory motion artifacts are less harmful for pulmonary CTA interpretation than insufficient opacification.

As a side note, it is also preferable that a test bolus injection is performed during shallow respiration rather than during breath holding, because this better reflects the early flow dynamics of a subsequent CTA.

6.7 Injection Strategies for CTA

Before considering specific injection strategies for CTA it is helpful to adopt the way of thinking about CTA injection protocols. Injection protocols (and of course the subsequent arterial enhancement) have a time dimension and thus should be understood as *injection rate* and *injection duration* rather than as *injection volume* and *injection rate* (the injection volume is not an important parameter in the setting of CTA, in contrast to parenchymal imaging).

The initial step in the design of injection protocols for CTA is then to consider the anticipated scan time. For *slow acquisitions* (in the range of 20 s or longer), traditional protocols yield reliable arterial enhancement. For example, one can use a standardized injection (e.g., 1.2–1.5 g I/s for an average individual) for the duration of the scan time. The scanning delay is set to the patient's t_{CMT}. Higher or lower flow rates (±20%) should be used in larger (>90 kg) and smaller (<60 kg) patients, respectively. With long scan times, biphasic or multiphasic injections lead to more uniform arterial enhancement over time [5,6].

For *fast acquisitions* (in the range of 10 s), the injection parameters and the choice of the scanning delay need to be adopted in order to achieve adequate arterial enhancement. Based on the first two rules of early contrast medium dynamics, one can apply two strategies to increase arterial enhancement for fast acquisitions – alone or in combination (Fig. 6.4): One can (1) increase the iodine flux (grams of iodine injected per unit of time), which will translate into a proportionally stronger enhancement. The iodine flux, as mentioned earlier, can be increased by the selection of a higher iodine concentration of the contrast medium, and/or by increasing the injection flow rate (Fig. 6.1). In addition, one can (2)

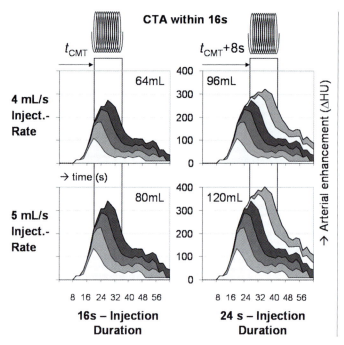

Fig. 6.4. Strategies to improve arterial enhancement for fast MDCTA. Two strategies to increase arterial enhancement when compared to a baseline 16-s injection at 4 mL/s (*upper left panel*) can be employed – either alone or in combination. Increasing the injection rate from 4 to 5 mL/s increases the enhancement approximately 20% (*lower left panel*). Increasing the iodine concentration from 300 to 400 mg/mL would achieve an even greater enhancement increase, without the need to increase the injection rate. Alternatively, one can also increase the injection duration and the scanning delay, taking advantage of the fact that enhancement increases with longer injection durations (*right upper panel*). Maximum enhancement can be achieved when both the injection rate (and/or the iodine concentration) as well as the injection duration are increased (*right lower panel*) simultaneously

also increase the scanning delay relative to a patient's t_{CMT}. This will also increase arterial enhancement, because of the continuing rise of opacification with longer injection duration. It is crucial, however, to also increase the injection duration in this case, because otherwise the arterial enhancement would not be maintained long enough [7].

For *very fast acquisitions* (equal to or less than 5 s), if one extends the example shown in Fig. 6.3, to a scan time of only 4 s, the solution is again to increase the iodine flux (to 2 g/s), and to increase both the scanning delay and the injection duration e.g. by 8 s. Specifically, this would translate into using a flow rate of 5 mL/s with 400 mg/mL CM, injected for 12 s (4+8), with a scanning delay of t_{CMT}+8 s.

Another truism which should not go unnoticed at this point is that one does not necessarily have to use the latest scanners at their maximum acquisition speed. Not only is this unnecessary, it may even be detrimental, because a very fast acquisition speed may not allow complete and sufficient opacification of a diseased arterial tree. This has been observed in mesenteric CTA and, most noticeably, in peripheral (lower extremity) CTA. For example, our current protocol for lower extremity CTA using a 64-channel scanner uses small pitch and slow gantry rotation settings aiming at a scan time of as long as 40 s for all patients, in order to prevent outrunning the bolus. The fixed scan time of 40 s is combined with biphasic injections with a total injection duration of 35 s.

6.8 Injection Strategies for Liver and Parenchymal Imaging

Because of the rapid acquisition times, MDCT allows a precise separation of different enhancement phases of the liver (early arterial, late arterial, and parenchymal). This is particularly important in the setting of suspected or known hypervascular liver lesions. The enhancement of hypervascular liver lesions follows arterial enhancement (Fig. 6.2). As a result, the lesion-to-background contrast can be maximized by increasing the iodine flux, and by timing the acquisition to the late-arterial phase of hepatic enhancement, which commences approximately 10 to 15 s after CM arrives in the aorta/hepatic artery [8]. The faster the CT acquisition, the longer the delay.

For imaging low-attenuation liver lesions, it is important to administer a sufficient total iodine dose (e.g., 600 mg/kg bodyweight), similar to what has been used in the past, with single detector-row CT. Also, timing is less critical, with a scanning delay of approximately 60–70 s after the beginning of the injection, or 40–50 s after CM arrival in the aorta. More specific protocol suggestions for hepatic and abdominal imaging are provided in the following chapters.

References

1. Fleischmann D (2002) Present and future trends in multiple detector-row CT applications: CT angiography. Europ Radiol 12:S11–S16
2. Dawson P, Blomley MJ (1996) Contrast agent pharmacokinetics revisited: I. Reformulation. Acad Radiol 3(2):S261–263
3. Foley WD, Mallisee TA, Hohenwalter MD, Wilson CR, Quiroz FA, Taylor AJ (2000) Multiphase hepatic CT with a multirow detector CT scanner. Am J Roentgenol 175:679–685
4. Gosselin MV, Rassner UA, Thieszen SL, Phillips J, Oki A (2004) Contrast dynamics during CT pulmonary angiogram: analysis of an inspiration associated artifact. J Thorac Imaging 19:1–7
5. Fleischmann D, Rubin GD, Bankier AA, Hittmair K (2000) Improved uniformity of aortic enhancement with customized contrast medium injection protocols at CT angiography. Radiology 214:363–371
6. Bae KT, Tran HQ, Heiken JP (2000) Multiphasic injection method for uniform prolonged vascular enhancement at CT angiography: pharmacokinetic analysis and experimental porcine model. Radiology 216:872–880
7. Fleischmann D (2003) Use of high-concentration contrast media in multiple–detector-row CT: principles and rationale. Eur Radiol 13(5):M14–M20
8. Awai K, Takada K, Onishi H, Hori S (2002) Aortic and hepatic enhancement and tumor-to-liver contrast: analysis of the effect of different concentrations of contrast material at multi-detector row helical CT. Radiology 224:757–763

7 Indications for PET-CT

P. Herzog and R.A. Schmid

7.1 Indications for PET/CT [1]

- Oncology: tumor detection and staging, therapy control
- Inflammation: search for occult inflammatory focuses
- Cardiac: myocardial viability, perfusion and function
- Neurology: selected neurodegenerative or inflammatory disorders, brain tumors and intractable epilepsy
- Vascular: detection of active atherosclerosis or vulnerable plaques (work in progress)

7.2 Introduction

Multidetector row CT (MDCT) has the capability to deliver excellent morphological imaging of almost every body section. Combining MDCT techniques with a functional imaging modality such as positron emission tomography (PET) or single photon emission computed tomography (SPECT) can add functional information to high-resolution morphological imaging. The combined acquisition of MDCT together with PET or SPECT in the same session and using the same scanner system has several advantages compared to using single modality scanners at two different time points.

One advantage is that the combined acquisition generates coregistered image data; each image voxel of the CT scan has a certain corresponding voxel in the PET or SPECT examination. Data derived from a combined system is superior to offline fused-image data from two separate systems because the patient is positioned differently in two separate investigations on separate systems [2].

Another advantage is that the data from the CT scan can be used for attenuation correction of the functional modality. PET or SPECT are both nuclear emission scans using radioactive tracer pharmaceuticals. Emission undergoes attenuation when penetrating the body tissue to the surface. This leads to a considerable attenuation of emissions if originating from central parts of the body compared to emissions originated from peripheral locations. In standalone PET or SPECT scanners a rotating radiation source containing radioactive material is used to obtain a low-quality transmission attenuation map for attenuation correction that can take up to 2 h of acquisition time when performing whole body scanning. In combined systems the CT scan can be used as an attenuation map for correction of the emission scan and can reduce scan time tremendously compared to external-source attenuation correction because a MDCT scan typically has an acquisition time of no more than a minute.

Today most combined systems are PET/CT systems rather than SPECT/CT systems. PET delivers a higher spatial resolution of typically 5 mm compared to SPECT with typically 20 mm. Both resolutions are, of course, inferior to the resolution derived from CT scanners with less than 1 mm resolution. Since the introduction of combined PET/CT systems, vendors have noticed a considerably lower demand for standalone PET scanners. It is estimated that 99% of all PET scanners sold in 2005 will be combined PET/CT systems.

Table 7.1. Indications for PET and PET/CT and the appropriate tracer substances

Oncology	Standard PET, most widely used	[18F]-Fluoro-deoxyglucose (FDG)
	High resolution bone scan	Fluorine [18F]
	Prostate cancer	[11C]-Choline
	Some FDG-negative tumors	O-(2-[18F]-Fluoroethyl)-L-tyrosine ([18F]-FET)
	Tumor hypoxia (e.g., prior to radiation therapy)	[18F]-Fluoromisonidazole ([18F]-FMISO)
Inflammation	Search for inflammatory focuses	[18F]-Fluoro-deoxyglucose (FDG)
Cardiac	Myocardial viability	[18F]-Fluoro-deoxyglucose (FDG) or [82Rb] or [62Cu]-Pyruvaldehyde-bis-[4N-thiosemicarbazone] (PTSM)
	Myocardial perfusion	Water $H_2^{15}O$ or Ammonia $^{13}NH_3$
	Myocardial function, dynamic acquisition	[18F]-Fluoro-deoxyglucose (FDG)
Neurology	Neurodegenerative	[18F]-Fluoro-deoxyglucose (FDG)
	Brain tumors	[18F]-Fluoro-deoxyglucose (FDG) or O-(2-[18F]-Fluoroethyl)-L-tyrosine ([18F]-FET)
	Epilepsy	[18F]-Fluoro-deoxyglucose (FDG)
Vascular	Active atherosclerosis or vulnerable plaques	[18F]-Fluoro-deoxyglucose (FDG)

7.3 Indications and Radiopharmaceuticals

Depending on the indication different radiopharmaceuticals are used as a tracer substance (Table 7.1). All radionuclides mentioned in Table 7.1, except for ^{82}Rb and ^{62}Cu, which are generator products, must be produced in a cyclotron and delivered to the PET/CT site in reasonable time because of their fast decay. The half-life of ^{18}F is 109.8 min; that of ^{11}C is 20 min. Tracer substances have to be labeled with the radionuclides to generate a radiopharmaceutical.

After injection of the radiopharmaceutical an in vivo beta$^+$ decay emits a positron and a neutrino. The emitted positron and an electron from some other atom in the body tissue undergo a nuclear reaction in which both subatomic particles are destroyed and two gamma rays with an energy of 511 keV are emitted in opposite directions. These gamma rays are then detected by the PET scanner and the exact location of the nuclear reaction can be determined. Locally increased tracer uptake causes a local increase of radiation emission, which subsequently causes a hotspot in the images reconstructed from PET emission data.

[18F]-FDG is the most widely used PET radiopharmaceutical (Fig. 7.1). It is transported via the selective GLUT-1 glucose transporter into the cells. There, the FDG is phosphorylated similarly to normal glu-

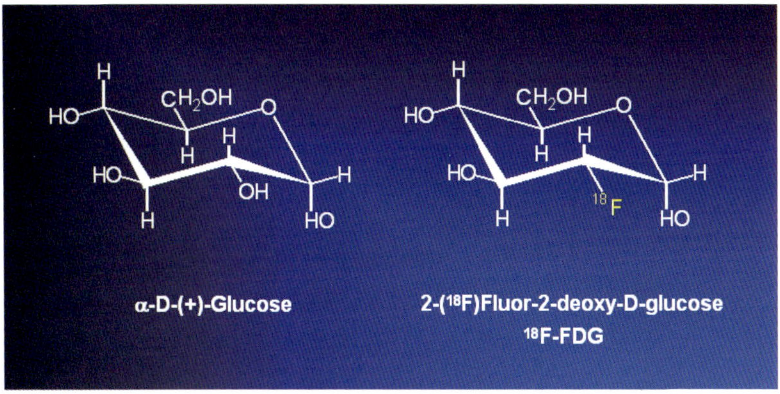

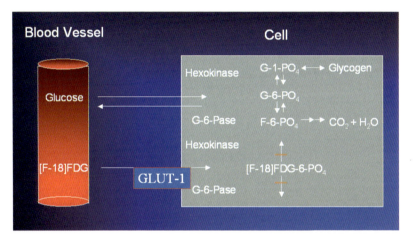

Fig. 7.1. Glucose and FDG. To label glucose an OH group is replaced by an ^{18}F atom

Fig. 7.2. Transport of FDG into the cell by GLUT1-transporter and intracellular trapping

cose. Enzymes involved in further glucose metabolism are very substrate-specific. They do not support FDG as a substrate, therefore the FDG can not leave the cell nor can it undergo further metabolism (Fig. 7.2). It is trapped in the cell until it decays. Expression and activity of GLUT-1 transporters is highly regulated. Malignant tumor cells, activated white cells, myocardiocytes and some nervous cells show an increased FDG-uptake. Therefore, FDG-PET can detect malignomas or inflammation (infectious as well as noninfectious such as active atherosclerosis) and show changes in metabolism in the brain or the heart muscle. In oncology most malignant tumors show an increased FDG-uptake

compared to nonaffected tissues. Renal cell carcinomas, prostate cancer or hepatocellular carcinomas as well as some soft tissue tumors do not show a reliable FDG-uptake. In these tumor entities FDG-uptake is dependent on the grade of differentiation. Less differentiated tumors show higher FDG-uptake. These tumors can be assessed by alternative radiopharmaceuticals.

7.4 Protocols and Patient Preparation

Patients undergoing FDG-PET imaging should have fasted six hours prior to the examination. Beverages containing carbo-

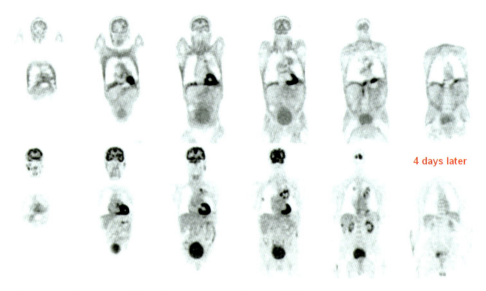

4 days later

Fig. 7.3. Male patient suffering from metastatic disease. The first PET scan (*upper row*) was acquired after the patient had breakfast, but told the investigators that he had fasted. PET scan showed only minor tumor activity (one hot spot in the mediastinum) while the CT showed large masses. After more intensive questions he admitted to his meal. Four days later a second PET scan was performed after fasting, which showed the realistic tumor metabolism with many mediastinal masses and pulmonary and hepatic metastasis

hydrates such as sugar should also not be consumed six hours prior to the examination. Diabetics should be prepared to have normoglycemic blood glucose levels. Before FDG-injection the blood glucose level should be checked in every patient because increased glucose levels can cause a false negative FDG-PET (Fig. 7.3).

After intravenous injection of 200 MBq FDG, 20 mg of Furosemid and 20 mg of butyl scopolamine followed by a saline flush should be injected. Then the patient should undergo a 45- to 60-minute period of rest in which the tracer is taken up into the cells. In certain tumor entities, such as sarcoma, the period of rest should be 90 min due to the slow FDG-uptake of these tumors, and more radioactivity, e.g., 270 MBq, should be injected to compensate for the longer decay before acquisition. Muscular activity should be avoided after FDG-injection because it leads into an increased glucose uptake into the muscles and can compromise readability [3] of the PET scan and increase exposure to radiation. The scopolamine that should be injected together

with the FDG avoids a first-pass uptake of the tracer in nonskeletal muscles. The Furosemid increases the urinary elimination of FDG, which has not been taken up into the cells and rinses the bladder with urine before PET acquisition. Therefore patients should empty the bladder before the PET scan. High amounts of radioactivity in the bladder can compromise the detection of hot spots in the pelvis, such as a rectum carcinoma. With non-FDG tracers Furosemid and scopolamin do not have to be administered. Contraindications, such as glaucoma or benign prostate hyperplasia to scopolamin and decreased blood potassium levels or cardiac insufficiency to Furosemid, must also be observed.

Acquisition of the PET/CT should be started with a topogram to plan the desired target volume identically to conventional MDCT. A standard oncological PET ranges from the base of the skull down to the middle of the upper leg. For special indications, the scan range can be enlarged to the full body, such as in melanoma, which can cause satellite lesions in any part of the

Table 7.2. Scan parameters for CT in PET/CT. Parameters may vary between different vendors or scanners with different numbers of detector rows

	Low dose CT (CTAC)	Diagnostic CT	CT angiography
Collimation	5 mm	1 to 5 mm	1 mm
Pitch	1.5	1	1.5
kVp	120	120	100
Tube current time product (mAs(	30 – 90	180 – 300	150 – 330
Pitch corrected tube current time product (eff. mAs)	20 – 60	120 – 200	100 – 220
Recon. algorithm	smooth	Dependent on indication	Smooth
Slice thickness	5 mm	1 to 6 mm	1.25
Slice increment	5 mm	Identical to slice thickness. Overlapping for MPR, etc.	0.8 mm
Field of view	Identical to physical PET axial FOV	Adapted to body size	Adapted to target volume
Contrast	None	120 cc at 3 cc/s	120 cc at 5 cc/s
Postprocessing	Used for CTAC	Coronal and sagittal MPRs	MIP dependent on indication

skin [4], or the scan range can be minimized, for example, in therapy control of a certain, previously detected index lesion. A low-dose spiral CT acquisition has to be performed prior to the PET scan to generate the attenuation correction map (CTAC) for the PET emission scan (see Table 7.2 for applicable scan parameters). The PET emission scan should be acquired in a 3D mode if available. While the CT is acquired in a spiral mode with continuous table movement, the PET is recorded with incremental, sequential table positions. Reasonable acquisition times for a single table position are 2 to 3 min. z-Axis fields of view (FOV) in PET scanners are between 10 and 20 cm. The table increment for 3D-acquisition should allow an overlap between adjacent table positions to improve image quality. Reasonable table increments for an 18-cm z-axis FOV 3D PET scanner are 10 to 12 cm.

The PET should be reconstructed with and without attenuation correction using an image matrix of at least 144×144 pixels.

Depending on the indication, a diagnostic normal-dose CT scan with contrast enhancement or a CT-angiography can be performed after the PET emission scan (see Table 7.2 for applicable scan parameters). The patient should undergo all parts of the examination in shallow breathing.

Scan parameters for the CT scan should always be adapted to the specific target volume and body size. For scanning the neck and thorax only, the mAs can be reduced compared to an abdominal scan. Slim patients need a lower dose than obese patients. PET/CT scanning is a high-dose examination, especially when doing whole body scanning combined with diagnostic CT or CT angiography (see Table 7.3) and indication should be established very care-

Table 7.3. Average effective radiation exposure for both sexes in PET/CT. Parameters may vary significantly between different vendors or different scan parameters

Scan	Effective dose (mSv) (200 MBq FDG)	Effective dose (mSv) (300 MBq FDG)
Topogram	< 0.1	< 0.1
Low-dose CT (CTAC)	4	4
PET	3.8	5.7
Whole-body CT	13.9	13.9
Total	21.8	23.7

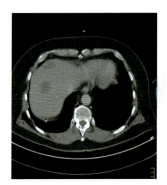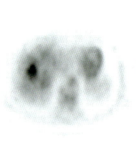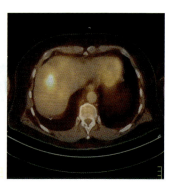

Fig. 7.4. Patient status post resected colon cancer and radio-frequency ablation (RFA) of a liver metastasis and again rising tumor markers. PET/CT shows an avital, successfully treated liver lesion ventrally in the liver and a new, centrally located liver metastasis with tumor metabolism. Proving that the first treated metastasis is avital PET enables RFA treatment of the second metastasis. CT alone could not reliably show which lesions are left to treat

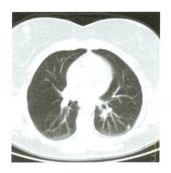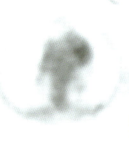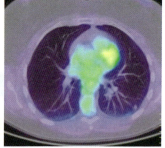

Fig. 7.5. CT shows an indeterminate pulmonary nodule. Negative FDG-PET shows nonmalignant etiology

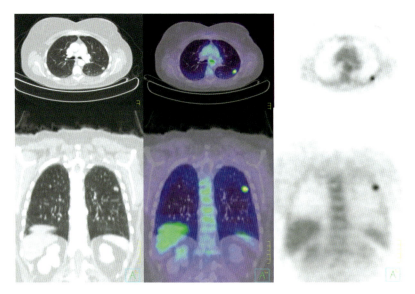

Fig. 7.6. CT shows an indeterminate pulmonary nodule. Positive FDG-PET shows malignoma

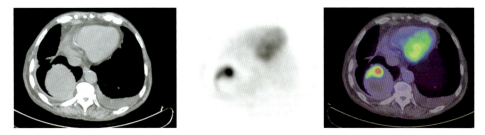

Fig. 7.7. PET/CT shows realistic extension of vital tumor tissue after neoadjuvant chemotherapy of lung cancer prior to surgery

fully especially in younger patients or in patients not suffering from a malignant disease.

7.5   Evaluation

PET/CT reading is the reading of coregistered PET and CT data. Coregistered data means that for any displayed image of one modality, a corresponding image with the same FOV, slice position, and plane orientation can be displayed. Simultaneously scrolling through both datasets is possible and every finding can be at the same time evaluated in both modalities. Additionally, an image fusion [5] can be achieved by superimposing color-coded PET data to grayscale CT data (Fig. 7.4) showing the metabolic activity of any CT-detected lesion. Using the PET in addition to the CT data can help to distinguish between benign and malignant lesions, such as in indeterminate pulmonary nodules (Figs. 7.5 and 7.6) [6]. Three-dimensional viewing is standard when evaluating PET/CT data. To quantify tracer uptake in PET/CT the standardized uptake value (SUV) can be calculated. The SUV is dependent on body size and weight of the patient, the specific amount of radioactivity detected in the target lesion, the amount of radioactivity administered, the half-life of the radionuclide used and the time after injection. In

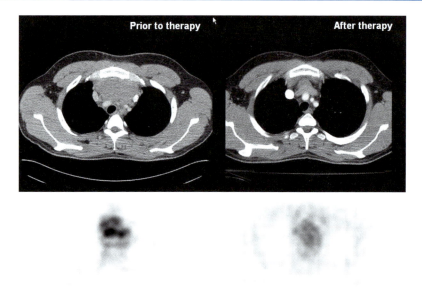

Fig. 7.8. CT as well as PET show the effect of chemotherapy in a patient suffering from lymphoma. While the CT documents the decrease in size, FDG-PET exhibits the decrease in tracer uptake

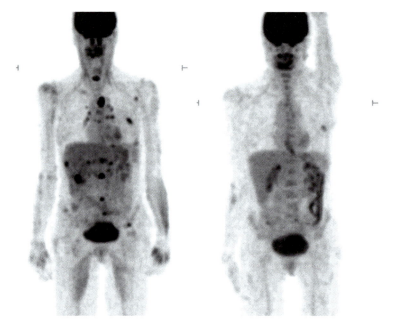

Fig. 7.9. PET on the left shows primary left side breast cancer as well as multiple metastases prior to chemotherapy. PET on the right shows early effect of chemotherapy: only the primary shows persistent tumor metabolism

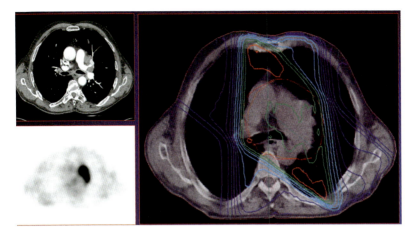

Fig. 7.10. PET/CT used for radiation therapy planning. CT shows tumor mass and suspicious lymph nodes. PET shows tumor but rules out affection of hilar lymph node and enables a more targeted therapeutic approach

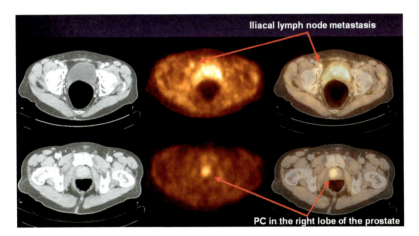

Fig. 7.11. C11-Choline PET/CT shows an example of prostate cancer and iliac lymph node metastasis

FDG-PET, an SUV of more than 2.5 is suspicious and of more than 3.0 is typical of malignoma.

PET/CT can help to determine still vital tumor portions after neoadjuvant chemotherapy and to limit surgery to the still vital portions of the tumor. It can also show that the disease is now operable (Fig. 7.7). PET/CT combining morphological and functional assessment is the ideal modality to monitor therapy response (Fig. 7.8) [7]. PET can show response to chemotherapy very early (Fig. 7.9) and can help to change an ineffective regimen as early as possible while remaining lesions can be accurately localized in CT to plan further therapy such as by radiation or surgery. PET/CT data can be used to plan radiation therapy (Fig. 7.10) and can help to limit the target volume to vital parts of the tumor or affected lymph nodes. Alternative tracers to FDG can be evaluated similarly to FDG (Fig. 7.11). SUV values typical for malignant or other pathologic findings have to be determined for each different tracer individually since the SUV is specific to tracer kinetics.

7.6   Conclusion

PET/CT has the potential to become the new high-end diagnostic imaging modality for various indications. Today PET/CT is most widely used in oncological imaging and detection of inflammatory disease but also for selected questions in neurology, cardiac and vascular imaging. New developments, especially in molecular imaging can further increase the spectrum of PET/CT indications. Availability and the high costs of the PET/CT examination are still limiting the use of PET/CT to certain centers. The comparatively high radiation exposure of whole body PET/CT scanning requires a very responsible establishment of indications for PET/CT examinations.

References

1. Reske SN, Kotzerke J (2001) FDG-PET for clinical use. Results of the 3rd German Interdisciplinary Consensus Conference, Onko-PET III, 21 July and 19 September 2000. Eur J Nucl Med 28(11):1707–1723

2. Osman MM, Cohade C, Nakamoto Y, Marshall LT, Leal JP, Wahl R (2003) Clinically significant inaccurate localization of lesions with PET/CT: frequency in 300 patients. J Nucl Med 44:240–243

3. Yeung HW, Grewal RK, Gonen M, Schoder H, Larson SM (2003) Patterns of (18)F-FDG uptake in adipose tissue and muscle: a potential source of false-positives. J Nucl Med 44:1789–1796

4. Mijnhout GS, Hoekstra OS, van Tulder MW, Teule GJJ, Devillé WLJM (2001) Systematic review of the diagnostic accuracy of 18F-fluorodeoxyglucose positron emission tomography in melanoma patients. Cancer 91:1530–1542

5. Wahl RL, Quint LE, Cieslak RD, Aisen AM, Koeppe RA, Meyer CR (1993) Anatometabolic tumor imaging: fusion of FDG PET with CT or MRI to localize foci of increased activity. J Nuc Med 34:1190–1197

6. Beyer T, Townsend DW, Brun T, Kinahan PE, Charron M, Roddy R, Jerin J, Young J, Byars L, Nutt R (2000) A combined PET/CT scanner for clinical oncology. J Nucl Med 41:1369–1379

7. Freudenberg LS, Antoch G, Schutt P, Beyer T, Jentzen W, Muller SP, Gorges R, Nowrousian MR, Bokisch A, Debatin JF (2003) FDG-PET/CT in re-staging of patients with lymphoma. Eur J Nucl Med Mol Imaging 31:325–329

II Brain

8 Acute Neurovascular Events: Bleeding and Ischemia Diagnosed by MSCT

B. Ertl-Wagner

Indications for CT in Patients with Acute Neurovascular Events

Indications for Nonenhanced Cranial CT (NECT)

- To rule out intracerebral hemorrhage.
- Delineation and extent of a cerebral ischemia.
- To discern early signs of cerebral ischemia, e.g., a hyperdense media sign or a loss of the insular ribbon.
- To evaluate and quantify space-occupying effects of an intracerebral hemorrhage or of a large cerebral infarction.
- To discern a possible noncommunicating hydrocephalus due to space-occupying infarctions in the posterior fossa.
- To rule out other differential diagnoses, such as subdural hematoma, epidural hematoma, subarachnoid hemorrhage, cerebral venous thrombosis or intracranial tumors.

Indications for CT Angiography

- To assess the site of the macrovascular occlusion.
- To determine the degree of collateral circulation.
- Therapy control of therapeutic interventions, e.g., intravascular thrombolysis or mechanical methods of recanalization.

Indications of CT Perfusion Imaging

- To determine the degree and extent of the perfusion deficit in the ischemic region (compare with Chap. 11 on perfusion CT by M. Wiesmann).

Patient Preparation and Positioning

Patient Preparation

- The patient should undergo informed consent about the risks of contrast medium application as is standard practice.
- Information regarding renal and thyroid function (creatinine and TSH values) should be obtained for contrast enhanced studies, if possible.
- Information about the patient's current medication should be available (e.g., metformine).
- A large peripheral venous access, e.g., in an antecubital vein, should be obtained.

Patient Positioning

- The patient should be positioned supine on the CT examination table.
- The patient's head should be positioned in the headrest.
- If the gantry cannot be tilted, it is advantageous to position the patient's head in 30° flexion in the head holder for an intracranial examination.

Topogram and Scan Range

- In intracranial examinations the lens should be outside the scan range, if at all possible, in order to reduce the dose to the radiation-sensitive lens.
- The gantry should therefore be tilted parallel to the base of the skull (German horizontal line) or the head should be positioned in 30° flexion in intracranial examinations.

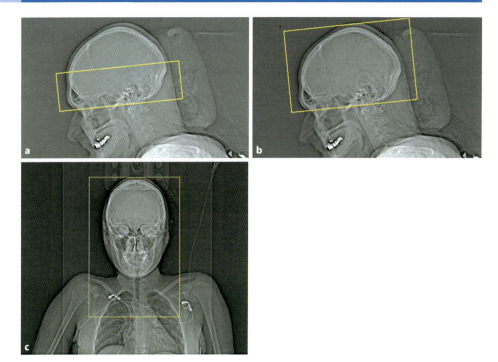

Fig. 8.1. a This lateral topogram demonstrates the scan range in a CT angiography of the circle of Willis. **b** This lateral topogram demonstrates the scan range of a combined arterial and venous protocol covering both the circle of Willis and the cerebral veins and sinuses. **c** This coronal topogram demonstrates the scan range of a CT-angiographic examination of the entire cervicocranial vasculature covering both the extracranial and the intracranial arteries

- For intracranial CT-angiographic examinations of the arterial vessels, the scan range should reach from cervical spine C2 to the mid-skull above the sella (see Fig. 8.1a).
- For combined CT-angiographic examinations of the arterial vessels, the scan range should reach from the lower end of the skull base to the vertex (see Fig. 8.1b).
- For CT-angiographic examinations of the entire cervicocranial vasculature, the scan range should extend from the aortic arch to the vertex (see Fig. 8.1c).

Scan Parameters

See Tables 8.1 and 8.2.

Tips and Tricks

- If an automated bolus tracking or a test bolus is not possible, a fixed delay can be used. A fixed delay of 35 s will usually provide an even contrast of both the intracranial arteries and the intracranial veins, while a fixed delay of 20 to 25 s should result in a predominantly arterial contrast.
- A simultaneous contrast of both the intracranial arteries and the intracranial veins can be advantageous in the emergency setting, if the patient´s symptomatology is not clear.
- If a carotid artery stenosis is suspected, the supraaortic arteries should be included in the scan range. It is then feasible to assess both a thrombembolic occlusion of an intracranial artery and the potential source of a thrombembolus in the carotid arteries.

Table 8.1. Scan parameters for CT angiography of the cranial vessels

Parameters	4–8 slice scanners	10–16 slice scanners	32–64 slice scanners
Scanner settings			
Tube voltage (kV)	120	120	120
Rotation time (s)	0.5	0.5	0.33–0.5
Tube current time product (mAs)	135–200	135–200	135–240
Pitch corrected Tube current time product (eff. mAs)	150–200	150–200	150–200
Collimation (mm)	1/1.25	0.625/0.75	0.6/0.625
Norm. pitch	0.9–1	0.9–1	0.9–1.2
Reconstr.-slice increment (mm)	1	0.6	0.5
Reconstr.-slice thickness (mm)	1.25[*]	0.75–1[*]	0.6–0.75[*]
Reconstruction Kernel	Standard	Standard	Standard
Contrastmedia application			
Concentration (mg iodine/mL)	300	300	300
Mono/Biphasic	Monophasic	Monophasic	Monophasic
Volume (mL)	120	120	120
Injection rate (mL/s)	4–5	4–5	4–5
Saline chaser (mL, mL/s)	30/4.0	30/2.5	30/4.0
Delay (s) • Circle of Willis	Autom. Bolus-Detection +7 s	Autom. Bolus-Detection +10 s	Autom. Bolus-Detection +10 s
• Combined arterial and venous	Fixed delay 35 s	Fixed delay 40 s	Fixed delay 40 s
• Entire craniocervical vessels	Autom. Bolus-Detection +4 s	Autom. Bolus-Detection +8 s	Autom. Bolus-Detection +8 s

[*] STS-MIPs in coronal and sagittal planes in addition to the axial slices are mandatory.

Table 8.2. Scan parameters for unenhanced CT of the brain

Parameters	4–8 slice scanners	10–16 slice scanners	32–64 slice scanners
Scanning parameters			
Tube voltage (kV)	120	120	120
Rotation time (s)	0.75	1.0	1.0
Tube current time product (mAs)	195–255[*]	190–250[*]	350[*]
Pitch corrected tube current time product (eff. mAs)	300[*]	290[*]	410[*]
Slice collimation (mm)	2.5	1.5	0.6
Norm. pitch	0.65–0.85	0.65–0.85	0.85
Contrast material			
Volume (mL)	N/A	N/A	N/A
Injection speed (mL/s)	N/A	N/A	N/A
Saline flush (mL, mL/s)	N/A	N/A	N/A
Delay arterial (s)	N/A	N/A	N/A
Delay portal-venous (s)	N/A	N/A	N/A

[*] CTDI must be lower than or equal to 60.00

- The source images of an intracranial CTA can often be very helpful in the evaluation of the location and extent of a cerebral ischemia, when the window and level settings are chosen accordingly.

Comments

Neurovascular events are among the most common presenting symptoms in the emergency setting. The classical role of CT used to be the exclusion of hemorrhage, while it was considered inferior in the diagnosis of cerebral ischemia. However, awareness of early CT signs in the mid-1990s led to an increasing role of CT in the diagnosis of early cerebral ischemia as well [1]. However, the determination of the exact extent of the ischemic region, the diagnosis of the site of the vascular occlusion and the extent of a possible diffusion-perfusion mismatch could not be assessed.

The introduction of multislice CT into clinical practice altered several limitations of CT by improving both the spatial and the temporal resolutions. It became possible to evaluate the entire cervicocranial vasculature in a high spatial resolution allowing the assessment of even subsegmental arterial occlusions [2,3].

When a patient presents with signs and symptoms of a neurovascular event, timing is usually critical in order to ascertain the administration of the proper therapeutic regimen in a timely fashion. Moreover, time frames for potential intravenous or intraarterial thrombolytic therapies need to be respected. The diagnostic workup should therefore be fast and focused.

In every patient presenting with an acute neurovascular event, an unenhanced cranial CT scan should be performed first. This CT scan is the basis to rule out an intracerebral hemorrhage, which often cannot be differentiated from a cerebral ischemia on clinical grounds alone. Moreover, the un-

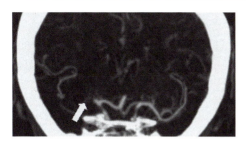

Fig. 8.2. Coronal sliding thin slab (STS) maximum intensity projections (MIP) demonstrate an acute occlusion of the right middle cerebral artery in the M1 segment (*arrow*)

enhanced CT scan can be used to evaluate early signs of cerebral ischemia such as the loss of the insular ribbon or the hyperdense media sign [1]. It is also the basis for evaluating potential complications of cerebral infarctions, such as a midline-shift in large space-occupying supratentorial infarctions or a noncommunicating hydrocephalus in infarctions of the posterior fossa.

When an intracerebral hemorrhage is ruled out, a CT angiography can be performed in the absence of contraindications to an administration of a contrast medium. It is usually advantageous to plan the CT angiography with a maximum of clinical information available. If the symptomatology of the patient is not clear and cerebral venous thrombosis is a potential differential diagnosis, a CT-angiographic protocol attaining an even contrast of both the intracerebral arteries and veins can be advantageous (2). The scan range should include the region between the lower part of the skull base and the vertex. If the patient's signs and symptoms point toward an intracranial arterial occlusion, the CT-angiographic examination can be focused on the Circle of Willis in order to demonstrate the exact site of occlusion. CTA can be very helpful to assess here, especially if Doppler/duplex sonography is not available in the emergency setting. It can be helpful to use CTA to evaluate the entire supraaortic arteries [4]. In addition to imaging the intracranial arteries, the carotid arteries can be assessed in this setting as well in order to rule out plaques as a source of thrombem-

bolism and/or hemodynamically relevant occlusions [4]. The scan range should then reach from the aortic arch to the Circle of Willis.

When evaluating an intracranial CT angiography, it is important to scrutinize every segment of the intracranial arteries. Most commonly, thrombembolic occlusions can be found in the middle cerebral artery (MCA) (Fig. 8.2). As the spatial resolution was pronouncedly improved with multislice CT, it is now possible to diagnose even small, subsegmental occlusions, e.g., in the M2 or M3 segments [5]. If the M1 segment of the MCA is occluded, care should be taken to differentiate whether the thrombembolic process also involves the intracranial carotid bifurcation (carotid-T), thus representing a carotid-T rather than a mere M1 occlusion.

While the clinical symptomatology can be very helpful in guiding the diagnostic evaluation of an intracranial CT angiography, the assessment should not be limited to the artery in question. In addition, every vascular segment needs to be analyzed. Vascular norm variations, such as an embryonic origin of the posterior cerebral artery PCA, should be noted, as these variations may favor unusual thrombembolic routes. In addition, other differential diagnoses such as intracranial aneurysms, need to be ruled out, even in the absence of a subarachnoid hemorrhage as these can present as a purely incidental – but highly relevant – finding in the intracranial CTA.

If a combined arterial and venous protocol was chosen, the cerebral veins and dural sinuses need to be scrutinized as well. Care should be taken to differentiate arachnoid granulations or hypoplasias of the sinus from cerebral venous or sinus thromboses. An engorgement of the smaller venous structures such as the bridging veins can be an indirect sign of a venous congestion due to a cerebral venous thrombosis.

The assessment of the CT-angiographic source images in a proper window and level setting may be helpful in evaluating the extent of the ischemic region, as the ischemia can usually be discerned positively in these contrast enhanced images, which allows

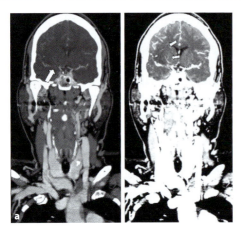

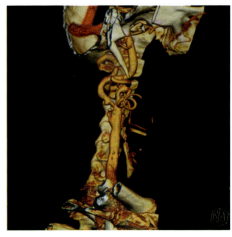

Fig. 8.3. a Coronal STS-MIP reformations demonstrate an acute thromboembolic occlusion of the right middle cerebral artery in the M1/M2 segments (*arrow*). **b** An adjustment of the window and level settings demonstrates the ischemic region in the same CT angiographic dataset (*arrows*)

Fig. 8.4. Volume rendering technique (VRT) reformations demonstrate a higher grade, complex stenosis of the internal carotid artery in a patient with an acute neurovascular event

to view a form of "blood volume images" (Figs. 8.3a,b) [6–8].

When evaluating the carotid arteries in the setting of an acute neurovascular event, several questions need to be answered. First, the CT angiography needs to be evaluated regarding the presence (or absence) of a hemodynamically relevant stenosis of the carotid artery (Fig. 8.4). These hemodynamically relevant stenoses will mostly be found in the proximal internal carotid artery (ICA) in close proximity to the carotid bifurcation. However, stenoses of the carotid artery can arise in more unusual locations as well, such as in the proximal portion of the common carotid artery (CCA) or in the distal part of the ICA. This again underscores the necessity to closely scrutinize all vascular segments when evaluating a supraaortic CT angiography. In addition, plaques along the carotid arteries should be described with an emphasis on plaque morphology, mentioning both the plaque configuration and the presence or absence of calcifications within the plaque. Moreover, the potential presence of an arterial dissection of either the carotid arteries or the vertebral arteries should be ruled out. Arterial dis-

sections in this region usually present as a tapering of the vascular lumen with a directly adjacent mural hematoma.

Multislice CT with CT angiography offers several pronounced advantages over other imaging modalities such as MRI and ultrasonography. First and foremost, multislice CT is usually readily available even in the emergency setting and can be performed in the range of seconds. Patient access is almost unlimited allowing imaging of even critically ill patients. Moreover, the cranial vessels can now be imaged at an exceedingly high resolution allowing a diagnostic evaluation of even small, subsegmental arteries. The analysis of the source images in a proper window setting moreover may allow an enhanced view of an early demarcation of the ischemic territory. In addition, the CT-angiographic evaluation can also be combined with a CT perfusion (see Chap. 11). Relative drawbacks of CT are the application of ionizing radiation (the dose of which can be reduced when optimized scan parameters are employed and when the scan rage is limited to the potentially diagnostically relevant region), and the inability to perform diffusion-weighted imaging and thus evaluate a diffusion-perfusion mismatch (8).

References

1. von Kummer R, Bourquain H, Bastianello S et al. (2001) Early prediction of irreversible brain damage after ischemic stroke at CT. Radiology 219:95–100
2. Klingebiel R, Zimmer C, Rogalla P et al. (2001) Assessment of the arteriovenous cerebrovascular system by multi-slice CT. A single-bolus, monophasic protocol. Acta Radiol 42:560–562
3. Ertl-Wagner BB, Hoffmann RT, Bruning R et al. (2004) Multi-detector row CT angiography of the brain at various kilovoltage settings. Radiology 231:528–535
4. Tomandl BF, Klotz E, Handschu R et al. (2003) Comprehensive imaging of ischemic stroke with multisection CT. Radiographics 23:565–592
5. Verro P, Tanenbaum LN, Borden NM, Sen S, Eshkar N (2002) CT angiography in acute ischemic stroke: preliminary results. Stroke 33:276–278
6. Nabavi DG, Kloska SP, Nam EM et al. (2002) MOSAIC: multimodal stroke assessment using computed tomography: novel diagnostic approach for the prediction of infarction size and clinical outcome. Stroke 33:2819–2826
7. Hill MD, Coutts SB, Pexman JH, Demchuk AM (2003) CTA source images in acute stroke. Stroke 34:835–837
8. Schramm P, Schellinger PD, Fiebach JB et al. (2002) Comparison of CT and CT angiography source images with diffusion-weighted imaging in patients with acute stroke within 6 hours after onset. Stroke 33:2426–2432

9 CTA of Intracranial Aneurysm

D. Morhard

Indications

MS-CTAs are indicated in the following situations:
- Acute and subacute subarachnoid hemorrhage in which a digital subtraction angiography (DSA) is not instantly available in addition to the unenhanced CT.
- Incidental aneurysm MS-CTA may be an alternative to the gold-standard DSA for the determination of location, size and neck ratio.
- AVMs in conjunction with other modalities.
- Stenosis of intracranial vessels.

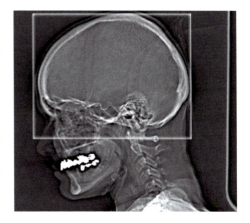

Fig. 9.1. Topogram with suggested maximum scan range for intracranial CTA

Patient Preparation and Positioning

Supine, arms bilaterally downward, use of headrest recommended, injection needle in cubital vein or central venous catheter with at an 18-gage lumen.

Topogram

See Fig. 9.1

Scan Parameters

See Table 9.1

Tips and Tricks

- 2D-reconstructions in three orientations (sagittal, axial and coronar planes) are obligatory, with a strongly recommended slice thickness between 1.0 and 1.3 mm.
- MIP reconstructions are felt to be better than MPR reconstructions.
- Interactive generation of VRT-images can be useful for the choice of surgical or endovascular treatment decision.
- Start scanning at C2, so as not to miss any of the intradural vertebral artery aneurysms.

Comments

The incidence of intracranial aneurysms is about 1.9%, depending on the population. The degree of subarachnoid hemorrhage (SAH) seen in CT can be staged by the Fisher grading system (Table 9.2) [5]. Clinical symptoms in most cases are the sudden onset of maximum headache, possibly with nuchal rigidity on middle-aged adult patients (the clinical severity of the SAH can

Table 9.1. Scan parameters

Parameters	4–8 slice scanners	10–16 slice scanners	32–64 slice scanners
Scanner settings			
Tube voltage (kV)	120	120	120
Rotation time (s)	0.5	0.5	0.33–0.5
Tube current time product (mAs)	135–200	135–200	135–240
Pitch corrected tube current time product (mAs)	150–200	150–200	150–200
Collimation (mm)	1/1.25	0.625/0.75	0.6/0.625
Norm. pitch	0.9–1	0.9–1	0.9–1.2
Reconstr.-slice increment (mm)	1	0.6	0.5
Reconstr.-slice thickness (mm)	1.25	0.75–1	0.6–0.75
Reconstruction Kernel	Standard	Standard	Standard
Scan range	Sutura sagittalis to Foramen magnum for strict intracranial aneurysm. Sutura sagittalis to arcus aortas in order to include the extracranial parts of VA and carotids.		
Scan direction	Caudocranial	Caudocranial	Caudocranial
Contrast media application			
Concentration (mg iodine/mL)	300–400	300–400	300–400
Mono/biphasic	Monophasic	Monophasic	Monophasic
Volume (mL)	80–120	80–100	80–100
Injection rate (mL/s)	3–4	3–4	3–4
Saline chaser (mL, mL/s)	30/3.0	30/3.0	30/3.0
Delay (s)	15–20 (12–15 for extracranial carotid and VA) or automatic bolus detection if available		

(among others) be assessed by the WFNS grading system, see Table 9.3).Twenty-five percent of all intracranial hemorrhages and almost all atraumatic subarachnoidal hemorrhages are caused by ruptured aneurysm. However, the most common cause of SAH is blunt head trauma. Depending on the aneurysm size and other factors (e.g., shape, localization, former SAH or former symptoms) the annual risk for an aneurysm rupture is estimated to be between 0.05% for aneurysms smaller than 10 mm and 6% for giant aneurysms (over 25 mm). For the most typical locations of intracranial aneurysms see Fig. 9.2. Additional risk factors for aneurysm hemorrhage include arterio-sclerosis, hypertension, and cigarette and alcohol abuse. The mortality for aneurysm induced SAHs is up to 50% in the first 30 days. The rebleeding risk from ruptured, untreated aneurysms is 20–50% (up to 15% in the first 24 h, then daily 1–3%).

Recent evaluations [1–4] show an overall sensitivity for intracranial aneurysm detection in acute subarachnoid hemorrhage of 85–95% when compared to DSA. Limitations for MS-CTA are small aneurysms with a maximum size between 1 and 3 mm, aneurysms in the posterior fossa and aneurysms in the cavernous sinus (supraophthalmic carotid aneurysms). Besides, negative DSA-findings for aneurysmal SAH is

Table 9.2. Fisher grading system of acute subarachnoidal bleeding

0	No blood detectable
1	Lumbar puncture positive, CT negative
2	Blood clot visible
3	Blood clots thicker than 3 mm
4	Intraventricular or intraparechnchymal hemorrhage

Table 9.3. World Federation of Neurologic Surgeons (WFNS) SAH grade

WFNS grade	Glasgow Coma Scale Score	Major focal deficit[*]
0 (intact aneurysm)	-	-
1	15	Absent
2	13–14	Absent
3	13–14	Present
4	7–12	Present or absent
5	3–6	present or absent

[*] Aphasia and/or hemiparesis or hemiplegia

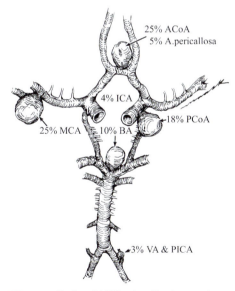

25% ACoA
5% A.pericallosa
4% ICA
18% PCoA
25% MCA
10% BA
3% VA & PICA

Fig. 9.2. Circle of Willis, localization and statistical distribution of cerebral aneurysm. Most common are aneurysms of the anterior communicating artery, and the A. cerebri media (MCA), followed by aneurysms at or near the origin of the posterior communicating artery (PCoA), and the basilar tip. Relatively seldom, especially difficult to detect are aneurysms of the posterior circulation in the infratentorial region

15–20% at first examination and below 5% when a patient is admitted for a second additional angiography (Fig. 9.3).

Important criteria to describe a finding of an aneurysm in CTA include the relationship of the aneurysm to the parent vessel (small neck or wide neck, fusiform, dissecting), the size and form of the aneurysm, presence or absence of a baby aneurysm, presence or absence or calcifications, thrombosis; and vessels originating from the aneurysm itself. To get this information, very detailed information is necessary. This description in turn will assist the decision, if (in incidental aneurysms) or by which means (in ruptured aneurysms) the treatment will be attempted. In general, endovascular treatment is carried out by filling the aneurysm with detachable platinum coils (e.g., GDC), delivered through a microcatheter. Aneurysms optimal for this endovascular treatment have a small neck and are located in the ACA, ICA or VA/BA territory. Endovascular stent application may be necessary, if an aneurysm is featuring a relatively broad neck. The neurosurgical treatment is performed

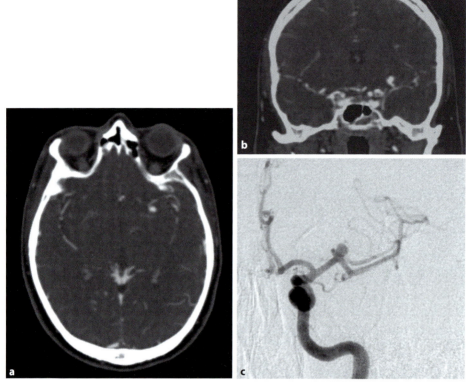

Fig. 9.3. a Left-sided, superior- and lateral-orientated MCA-bifurcation aneurysm with a maximum dome size of 4 mm and a neck size of 2 mm in a patient with mild acute SAH. This image demonstrates the good delineation of neck and dome (16-row MSCT, axial MIP-reconstruction with 1.3-mm thickness and 1.0-mm increment). **b** Coronar MIP-reconstruction (1.3×1.0 mm) of the same patient showing the superiolateral orientation of the aneurysm. **c** DSA (matrix 1024×1024), selective injection of left internal carotid artery, pa-orientated and zoomed of the same patient. DSA demonstrates the good correlation between MS-CTA and DSA

with the placement of a clip along the neck of the aneurysm. Candidates optimal for this procedure are located in the MCA or ACA territory. Regardless of the aneurysm, treatment prevention and treatment of secondary complications like vasospasm via hyperdynamic therapy are also often necessary.

Important differential diagnoses of the subarachnoidal hemorrhage are all forms of nonaneurysmal SAH (occult trauma, vasculitis, dissection, perimesencephalic nonaneurysmal SAH, vascular malformation, neoplasm). These forms can exhibit low density in brain scans representing diffuse cerebral edema, and may have high density CSF (e.g., following intrathecal contrast).

The protocol can be extended to assess suspected arteriovenous malformations (AVM). In these cases, CTA can give information on the major feeding vessels, the AVM nidus site and size, and the superficial or deep draining veins. All of these are important to the grading of the AVMs, which are done in most institutions by the grading system of Spetzler and Martin (see Table 9.4). However, for the treatment decision to recommend treatment by either gamma knife radiation, endovascular occlusion,

Table 9.4. Spetzler and Martin grading system for AVMs

Size of AVM	Eloquence of adjacent brain	Venous drainage
Small (<3 cm), 1 point	Noneloquent, 0 points	Superficial only, 0 points
Medium (3–6 cm), 2 points	Eloquent, 1 point	Deep drainage, 1 point
Large (>6 cm), 3 points		

surgery or combinations thereof, the invasive selective multiplanar DSA presently remains the method of choice.

References

1. Morhard D, Bruening R, Ertl-Wagner B, Reiser M, Brueckmann H (2004) MS-CTA vs. DSA in acute subarachnoidal haemorrhage. RSNA Book of Abstracts, p 688
2. Jayaraman MV, Mayo-Smith WW, Tung GA, Haas RA, Rogg JM, Mehta NR, Doberstein CE (2004) Detection of intracranial aneurysms: multi-detector row CT angiography compared with DSA. Radiology 230(2):510–518
3. Pedersen HK, Bakke SJ, Hald JK, Skalpe IO, Anke IM, Sagsveen R, Langmoen IA, Lindegaard KE, Nakstad PH (2001) CTA in patients with acute subarachnoid haemorrhage. A comparative study with selective, digital angiography and blinded, independent review. Acta Radiol 42(1):43–49
4. Kato Y, Katada K, Hayakawa M, Nakane M, Ogura Y, Sano K, Kanno T (2001) Can 3D-CTA surpass DSA in diagnosis of cerebral aneurysm? Acta Neurochir (Wien) 143(3):245–250
5. Fisher CM (1975) Clinical syndromes in cerebral thrombosis, hypertensive haemorrhage and ruptured saccular aneurysm. Clin Neurosurg 22:117–147

10 Imaging of the Cerebral Veins and Sinuses with MS-CT

B. Ertl-Wagner

Indications for Cerebral CT-Venography

- To diagnose or rule out cerebral venous thromboses (CVT).
- To precisely evaluate the site and extent of a cerebral venous occlusion in CVT.
- To evaluate the degree of compression of the cerebral veins and sinuses in patients with an intracranial neoplasm, especially in patients with meningioma.
- To non-invasively evaluate the venous drainage in patients with cerebral arteriovenous malformations.

Patient Preparation and Positioning

Patient Preparation

- The patient should undergo informed consent about the risks of contrast medium application as is standard practice.
- Information regarding renal and thyroid function (creatinine and TSH) should be obtained.
- Information about the patient's current medication should be available (e.g., metformine).
- A large peripheral venous access, e.g., in an antecubital vein, should be obtained.

Patient Positioning

- The patient should be positioned supine on the CT examination table.
- The patient's head should be positioned in the headrest.

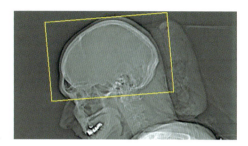

Fig. 10.1. This lateral topogram demonstrates the normal scan range for a CT-angiographic evaluation of cerebral veins and sinuses

- If the gantry cannot be tilted, it is advantageous to position the patient's head in 30° flexion for an intracranial examination.

Topogram and Scan Range

- The scan range should reach from the lower end of the skull base to the vertex (see Fig. 10.1).
- The upper boundary of the scan range always needs to include the entire superior sagittal sinus; care should be taken to include the most cranial portion of the skull.
- The lower boundary of the scan range should include the sigmoid sinus.
- The scan range should include the petrous bones in order to evaluate a possible mastoiditis in the setting of septic CVT.
- It is usually not necessary to include the entire jugular veins in the scan range, since these can be imaged with Doppler and duplex sonography. However, should doubt prevail, the neck region can also be included to image the cervical veins.

Scan Parameters

See Table 10.1.

Tips and Tricks

- Cerebral venography can usually be quite reliably and easily performed with a fixed delay of 40 to 45 s and a bolus of contrast medium of 120 mL.
- If the patient's symptomatology is not clear, a simultaneous contrast of both the intracranial arteries and the intracranial veins can be helpful, especially in the emergency setting. A slightly reduced delay of about 35 s will usually provide an even contrast of both the intracranial arteries and the intracranial veins.
- Care should be taken to evaluate the petrous bones, especially in the setting of a CVT of the sigmoid and transverse sinuses, as these can potentially represent septic thromboses resulting from a purulent mastoiditis.
- It is important to differentiate mere hypoplasia of the transverse sinus, which is a common variant, from true CVT. Moreover, arachnoid granulations need to be recognized and differentiated from CVT.
- The nonenhanced cranial CT should always be scrutinized as well, since the location, extent and contour of edema and/or hemorrhage as secondary signs of a cerebral venous thromboris can provide important information about the potential site of the venous occlusion.

Comments

The most common indication to image the intracranial veins and sinuses is to rule out CVT. CVT can present with relatively unspecific signs and symptoms, which vary substantially from asymptomatic to severe symptoms requiring intensive care treatment. Other differential diagnoses are often contemplated by the referring clinician as well [1,2]. Please keep in mind that CVT is a disease with a mortality of up to 10% even in the presence if intensive care and the standard practice of iv. Heparine.

The computed tomographic evaluation of CVT usually consists of a nonenhanced CT (NECT) scan followed by a CT-angiographic examination. The NECT should always be carefully examined as the presence of edema and/or hemorrhage as well as its respective size, location and shape can provide important information regarding the extent and location of the venous occlusion. However, a normal NECT does not rule out the presence of CVT.

Therefore, a CT-angiographic examination of the cerebral veins and sinuses is usually performed next. The scan range should always include the entire cerebral venous vasculature. It is therefore important to carefully include the uppermost point of the vertex in order to image the entire superior sagittal sinus. Coronar and sagittal reconstructions are important here and should be performed routinely. The lower boundary of the scan range should include the skull base with the petrous bones and the entire posterior fossa.

A fixed delay of 40 to 45 s usually results in a homogeneous contrast of the intracranial venous vessels. In our experience, it is frequently helpful to attain a mixed arterial and venous contrast as the symptomatology of the patient is often not specific for a venous pathology. A fixed delay of 35 s usually provides a homogeneous contrast of both the arteries and the veins, when a bolus of 120 mL of contrast medium is applied [3,4]. The scan direction should usually "follow the flow." Thus, when imaging the cerebral veins and sinuses, the direction of acquisition should be craniocaudal.

When evaluating a CT-venographic examination in a patient with suspected CVT, it is important to look for the site and the extent of the venous occlusion (Fig. 10.2). As mentioned above, the site of parenchymal edema and/or hemorrhage can provide important information regarding the occluded vessel. The CT-venographic examination generally allows a direct visualiza-

Table 10.1. Scan parameters for MSCT-imaging of the cerebral veins and sinuses

Parameters	4–8 slice scanners	10–16 slice scanners	64 slice scanners
Scanner settings			
Tube voltage (kV)	100–120 [6]	100–120 [6]	100–120 [6]
Rotation time (s)	0.5	0.5	0.33–0.5
Tube current time product (mAs)	150–200	150–200	150–200
Pitch corrected tube current time product (eff. mAs)	150–200	150–200	150–200
Tube current (mAs)	100–200	100–200	100–200
Collimation (mm)	1	0.75	0.65
Norm. pitch	1	1	1
Reconstr.-slice increment (mm)	0.75–2	0.6–2	0.5–2
Reconstr.-slice thickness (mm)	1–3 mm	1–3 mm	1–3 mm
Reformation technique	Sliding thin slab (STS) MIP	STS-MIP	STS-MIP
Scan range	Base of skull to vertex	Base of skull to vertex	Base of skull to vertex
Scan direction	Craniocaudal	Craniocaudal	Craniocaudal
Reconstruction kernel	Standard	Standard	Standard
Contrast media application			
Concentration (mg iodine/mL)	300	300	300
Mono/Biphasic	Monophasic	Monophasic	Monophasic
Volume (mL)	120	120	120
Injection rate (mL/s)	4–5 [7]	4–5 [7]	4–5 [7]
Saline chaser (mL, mL/s)	30/4.0	30/4.0	30/4.0
Delay (s) • Venous • Combined arterial and venous	Fixed delay 40–45 s Fixed delay 35 s or Autom. Bolus-Detection +12 s	Fixed delay 40–45 s Fixed delay 35 s or Autom. Bolus-Detection +12 s	Fixed delay 40–45 s Fixed delay 35 s or Autom. Bolus-Detection +12 s

tion of the thrombotic material within the occluded (or partially thrombosed) cerebral vein or sinus, which is referred to as the cord sign [5]. While the surrounding vessel is filled with contrast material, the thrombotic material is relatively hypodense compared to the contrast enhanced sinus often described as the empty triangle sign (Fig. 10.3).

It is important to differentiate CVT from simple arachnoid granulations. In contrast to the more amorphous structure of a venous thrombus that tends to fill large parts of the venous structure, an arachnoid granulation usually has a density resembling that of fat, is comparatively small and round, and is well demarcated. Arachnoid granulations moreover tend to be lobulated

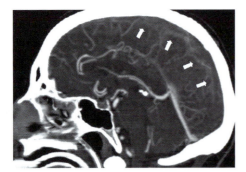

Fig. 10.2. Sagittal sliding thin slab (STS) maximum intensity projections (MIP) demonstrate a complete thrombotic occlusion of the superior sagittal sinus

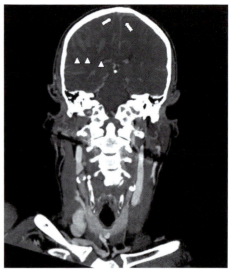

Fig. 10.3. Coronal STS-MIP reformations demonstrate an occlusion of the superior sagittal sinus (*arrows*). Note the presence of edema and hemorrhage on the right-hand side (*arrowheads*). In this case, the entire cervicocranial vascular system was examined, as the thrombus extended into the internal jugular vein

and can be found anywhere, but predominantly in characteristic locations such as the transverse and superior sagittal sinus. In addition, it is crucial to differentiate mere hypoplasia of the sinus from true venous thrombosis. The transverse sinus can commonly display an asymmetric configuration with relative hypoplasia of one side, just constituting a normal variant [2]. Care should be taken not to mistake such a normal variant for a thrombosed vessel. In this setting, it is important to look for direct manifestations of the thrombus, i.e., to look for thrombotic material within the vessel. It can moreover be helpful to search for indirect signs of venous thrombosis such as edema or hemorrhage of the brain parenchyma.

A CT-angiographic examination of the cerebral veins and sinuses with modern multislice CT scanners now allows for the visualization of even small venous structures such as bridging veins or the internal cerebral veins. However, despite promising reports, the sensitivity of MDCT to detect or exclude superficial venous thrombosis is not certain. Also, in order not to miss the diagnosis of a selective thrombosis of these veins, it is important to be familiar with the intracranial venous anatomy and to actively search for the small vascular structures. Again, the presence and location of edema and/or hemorrhage within the brain parenchyma can provide important clues regarding the site of the thrombosis.

CT-venographic examinations with multislice CT can moreover provide information regarding the degree of venous congestion. Three-dimensional reconstructions may help in selected cases to improve the visualization of a thrombus (Fig. 10.4). The smaller venous structures draining into the thombosed vessel are commonly enlarged as a result of the obliterated venous lumen. In addition, in the setting of a more longstanding venous obstruction, the degree of collateral circulation can be assessed. This can also constitute important information in the setting of a compression of a cerebral sinus, which can often occur in the setting of meningiomas (Fig. 10.5). The superior sagittal sinus is an especially common site of venous compression, secondary to perifalcine meningiomas. In this setting, the degree of venous compression and the presence or absence of a collateral circulation should be described.

When a thrombosis of the sigmoid and/or transverse sinus is found, it is especially

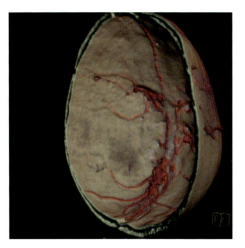

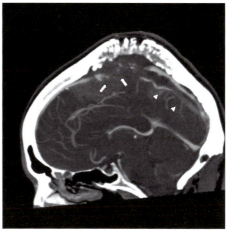

Fig. 10.4. Volume rendering technique images of the same patient demonstrate a congestion of the small vessels draining into the thrombosed superior sagittal sinus

Fig. 10.5. Sagittal STS-MIP reformations in a patient with a transosseous meningioma demonstrate a compression of the superior sagittal sinus by the tumor (*arrows*). A collateral circulation is present (*arrowheads*)

important in children and young adults to also assess the petrous bones for the potential presence of a mastoiditis, as these thromboses commonly represent septic processes as a consequence of a mastoidal infection. The dataset should be reconstructed in a bone kernel in this setting in order not to miss this important additional information. Finally, it has to be mentioned that the detection and exclusion of recurrent/remitting CVT may still represent a diagnostic problem both in venous CT and MRI.

In summary, CT angiography of the cerebral veins and sinuses with multislice CT provides an excellent tool in the diagnosis of CVT. It not only directly depicts the presence and location of the venous thrombus, but also demonstrates the degree of venous congestion and/or collateralization and may provide important additional information, e.g., regarding the presence of an inflammatory process in the mastoid.

References

1. Hagen T, Bartylla K, Waziri A, Schmitz B, Piepgras U (1996) Value of CT-angiography in diagnosis of cerebral sinus and venous thromboses. Radiologe 36:859–866
2. Haage P, Krings T, Schmitz-Rode T (2002) Nontraumatic vascular emergencies: imaging and intervention in acute venous occlusion. Eur Radiol 12:2627–2643
3. Klingebiel R, Zimmer C, Rogalla P et al. (2001) Assessment of the arteriovenous cerebrovascular system by multi-slice CT. A single-bolus, monophasic protocol. Acta Radiol 42:560–562
4. Ertl-Wagner B, Hoffmann RT, Bruning R, Dichgans M, Reiser MF (2002) Diagnostic evaluation of the craniocervical vascular system with a 16-slice multi-detector row spiral CT. Protocols and first experiences. Radiologe 42:728–732
5. Casey SO, Alberico RA, Patel M et al. (1996) Cerebral CT venography. Radiology 198:163–170
6. Ertl-Wagner BB, Hoffmann RT, Bruning R et al. (2004) Multi-detector row CT angiography of the brain at various kilovoltage settings. Radiology 231:528–535
7. Cademartiri F, van der Lugt A, Luccichenti G, Pavone P, Krestin GP. Parameters affecting bolus geometry in CTA: a review. J Comput Assist Tomogr 26:598–607

11 Brain Perfusion

M. Wiesmann

Indications

- Acute ischemic cerebral infarction.
- Chronic stenosis of supraaortic or intra-cranial arteries.
- Currently evaluated indications include vasospasm after subarachnoid hemorrhage and evaluation of cerebral neoplasms.

Patient Preparation

Large-caliber cubital venous access is recommended (preferably 16 or 18 G).

Patient Positioning

- Supine, arms downward, use of headrest recommended.
- If tilting the gantry during continuous scan mode is not possible, the head of the patient should be inclined to protect the lenses from radiation.

Topogram/Scan Range

See Fig. 11.1.

Table Scan Parameters

See Table 11.1.

Tips and Tricks

- Instruct the patient before the acquisition to lie still although the bolus injec-

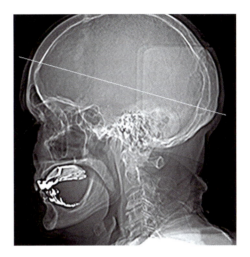

Fig. 11.1. Perfusion studies in acute stroke are centered at the level of the basal ganglia to include portions of those vascular territories most likely affected from major vessel occlusion (i.e., anterior, middle, and posterior cerebral arteries)

tion of contrast material may cause discomfort.
- Injection of a saline chaser following the contrast media improves image quality.
- If the first study is negative, up to two additional perfusion studies can be performed to cover other clinically suspected brain areas.

Comments

Perfusion CT allows accurate quantitative assessment of brain tissue perfusion, is well tolerated, and is not time-consuming. It has become a valuable tool in the imaging of acute stroke for two reasons: (1) areas of impaired perfusion can be de-

Table 11.1. Scan parameters for MSCT measurement of brain perfusion

Parameters	4–8 slice scanners	10–16 slice scanners	32–64 slice scanners
Scanner settings			
Tube voltage (kV)	80	80	80
Tube current (mAs)	120–240	120–240	120–240
Collimation (mm)	2×10 / 4×8	2×10 / 4×8	2×10 / 4×8
Norm. pitch	0	0	0
Rotation time (s)	1.0	1.0	1.0
Reconstruction increment (mm)	0	0	0
Reconstruction thickness (mm)	10	12	12
Convolution kernel	Special	Special	Special
Specials	Dynamic scan: 45 scans (1 scan/s)	Dynamic scan: 45 scans (1 scan/s)	Dynamic scan: 45 scans (1 scan/s)
Contrast media application			
Concentration (mg iodine/ml)	370–400 mg/mL	370–400 mg/mL	370–400 mg/mL
Mono/Biphasic	Monophasic	Monophasic	Monophasic
Volume (mL)	40	40	40
Injection rate (mL/s)	5–10	5–10	5–10
Saline chaser (mL, mL/s)	40/5.0	40/5.0	40/5.0
Delay (s)	5 (fixed)	5 (fixed)	5 (fixed)

tected right after the onset of stroke, and (2) there is evidence that if the information from a normal brain CT and perfusion parameter maps are combined, it is possible to discriminate between irreversibly damaged and potentially salvageable tissue [1,2]. Perfusion CT can therefore support therapeutic strategies based on individual assessment of brain perfusion in stroke patients rather than using rigid time intervals related to the onset of symptoms [3].

Strokes are the third leading cause of death after cardiovascular diseases and cancers as well as a leading cause of serious disability. Thrombolysis, administered either intravenously or intraarterially, has been approved as an effective therapy for acute human stroke. It is intended to rescue the penumbra and to reduce the final infarct size, and thus the resulting handi-

cap. At present, the selection of patients for thrombolytic therapy is mainly related to the time interval since the onset of symptoms (less than 3 to 6 h, depending on the applicable protocol), the absence of cerebral hemorrhage, and the infarct size (cerebral hypodensity on CT extending to less than one-third of the middle cerebral artery region). However, even with such restrictive criteria not all patients selected benefit from thrombolytic therapy and thrombolysis itself bears a significant risk of intracranial bleeding. Therefore it has been proposed to take into consideration the individual hemodynamic situation of stroke patients.

To derive functional information on the hemodynamic status of the brain, sequential CT slices are acquired in cine mode during intravenous contrast administration. For each pixel, time-density profiles

12 Sinuses and Facial Skeleton

F. Dammann

Indications

- Inflammatory disease (sinusitis, polyposis, mukocele, orbital or intracranial complications).
- Preoperative planning (FESS functional endoscopic sinus surgery: identify anatomic variations, potentially dangerous situations).
- Midfacial or cranial trauma, congenital deformations, tumor disease (benign and malignant lesions, T-staging, follow-up).
- Preoperative workup for corrective surgery, planning of computer-aided surgery (image fusion, surgical simulation, navigation, robotics) and manufacturing of medical models (stereolithography models for preoperative simulation).

Patient Preparation

No special preparation necessary; i.v. access if CM administration needed.

Patient Positioning

- Supine (all scans are performed in the axial plane), arms downward, use headrest.
- Additional prone position of the patient is only indicated for the diagnosis of orbital floor fractures when using multislice CT with less than 16-row scanning to obtain direct coronal images.

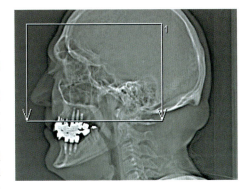

Fig. 12.1. Examination region including the frontal sinus to the alveolar ridge (including the chin, resp., when the mandibula is involved in facial trauma or surgical procedure)

Topogram/Scan Range

See Fig. 12.1.

Table Scan Parameters

See Table 12.1.

Tips and Tricks

Orthogonal positioning of the patient's head simplifies the image interpretation.

Multiplanar reformations (potentially also including angulated axial slices) that are anatomically adjusted in all three dimensions can be performed on patients for whom optimal positioning cannot be achieved.

Table 12.1. Scan and reconstruction parameter of CT of the paranasal sinuses and the midface

Parameters	4–8 slice scanners	10–16 slice scanners	32–64 slice scanners
Scanner settings			
Tube voltage (kV)	120	120	120
Rotation time (s)	<1	<1	<1
Tube current time product (mAs)	20/200*	20/90–200*	20/90–200*
Pitch corrected Tube current time product (eff. mAs)	20/220*	20/140–200*	20/140–200*
Collimation (mm)	1–1.25	0.625–0.75	0.6–0.625
Norm. pitch	0.9	0.6–1.0	0.6–1.0
Reconstruction increment (mm)	0.6	0.5	0.5
Reconstruction slice thickness (mm)	1.0–1.25	0.75–1	0.6–0.75
Convolution kernel	Bone	Bone	Bone
Specials	Multiplanar reformations, fac. 3D reformations fac. soft tissue ref.	Multiplanar reformations, fac. 3D reformations fac. soft tissue ref.	Multiplanar reformations, fac. 3D reformations fac. soft tissue ref.
Scan range	Frontal sinus/ alveolar ridge (mandibula)	Frontal sinus/ alveolar ridge (mandibula)	Frontal sinus/ alveolar ridge (mandibula)
Scan direction	Craniocaudal	Caudocranial	Craniocaudal
Contrast media application	No	No	No

* mAs values exceeding 100 mAs should be reserved for the diagnosis of tumor disease or complications of sinusitis when i.v. contrast material has to be administered. For the examination of the sinuses for trauma and benign sinus disease a low-dose protocol seems sufficient (see text).

A low-dose setting (20–50 mAs) is recommended for the majority of standard sinus CT.

Comments

Standard midfacial and/or sinus CT includes both axial and coronal images as proposed by Zinreich et al. [1]. Coronal images (Fig. 12.2) are considered to be more important for preoperative planning because they show the shape and relationship of most anatomic landmarks closest to the intraoperative aspect (cribriform plate, ostiomeatal complex, orbital walls). Axial slices (Fig. 12.3) help to define the localization and extent of disease (trauma, benign or malignant diseases) in the anterior–posterior direction, especially when the ethmoid cells, the sphenoid sinus, or the orbit is involved.

When using multislice CT, coronal reformations that are directly reconstructed out of the spiral raw data or calculated from a thin-slice axial data set can replace the direct coronal scan. For planning the position and range of coronal reformations,

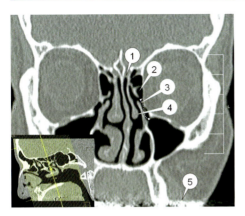

Fig. 12.2. Coronal image: 64-row CT, 50 mAs, 120 kV, direct coronal reformation, slice thickness 1 mm. Clear depiction of anatomical details: cribriforme plate (1), ostiomeatal complex (2–4), including the bulla ethmoidalis (2), the uncinate process (3), the middle turbinate (4), and the maxillary infundibulum (*dashed line*) extending from the maxillary ostium (*dot*) to the hiatus semilunaris (*arrow head*). No stair step artifacts. Dental metal artifacts do not superimpose the midface but are horizontally oriented (5), corresponding to the axial scan direction

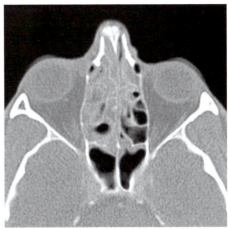

Fig. 12.3. Axial image: 4-row CT, 20 mAs, 120 kV, slice thickness 2 mm. Chronic sinusitis with bilateral involvement of the anterior and posterior ethmoid and the sphenoid sinus

a sagittal view should be used (Fig. 12.2). The angulation of coronal reformations should be adjusted perpendicularly to the maxillary plate. The advantages of coronal reformations include the absence of dental metal artifacts that may superimpose relevant anatomical structures of the midface in direct coronal scans, the more comfortable position of the patient, and the reduction of the exposure dose and examination time by 50% as compared with a conventional two-scan CT examination. Direct coronal scans may still be indicated for the diagnosis of non- or slightly dislocated orbital floor fractures that can be missed on coronal reformations derived from axial CT scans with a less than 16-row scanner due to stair step artifacts.

A low-dose setting (20–50 mAs) is recommended for the majority of standard sinus CT examinations because predominantly young patients suffering from benign diseases are involved and high levels of image noise can be tolerated due to the high contrast of tissue versus air. The surface dose can be reduced to 3–4 mGy and the effective dose to 0.1–0.2 mSv when using 20 mAs [2]. A medium dose setting (100 mAs) is recommended for diagnosis of trauma and tumor disease, complications of inflammatory diseases (e.g., orbital or intracranial involvement), and for 3D applications (e.g., SSD, volume rendering, and medical modeling).

I.v. Contrast

I.v. contrast does not add relevant diagnostic information in the majority of sinus CT examinations, but may be helpful to delineate the extent of benign or malignant lesions that pass over the bony borders of the paranasal sinuses. In these cases a monophasic c.m. application of 50 mL with a scan delay of 90–120 s and a medium dose setting (100–150 mAs) is recommended. Beside standard bone reformations (Table 12.1) additional soft tissue data sets (slice thickness and increment 3–5 mm, medium-soft convolution filter, window 350/50) are calculated.

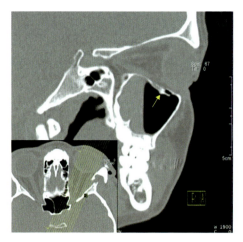

Fig. 12.4. Orbital floor fracture with slight dislocation (*arrow*) and maxillary sinus hemorrhage. Sagittally angulated reformation (slice thickness 1 mm, derived from axial scan: 16-row CT, 0.75-mm slice thickness, pitch 1.0, reconstruction increment 0.5 mm, 100 mAs, 120 kV)

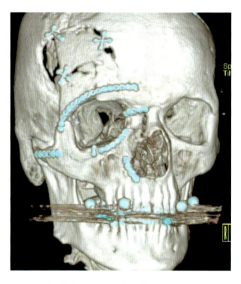

Fig. 12.5. Osteosynthesis of complex midfacial fractures, corrective surgery planned. Volume rendering of 64-slice CT (100 mAs, 120 kV, 0.6 mm collimation, pitch 1.0, reconstruction slice thickness 0.6 mm, increment 0.4 mm, intermediate convolution filter)

3D Reconstructions

In trauma diagnosis of the facial skeleton additional sagittally angulated reformations that are adjusted to the optical nerve axis may provide additional information in orbital floor trauma (Fig. 12.4). In trauma diagnosis the slice thickness of any multiplanar reformation should not exceed 2 mm. Three-dimensional reformations (SSD, volume rendering) allow for an intuitive understanding of complex midfacial fractures (Fig. 12.5). An additional axial thin-slice data set using an intermediate or slightly soft convolution filter is recommended as the basis for 3D reformations with reduced image noise. In contrast, edge-enhancing filters are recommended for the manufacturing of precise medical models.

Differential Diagnosis

CT is the most reliable imaging modality to diagnose midfacial trauma. It allows for a detailed analysis of the involved structures. Reports should be formulated according to the international trauma classifications (LeFort, AO classification) when applicable (Table 12.2). CT is also accepted as the gold standard for paranasal sinus imaging in benign inflammatory disease, i.e., chronic sinusitis. Reports should address the extent of the disease and the presence of anatomical variations that may potentially entail sinusitis or that may be critical for endoscopic surgery [3,4]. Ill-defined soft tissue is generally designated as soft-tissue opacification since CT does not allow further differentiation. MRI is superior to CT for soft tissue evaluation. Hence, MRI should be used preferentially to CT for tumor diagnosis (Table 12.3) and in complications of inflammatory disease [5,6].

Table 12.2. LeFort facial fractures [7]

LeFort 1	Horizontal fracture of the alveolar process of the maxilla (teeth contained in the detached fragment)
LeFort 2	Fracture of the body of the maxilla with pyramidal shape of the detached maxillary fragment; fracture extends into the floor of the orbit, the hard palate including the pterygoid process and the nasal cavity
LeFort 3	Entire maxilla and one or more facial bones are completely detached from the craniofacial skeleton; includes fracture of the zygomatic arch

Table 12.3. Staging criteria for maxillary sinus squamous cell carcinoma [8]

T1	Tumor limited to mucosa with no erosion or destruction of bone
T2	Tumor causing bone erosion or destruction including extension into the hard palate and/or middle nasal meatus, except extension to posterior wall of maxillary sinus and pterygoid plates
T3	Tumor invades any of the following: bone of the posterior wall of maxillary sinus, subcutaneous tissues, floor or medial wall of orbit, pterygoid fossa, ethmoid sinuses
T4a	Tumor invades anterior orbital contents, skin of cheek, pterygoid plates, infratemporal fossa, cribriform plate, sphenoid or frontal sinuses
T4b	Tumor invades any of the following: orbital apex, dura, brain, middle cranial fossa, cranial nerves other than maxillary division of trigeminal nerve, nasopharynx, or clivus

References

1. Zinreich SJ, Kennedy DW, Rosenbaum AE, Gayler BW, Kumar AJ, Stammberger H (1987) Paranasal sinuses: CT imaging requirements for endoscopic surgery. Radiology 163:769–775
2. Dammann F, Bode A, Heuschmid M, Kopp A, Georg C, Pereira PL, Claussen CD (2000) Multislice spiral CT of the paranasal sinuses: first experiences using various parameters of radiation dosage. Fortschr Röntgenstr 172:701–706
3. Ludwig JJ, Taber KH, Manolidis S, Sarna A, Hayman A (2002) A computed tomographic guide to endoscopic sinus surgery: axial and coronal views. J Comput Assist Tomogr 26:317–322
4. Sarna A, Hayman A, Laine FJ, Taber KH (2002) Coronal imaging of the osteomeatal unit: anatomy of 24 variants. J Comput Assist Tomogr 26:153–157
5. Som PM, Shapiro MD, Biller HF, Sasaki C, Lawson W (1988) Sinonasal tumors and inflammatory tissues: differentiation with MR imaging. Radiology 167:803–808
6. Som PM, Dillon WP, Sze G, Lidov M, Biller HF, Lawson W (1989) Benign and malignant sinonasal lesions with intracranial extension: differentiation with MR imaging. Radiology 172:763–766
7. Hunter TB, Peltier LF, Lund PJ (2000) Musculoskeletal eponyms: who are those guys? Radiographics 20:819–836
8. American Joint Committee on Cancer (2002) Cancer staging handbook, 6th edn. Greene FL et al. (eds). Springer, Berlin Heidelberg New York

13 Nasopharynx, Oropharynx, and Oral Cavity

M. Keberle

Indications

- Staging of malignant tumors.
- Suspected arrosion of the skull base, the hard palate or the mandible.
- Parapharyngeal masses, inflammatory processes such as para- or retropharyngeal abscesses.
- Detection and differentiation of benign lesions.

Patient Preparation

Remove dental prostheses, etc., instruct patient to perform quiet breathing and not to swallow, supine, arms (and shoulders) downward.

Topogram

See Fig. 13.1a,b.

Scan Parameters

See Table 13.1.

Example of Axial and Coronal Scans

See Fig. 13.2a,b.

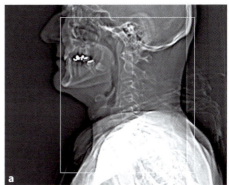

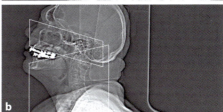

Fig. 13.1. a Topogram covering the entire pharynx and neck (for the majority of scanners, a gantry angulation is no longer possible). **b** Topogram showing two spirals avoiding dental artifacts (possible with a 4-row scanner)

Reconstructions

Coronal multiplanar reconstruction (MPR) in both soft tissue and bone kernel is obligatory if an infiltration of the skull base or the hard palate is suspected. Moreover, coronal MPR is extremely helpful for evaluating of the floor of the mouth.

Table 13.1. Scan parameters

Parameters	4–8 slice scanners	10–16 slice scanners	32–64 slice scanners
Scanner settings			
Tube voltage (kV)	120	120	120
Rotation time (s)	0.75–1	0.75–1	0.75–1
Tube current time product (mAs)	180	180	180
Pitch corrected tube current time product (eff. mAs)	140–230	140–230	140–230
Collimation (mm)	1/1.25 (lower spiral[b]: 2.5)	1.25/1.5	0.6/0.625
Norm. pitch	1–1.3	1–1.3	1–1.5
Reconstr.-slice increment (mm)	3 For recons 1.0	2–3 For recons: 1.0	2–3 For recons: 0.6
Reconstr.-slice thickness (mm)	3–5 For recons: 1.5	3 For recons: 1.5–2	3 For recons: 0.75–1
Convolution kernel	Standard (and bone[a])	Standard (and bone[a])	Standard (and bone[a])
Scan direction	Caudocranial	Caudocranial	Caudocranial
Contrast media application	Yes	Yes	Yes
Concentration (mg iodine/ml)	300	300	300
Volume (mL)	100	100	100
Injection rate (mL/s)	1.5–2.0	1.5–2.0	1.5–2.0
Saline chaser (mL, mL/s)	No	No	No
Delay (s)	50 (fixed) (40[b])	55 (fixed)	55 (fixed)

[a] For coronal MPR with bone kernel it is obligatory to exclude tumor infiltration of the skull base.

[b] In the case of many dental fillings, two spiral acquisitions with different angulations are necessary (a shorter delay is also required for contrast injection)

Criteria of Good Image Quality

1. High-quality axial scans (absence of blurring, absence of gross motion artifacts).
2. High-quality coronal MPR. To evaluate the skull base, bone kernel reconstructions are also necessary (maximum thickness: 3 mm).
3. Good contrast enhancement of vessels and lesions (see Tips and Tricks).

Tips and Tricks

In the case of severe dental artifacts, a 4-row-scanner allows one to acquire two spiral data sets that may be angulated conversely to avoid the teeth. The first spiral covering the neck should be performed with a collimation of 2.5 mm. However, the second spiral covering the nasopharynx must be performed with a collimation of 1.0 mm in order to obtain high-quality MPR of the skull base (see Table 13.1 showing the scan parameters).

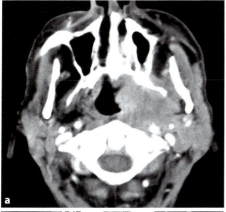

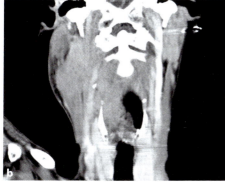

Fig. 13.2. a Huge nasopharyngeal carcinoma with infiltration of the parapharyngeal fat spaces and around the ICA (soft tissue window, axial). Note the importance of good vessel enhancement. The coronal MPR (**b**) shows the entire longitudinal extension of the mass

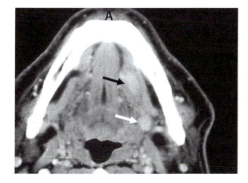

Fig. 13.3. Squamous cell carcinoma of the floor of the mouth with pronounced contrast enhancement (*black arrow*) and with infiltration of the sublingual fat; ipsilateral lymph node metastasis (*white arrow*), also with infiltration of fatty tissue

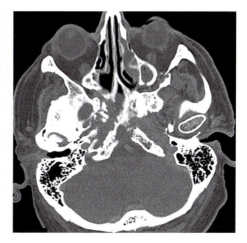

Fig. 13.4. T4-carcinoma of the nasopharynx with bony infiltration of the clivus (bone window, axial MPR)

Remember: the thinner the collimation the less prominent the artifacts.

During a "diagnostic window" – between 50 to 75 s after starting the injection of the contrast agent – both, an excellent tumor contrast (tumor rim versus surrounding muscle or fat) and good vessel enhancement ($\geq$ 150 HU; ROI measurement within the carotid artery) can be achieved (Table 13.1) [1].

Comments

Tumor Staging

The most frequent indication for CT of the nasopharynx, the oropharynx, or the oral cavity is to do local tumor staging in cases where the histology is already proven. The incidence of pharyngeal cancer is almost 10/100,000 inhabitants, mostly affecting men between 50–70 years of age [2,3]. Classical signs indicating a neoplastic lesion are tumor mass effect with distortion of normal anatomy, e.g., with asymmetrical lumen narrowing of the airway (Fig. 13.2), atypical and pronounced contrast enhancement, as well as infiltration of fat spaces (Fig. 13.3), and finally the direct destruction of bone (Fig. 13.4) [2,4]. Due to impor-

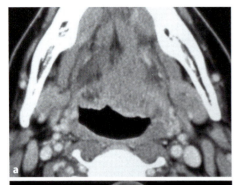

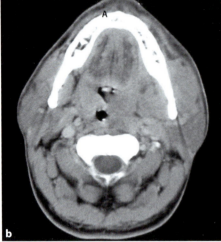

Fig. 13.5. Sharply delineated carcinoma of the base of the tongue (**a**) and ill-defined parapharyngeal abscess with central necrosis (**b**)

Table 13.2. TN-Staging of carcinoma of the nasopharynx, oropharynx and the oral cavity [6]

T- and N-stages of oropharyngeal carcinomas and/or carcinomas of the oral cavity	
T1	≤ 2 cm
T2	> 2–4 cm
T3	> 4 cm
T4a	Infiltration of the larynx, extrinsic muscles of the tongue, medial lamina of the pterygoid process, hard palate, and/or mandible
T4b	Infiltration of the lateral lamina of the pterygoid process, lateral pterygoid muscle, skull base, and/or internal carotid artery
N1	Unilateral single lymph node metastasis, ≤3 cm
N2a	Single unilateral lymph node, 3–6 cm
N2b	Multiple unilateral lymph nodes, ≤6 cm
N2c	Bilateral (or contralateral) lymph node(s), ≤6 cm
N3	>6 cm
T- and N-stages of nasopharyngeal carcinomas	
T1	Limited to the nasopharynx
T2	Infiltration of the oropharynx and/or nose
	T2a without parapharyngeal infiltration
	T2b with parapharyngeal infiltration
T3	Infiltration of skull base and/or paranasal sinuses
T4	Intracranial extension and/or infiltration of cranial nerves, the infratemporal fossa, the hypopharynx, the orbit, and/or the masticator space
N1	Unilateral cervical lymph node(s), ≤6 cm
N2	Bilateral cervical lymph nodes, ≤6 cm
N3a	>6 cm
N3b	Supraclavicular lymph node metastasis

tant therapeutical implications, such as the ability to resect, it is important to detect bony infiltration. Coronal MPR in both soft tissue and bone kernel are obligatory if an infiltration of the skull base is suspected. For detailed staging criteria please refer to Table 13.2 [5].

Regarding bony erosions CT is known to be superior to MRI, but regarding perineural tumor spread through skull base foramina and/or dural infiltration MRI is superior to CT [4,6]. Therefore, a combination of CT and MRI is often necessary in the complete assessment of nasopharyngeal carcinoma. Moreover, MRI better distinguishes if a lateral infiltration of the parapharyngeal fat space exists, and this way better distinguishes between the T2a- and

T2b-stages of nasopharyngeal carcinomas (Table 13.2).

Inflammatory Processes

In contrast to focal cancer, inflammatory processes, such as an abscess or a phlegmone, tend to be more diffuse (Fig. 13.5). Furthermore, inflammatory processes extend towards more deeply located submucosal and parapharyngeal fat spaces so that their entire extension is hard or impossible to evaluate clinically. The latter also holds true for primary parapharyngeal lesions, e.g., neoplasms, which are entirely located beneath an intact mucosa, so that a pathology other than carcinoma is very likely [2]. Deep extension or location can be easily evaluated with CT, especially if the mandible is involved [4]. MRI, however, is superior in case of severe dental artifacts and to differentiate any focal lesion from strongly contrast-enhancing lymphatic tissue at the level of the base of the tongue and the tonsils [2,7].

Lymph Nodes

Cervical lymph node metastases have a significant impact on the patient's prognosis. Thus, N-staging in patients with head and neck cancer is very important, and can be easily performed simultaneously (together with the T-staging) (Table 13.2).

A combination of good vessel enhancement (for N-staging) and excellent tumor contrast (for T-staging) can be achieved with a single contrast bolus during spiral CT of oro- and/or nasopharyngeal carcinomas (Table 13.1) [1].

References

1. Keberle M, Tschammler A, Hahn D (2002) Single-bolus technique for spiral CT of laryngopharyngeal squamous cell carcinoma: comparison of different contrast material volumes, flow rates, and start delays. Radiology 22:171–6
2. Mukherji SK, Weissmann JL, Holliday RA (2003) Pharynx. In: Som PM, Curtin HD (eds) Head and neck imaging (4th edn). Mosby, St. Louis
3. Ferlay J, Bray F, Sankila R, Parkin DM (1999) EUCAN: Cancer incidence, mortality and prevalence in the European Union 1995, version 2.0. IARC CancerBase No. 4. IARC Press, Lyon
4. Smoker WRK (2003) The oral cavity. In: Som PM, Curtin HD (eds) Head and neck imaging (4th edn). Mosby, St. Louis
5. UICC Union international contre le cancer (2002) TNM-Atlas. Springer, Berlin Heidelberg New York
6. Casselman JW (1994) The value of MRI in the diagnosis and staging of nasopharyngeal tumors. J Belge Radiol 77:67–71
7. Lenz M, Hermans R (1996) Imaging of the oropharynx and the oral cavity. Part II: Pathology. Eur Radiol 6:536–549

14 MDCT of the Hypopharynx and Larynx

R. Bruening

Indications

- Suspected tumor/mass of the hypopharynx or larynx.
- Unclear findings on endoscopy.
- Trauma to the laryngeal cartilages.

Patient Preparation, Patient Positioning, Topogram/Scan Range

- The patient should be positioned supine on the CT examination table.
- Information regarding renal and thyroid function (creatinine and TSH values) should be obtained for contrast-enhanced studies.
- The patient's head should be positioned in the headrest.
- Patient is instructed to resist swallowing or coughing for the moment of image acquisition.

Table Scan Parameters

See Table 14.1.

Tips and Tricks

- Patient instruction is important to get motion free data of the larynx: practice with the patient on the table before the topogram and inform the patient of the estimated length of scan. Breath-hold imaging is usually better tolerated by patients compared to phonation.

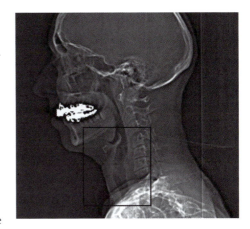

Fig. 14.1. Topogram. The scan range should include the region from the mandible to the jugulum as indicated

- If an automated bolus tracking or a test bolus is not feasible, a fixed delay of 70 s can be used.

Comments

The most common indications to perform cross-sectional imaging of the hypopharynx and larynx include the detection and staging of squamous cell carcinoma and their differential diagnosis, nonsquamous cell tumors and laryngoceles, as well as traumatic lesions. In numerous institutions MDCT now is the first imaging modality of choice for a suspected mass, while MRI is reserved for evaluating lesions close to the cartilage or the ventricle (Fig. 14.1) (1).

Imaging of the larynx, however, must be coordinated with the clinical exam.

Table 14.1. MSCT imaging parameters for the optimized study of the larynx. Generally all laryngeal helical acquisitions should use the breath-hold technique. In special instances, the Valsalva maneuver or phonation may also be required

Parameters	4–8 slice scanners	10–16 slice scanners	32–64 slice scanners
Scanning parameters			
Tube voltage (kV)	120	120	120
Rotation time (s)	0.5	0.5	0.5
Tube current time product (mAs)	200–225	135–225	135–225
Pitch corrected tube current time product (eff. mAs)	150	150	150
Slice collimation (mm)	1/1.25	0.625/0.75	0.6/0.625
Norm. pitch	1.375–1.5	0.9–1.5	0.9–1.5
Reconstruction increment (mm)	1	0.5	0.5
Reconstruction thickness (mm)	1.25, 3	0.75–1.3	0.75–1.3
Contrast material: indication (e.g., arterial phase scan)			
Volume (mL)	110	100	110
Injection speed (mL/s)	3	3	3
Saline flush (mL, mL/s)	40, 3	40, 3	40, 3
Delay arterial (s)			
Delay portal–venous (s)	70	80	80–90

The information acquired at imaging usually emphasizes the deeper tissues, while the superficial assessment of the laryngeal structures and the laryngeal mucosa and the histology is done by endoscopy. To emphasize the role of imaging in this specific anatomic area, knowledge of the anatomy is key to understanding the extension of a lesion.

Anatomy

The larynx is subdivided into three compartments: the supraglottic, the glottic and the subglottic level. These levels are defined by distinct anatomic landmarks:

- The hypopharynx borders the larynx from above. The major borderline between them is the aryepiglottic fold, where the lateral piriform recessus is part of the hypopharynx. The hypopharynx also includes the postcrycoid area and the posterior pharyngeal wall caudally of the level of the base of the tongue.
- The laryngeal structures above the ventricle of the larynx and below the hypopharynx are the supraglottic level.
- The glottic larynx refers only to the true folds. It has been defined as stretching from the ventricle to a plane approximately one centimeter below the ventricle. Here, the glottis merges with the subglottis (the lower part of the larynx).
- The subglottis extends from the lower margin of the glottis to the inferior margin of the cricoid cartilage.

The true vocal folds (cords) play a major role in speech generation (glottic level). They stretch across the lower larynx and are in the horizontal or axial plane. There is

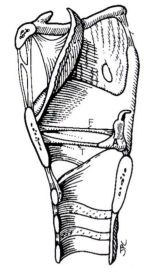
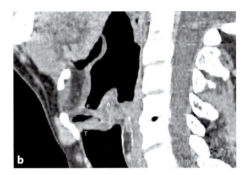

Fig. 14.2. Anatomical drawing. **a** The three levels of the larynx are shown from a lateral view. The true vocal cord is labeled *T*, the false vocal cord *F*, while the arythenoid cartilage is marked *A* (drawing modified from [4]). **b** Sagittal reconstruction of MDCT data set (4 row). A 1-mm collimated acquisition is reformatted in overlapping 3-mm sagittal planes. Imaging during breath hold (normal anatomy)

a small cease just above the true vocal folds called the ventricle. Immediately above the ventricle and true folds is a second pair of folds called the false vocal folds (Fig. 14.2) (4). Another important anatomic term is the anterior commissure. This is the point where the true folds converge bilaterally and insert anteriorly into the thyroid cartilage.

Cartilages define the structures of the larynx and help to orient the levels in the larynx. The cricoid is at the level of the glottis and subglottis. The upper posterior edge of the cricoid cartilage is actually at the level of the true folds and supports the tiny arythenoid cartilages (Fig. 14.2). The lower edge of the cricoid cartilage represents the lower boundary of the larynx and, therefore, the lower edge of the subglottis.

The key muscle is the thyroarytenoid muscle, best seen in the coronal plane (Fig. 14.3b). This forms the bulk of the true folds and extends from the arytenoid up to the anterior part of the thyroid cartilage at the anterior commissure. Deep and lateral to the throarythenoid muscle is the para-

glottic space, normally filled with fatty tissue. In the case of tumor infiltration the paraglottic space becomes obliterated (Fig. 14.4) and in more advanced cases this tumor infiltration also restricts movement of the vocal cords.

Generally, advanced postprocessing techniques, such as 3D volume rendering, are too time consuming and so far considered to be of limited use for the physician reading laryngeal images. However, image reconstruction techniques, such as MPRs (reconstructed thickness with an overlap of 2–6 mm), yield improved diagnostic results.

In general, for best results, a visualization procedure using standard MPR in all three planes is recommended.

Pathology

Over 90% of all masses in the region of the hypopharynx and larynx are squamous cell carcinomas. As a rule, these carcinomas arise from the mucosal surface, thus the clinical diagnosis is usually already made

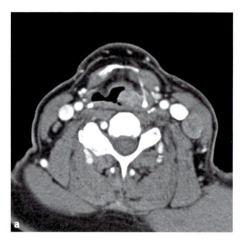
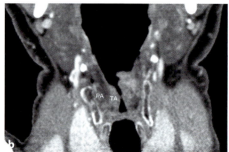

Fig. 14.3. Small supraglottic carcinoma originating from the aryepiglottic fold. Extension of the lesion in the left preepiglottic space best seen in the axial plane (**a**). The craniocaudal extend is best observed in the coronal reconstruction (**b**)

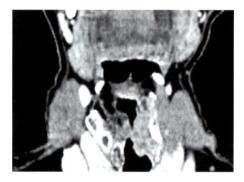

Fig. 14.4. T3-lesion on the left with infiltration of the paraglottic space (PA) in a 75-year-old man (coronal reconstruction)

at the time of imaging and is relatively easily confirmed by endoscopic biopsy. However, endoscopy only confirms mucosal spread. The submucosal extend and the deep extend of the tumor is a question for the radiologist (2).

Tumors of the hypopharynx most often arise in the piriform sinus (65%). Other locations include the postcricoid area (20%) and the posterior pharyngeal wall (15%). While the more lateral tumors tend to infiltrate into the soft tissues of the neck, laryngeal carcinomas arise from the su-

praglottic region in 30%, the glottic region in 65%, and from the subglottic region in 5%.

The most common location for the supraglottic tumors are the aryepiglottic fold and the epiglottis (Fig. 14.5). While these lesions in the more advanced stage are usually inseparable from hypopharyngeal tumors arising from the piriform sinus, an exact staging still makes sense. In MDCT, these masses can be identified with moderate contrast enhancement. Obscuration of the fat planes indicates the lateral paraglottic infiltration (Fig. 14.4). Typical patterns of infiltration are anteriorly toward the epiglottis and into the preepiglottic fat. They are best seen in axial and lateral reconstructions. Alternatively, tumors infiltrate laterally by direct involvement of the piriforme sinus and caudally towards the glottic level of the larynx. Supraglottic tumors arising from the epiglottis usually initially infiltrate the preepiglottic fat and both surfaces of the epiglottis (Fig. 14.5, Table 14.2).

Tumors of the glottis typically arise from the vocal cords in the anterior and second third of the cords. Spread is initially seen towards and through the anterior commissure. Lesions of the anterior commissure may extend either into the thyroid cartilage

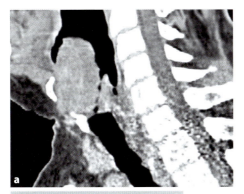

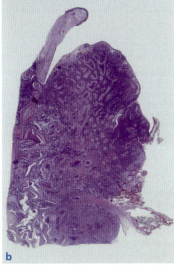

Fig. 14.5. a Large carcinoma infiltrating the entire epiglottis with both surfaces in a 58-year-old man. **b** Histology shows that the base of the epiglottic cartilage has been largely destroyed (arrow)

or through the cricothyroid membrane into the soft tissues of the neck. In later stages tumors may extend into the thyroarytenoid muscle, the deep paraglottic space and the cartilage (3), and towards the supra- and subglottic space. Coronal reformations are recommended to exclude tumor extend towards the subglottic space, which is relatively common in tumors of the glottic level. This subglottic spread is difficult to detect on endoscopy, therefore CT can help to avoid underestimation of tumor size (Table 14.3).

Primary subglottic carcinomas are uncommon. Patterns of spread may include direct infiltration of the adjacent organs like the esophagus, trachea, or thyroid gland.

Unusual malignant tumors of the larynx include chondrosarcomas and lymphomas. They are not differentiable from squamous cell carcinomas by contrast enhancement, but chondrosarcomas often feature the typical calcifications, a feature almost never seen in squamous cell carcinomas. Both entities, chondrosarcomas and lymphomas, do not arise from the mucosa, but are located entirely submucosally.

A laryngocele can also present as a submucosal swelling, but is actually totally benign. Laryngoceles can contain air or fluids. Internal laryngoceles are located within the larynx and extend superiorly in the paraglottic space. External laryngoceles extend outside through the thyrohyoid membrane and may form a swelling at the lateral neck. Laryngoceles result from an obstructive dilatation of the appendix of the ventricle. Even if laryngoceles are benign, they may be associated with a malignancy at the level of the true (or false) vocal cords. Therefore, careful evaluation of this level is important.

Most patients with an acute trauma of the upper airway do not undergo CT evaluation, but are referred directly to endoscopy or surgery. CT plays a role in identifying fragments of cartilage exposed into the airway. If these are not removed, chondritis can follow. On CT examination, the integrity of the thyoid cartilage, the integrity of the cricoid, and the position of the aretheniods should be carefully observed. While thyroid cartilage fractures can be vertical, horizontal, or in multiple fragments, the cricoid cartilage fractures are usually seen as bilateral fractures of the cartilage ring.

Table 14.2. Staging of supraglottic carcinoma

T1:	Tumor limited to one region:
	- Epiglottis
	- Aryepiglottic fold
	- False vocal cords
T2:	Tumor invades more than one region:
	Normal vocal cord movement
T3:	Infiltration of vocal cord:
	Postcricoidal region or preepiglottic
T4:	Distant tumor extension (e.g., oropharynx)

Table 14.3. Staging of glottic carcinoma

T1:	Tumor limited to vocal cord, normal movement
T2:	Tumor extends to supra- or subglottis with normal or limited movement
T3:	Fixation of vocal cord
T4:	Invasion of cartilage or extension to distant

References

1. Bruening R, Sturm C, Reiser M (2001) Staging of laryngeal cancer using multi-slice CT. In: Reiser MF, Takahashi M, Modic M, Bruening R (eds) Multislice-CT. Springer, Berlin Heidelberg New York, pp 93–98
2. Becker M, Zbären P, Lang H, Stoupis C, Porcellini B, Vock P (1995) Neoplastic invasion of the laryngeal cartilage: comparison of MR imaging and CT with histopathologic correlation. Radiology 194:661–669
3. Curtin HD (1995) Importance of imaging demonstration of neoplastic invasion of laryngeal cartilage. Radiology 194:643–644
4. Curtin HD (1996) The larynx. In: Som PM, Curtin HD (eds) Head and neck imaging. Mosby, pp 612-710

IV Chest

15 Multidetector CT-Diagnosis of Infectious Pulmonary Disease

M. Horger

Indications for MDCT-Diagnosis

1. Characterization of pulmonary infiltrates unclear/suspected in chest X-ray.
2. Evaluation of metapneumonic or parapneumonic complications (abscess, empyema, mediastinitis).
3. Unfavorable course of pneumonia in pediatric patients (e.g., necrotizing pneumonia).
4. Early diagnosis of (atypical) pneumonia in immunocompromised patients.
5. Evaluation of accompanying manifestation in lung tuberculosis.
6. Biopsy of lung infiltrates under CT-guidance.

Scan Parameters

See Table 15.1.

Tips and Tricks

- For detection and characterization of pulmonary infiltrates, inspiratory images performed at full inspiration alone are usually sufficient.
- Expiratory scans may be particularly useful to determine if a pattern of mosaic attenuation is primarily caused by airway disease, vascular disease, or infiltrative lung disease.
- In patients following hematopoietic stem cell transplantation (HSCT), expiratory images also help in early detection of air trapping caused by bronchiolitis obliterans. Consequently, expiratory images are performed only optionally.

- Most CT images are obtained with the patient in the supine position. Images with the patient prone can also be obtained occasionally for differentiation of lung infiltrates from dependent atelectasis.
- At follow-up, low-dose high-resolution CT, which refers to the use of a reduced tube current (e.g., 30–40 mAs) for obtaining high-resolution CT images of the lung, should be used in order to reduce radiation dose. Our experience corresponds with that of other researchers, in that anatomic detail is almost equivalent between low-dose and standard high-resolution CT [1,2].

Comments

Chest radiography is the most commonly used imaging tool in the diagnosis of infectious pulmonary disease due to its availability and excellent cost benefit ratio. However, its reliability is limited by significant interobserver variability in radiographic interpretation [3]. The adjunct diagnostic role of computed tomography (CT) and especially that of high-resolution CT is meanwhile well established. A better detection and characterization of pulmonary infiltrates is possible using CT. This is essential particularly in early diagnosis of pneumonia in immunocompromised patients or in the diagnosis of therapy refractory pulmonary infections. Nevertheless, the value of multidetector CT technology in thoracic imaging has not yet been widely investigated, with very few reports in the literature [4]. The first MDCT results, using thin-collimation protocols and high-spatial

Table 15.1. Multislice spiral computed tomography protocols for HRCT. Investigations on different MDCT scanners

Parameters	4–8 slice scanners	10–16 slice scanners	32–64 slice scanners
Scanner settings			
Initial CT			
Tube voltage (kV)	120	120	120
Rotation time (s)	1.0	0.5	0.5
Tube current time product (mAs)	65–80	65–80	60–70
Pitch corrected tube current time product (eff. mAs)	100–120	100–120	100–120
Collimation (mm)	1	1	0.75
Norm. pitch	0.65	0.65	0.57
Reconstruction increment (mm)	4 (1)	4 (0.8)	4 (0.6)
Reconstr.-slice thickness (mm)	4 (1.25)	4 (1.0)	4 (0.75)
Convolution kernel	High-res	High-res	High-res
Specials	Breath hold in full inspiration	Breath hold in full inspiration	Breath hold in full inspiration
Scan range	Upper aperture/ diaphragm	Upper aperture/ diaphragm	Upper aperture/ diaphragm
Scan direction	Caudocranial	Caudocranial	Caudocranial
Contrast material application	None	None	None
Follow up CT (selected parameters)			
Tube voltage (kV)	120	120	120
Tube current (mAs)	30–40	30–40	30–40
Postprocessing	MPR, thin-sliding MIP	MPR, thin-sliding MIP	MPR, thin-sliding MIP

reconstruction algorithms have shown that image quality is nearly comparable with that of incremental HRCT, with the advantage of gapless acquisition and potential to multiplanar reformations (MPR). Using thin-collimation protocols and suitable high-resolution reconstruction algorithms (kernel), follow up CT diagnosis can also be performed in low-dose technique by acceptable image quality.

Anatomy

Lung parenchyma consists of a network of connective tissue called the lung intersti-tium and peripheral air-filled preformatted spaces. The interstitium of the lung can be divided into a central compartment that surrounds the bronchovascular bundles and the peripheral interstitium that includes the interlobular septa and the subpleural interstitium. The secondary pulmonary lobule represents the smallest unit of lung structure marginated by connective tissue septa. The interlobular septa are not usually visible unless abnormal (with >0.1-mm thickness they become visible in HRCT). Structures of 0.2–0.3 mm can be routinely identified on HRCT when they are perpendicular to the plane of imaging. Within the lung parenchyma, the bronchi and pulmonary artery branches are closely associated and branch in parallel. The 1.0-mm diameter bronchiole supplying the lobule has an approximately 0.15-mm wall, just at the limit of HRCT and can not always be visualized. Postprocessing techniques such as multiplanar reformation (MPR), minimal- or maximal-intensity projection (MIP), or shaded-surface display (SSD), acquired with or without ECG-gaiting (prospectively, or retrospectively) have little impact on the diagnosis of pulmonary infection. However, anatomic relation of some pulmonary infiltrates to the bronchial tree, respectively to the vascular structures may sometimes be beneficial for diagnosis, particularly in guiding biopsy or surgery (e.g., in solitary pulmonary mycetoma).

MDCT Imaging of Pneumonia

Community-acquired pneumonia (CAP) is the most common cause of parenchymal lung disease in immunocompetent patients. Most frequent causes of CAP are bacterial pneumonias, which show a pattern of lobar pneumonia or bronchopneumonia, and are usually diagnosed by conventional chest radiographs. CT findings consist of areas of airspace consolidation that may be segmental or nonsegmental in distribution. CT-diagnosis is useful in particular cases because it sometimes reveals lung infiltrates not visualized in the chest radiographs, and can assure the existence of cavitation or other complications. Mycoplasma pneumonia, another frequent pathogen, has variable radiographic appearances, which are nonspecific. In CT, however, common findings consist of centrilobular branching structures and nodules, bronchial wall thickening, airspace consolidation, and ground-glass attenuation with lobular distribution, which correlate well with histologic specimens showing bronchiolitis and lobular consolidation. Legionella pneumonia presents with segmental peripheral consolidations that spread rapidly producing opacification of one or more lobes (Fig. 15.1). They become bilateral in many cases. Depending on the

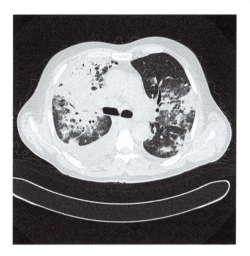

Fig. 15.1. 67-year-old patient presenting with signs of acute pulmonary infection. Axial MDCT image shows bilateral large lung infiltrates, in part (right lung) with lobar extension. Cultures from bronchiallavage revealed Legionella pneumonia

clinical setting, in which pulmonary infection occurs, it might sometimes be necessary to perform CT diagnosis for exclusion of other causes of bilateral opacified lungs. There are also unusual patterns of CAP such as round pneumonia and bilateral, multilobar pneumonia. Round pneumonia requires mostly CT diagnosis, in order to exclude malignancy. Positive airspace bronchogram and rush size and growth kinetics suggest pneumonia. But differentiation from other pathological entities such as lymphoma (maltom) or hemorrhage sometimes proves difficult at the time the first CT is performed. CT survey is necessary in such cases.

Nosocomial pneumonias (NP) are mostly due to aerobic Gram-negative bacilli (enterobacteria, *E. coli*, *Pseudomonas aeruginosa*). Their radiographic pattern may be quite variable, consisting mostly of bilateral diffuse, or multiple foci of consolidation. CT may be of great help in some cases when the chest films are inconclusive, especially in patients with ARDS.

Pleural effusion, empyema, and more seldom lung gangrene are complications of pneumonia, which occur mostly in patients

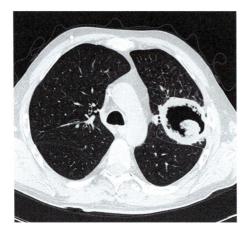

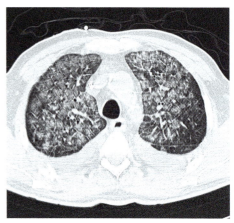

Fig. 15.2. 58-year-old male patient with GvHD following PBSCT by aplastic anemia, actually complaining about fever and cough. Large nodule with central cavitation is seen in the left lung upper lobe. Note also the accompanying pulmonary sequester due to infarction by vascular invasion

Fig. 15.3. 56-year-old male patient with progressive dyspnoea and fever, following HSCT by acute myelogenous leukemia. Axial MDCT image shows GGO and reticulation with delineation of secondary pulmonary lobules. Fine centrilobular nodules are also present. The patient succumbed to CMV pneumonia a few days later

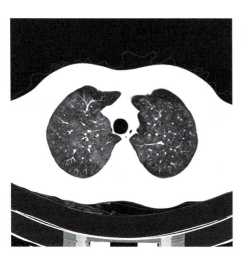

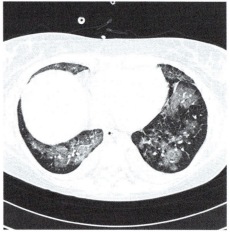

Fig. 15.4. 37-year-old male HIV+ patient complaining about progressive dyspnoea. Axial CT image shows diffuse GGO with focal sparing of the subpleural lung parenchyma. PCP was diagnosed by bronchial alveolar lavage

Fig. 15.5. 23-year-old female patient with T-cell non-Hodgkin lymphoma presenting with fever and dyspnoea. Axial MDCT image reveals patchy GGO in both lung lower lobes. Adenovirus pneumonia was diagnosed by bronchial alveolar lavage. The patient also developed an ADV colitis over the next few days

with a late-onset of antimicrobial therapy, or in immunosuppressed patients.

In children, the primary role of CT in bacterial pneumonia is when children fail to respond to treatment, and complications are suspected. Following intravenous contrast material administration, lung abscesses, characterized by an air–fluid level and a reactive rim, as well as necrotizing pneumonias characterized by nonenhancement, can be correctly diagnosed. Furthermore, aspiration, or drainage of lung abscesses can be performed optimally under CT-guidance.

Infectious complications are the major risk during neutropenia induced by high-dose chemotherapy and the lung is the most frequently involved organ. The use of CT, especially HRCT, for investigation of the lungs in HSCT recipients has been investigated extensively.

Candida species, the most frequent microorganisms, are mainly associated with ground-glass opacities (GGO) and ill-defined nodules, and are rarely associated with consolidation. The Aspergillus species, the second most frequent microorganisms, is mainly associated with ill-defined nodules, or focal consolidations (Fig. 15.2). A marginal GGO ("halo" sign), or the occurrence of the "crescent" sign or cavitation at follow-up are suggestive of pulmonary infection with angiotropic fungi [5]. In approximately 30% of cases of invasive aspergillosis, the fungus invades the airways, where the abnormalities in CT have a peribronchial or peribronchiolar distribution ("tree in bud"). The most common pathogens responsible for early phase complications after HSCT are cytomegalievirus (CMV) (Fig. 15.3) and Pneumocystis carini (PCP) (Fig. 15.4). The HRCT-manifestations of CMV pneumonia are known to be polymorphous consisting mainly of ground-glass opacities, airspace consolidations, nodular or a reticulonodular pattern, which in a specific clinical context are suggestive of this diagnosis, but not specific. The most characteristic finding in HRCT for patients with PCP is GGO, which can be diffuse, predominantly perihilar, or have a mosaic pattern with sparing of ad-

jacent secondary pulmonary lobules. Viral pneumonias, such as those caused by herpes simplex, hemophilus influenza, respiratory sincitial virus, adenovirus (ADV) (Fig. 15.5), and others are difficult to diagnose on conventional radiographs [6,7]. Differentiation from other complications (e.g., hemorrhage, pulmonary edema, idiopathic pneumonia syndrome, diffuse alveolar damage, or cryptogenic organizing pneumonia) induced by high-dose chemotherapy or HSCT, requires CT-diagnosis in most cases.

In conclusion, CT, particularly HRCT, plays a pivotal role in the diagnosis of pulmonary infection, due in the first line to the continuous progress in the characterization of atypical pulmonary infiltrates and their complications by the community of chest radiologists. MDCT technology makes a gapless chest CT investigation in HR-like quality possible, and therefore increasingly represents a substitute to incremental HRCT.

References

1. Rotondo A, Guidi G, Catalano O et al. (1994) High resolution computerized tomography in the study of the lung parenchyma: possibility of a low-dose protocol. Radiol Med 35:603–607
2. Lucaya J, Piqueras J, Garci-Pena P et al. (2000) Low-dose high-resolution CT of the chest in children and young adults. AJR 175:985–992
3. Albaum MN, Hill LC, Murphy M et al. Interobserver reliability of the chest radiograph in community-acquired pneumonia. Chest 11:343
4. Schoepf UJ, Bruening RD, Hong C et al. (2001) Multislice helical CT of focal and diffuse lung disease: comprehensive diagnosis with reconstruction of contiguous and high-resolution CT sections from a single thin-collimation scan. AJR 177:179–184
5. Soubani AO, Chandrasekar PH (2002) The clinical spectrum of pulmonary aspergillosis. Chest 121:1988–1999
6. Matar LD, McAdams HP, Palmer SM et al. (1999) Respiratory viral infections in lung transplant recipients: Radiologic findings with clinical correlation. Radiology 213:735–742
7. Worthy S, Flint J, Müller N (1997) Pulmonary complications after bone marrow transplantation: high-resolution CT and pathologic findings. Radiographics 17:1359–1371

16 Parenchymal Changes of the Lung

R. Eibel

Indications

Routine Chest

- Mediastinal and axillary lymph nodes.
- Tumors of the anterior, medial, and posterior mediastinum.
- Staging.
- Abscesses.
- Thoracic abnormalities.

HR-Chest (Helical)

- Diffuse lung diseases.

Combi Thorax

Evaluation of the lung tissue in conjunction with detailed analysis of the mediastinal structures.
- Sarcoidosis.
- To evaluate bronchogenic carcinoma or other.

HR-Chest (Sequential in Supine and Prone Position)

- Asbestosis.

Examination is in supine and prone positions, arms elevated over the head. The examined region should reach the lung apices to below the diaphragm. Scanning in the supine and prone position is recommended here to differentiate between initial lung fibrosis and hydrostatic subpleural dystelectasis.

Scan parameters for the detection of aspergillosis should include 0.5–1.0-mm collimation, 120 kV, 100 eff. mAs, a table feed of 10 mm, reconstruction thickness of 1 mm, kernel: high resolution, and a rotation time of at least 0.5 s. Contrast material is not necessary.

HR-Chest (Inspiration/Expiration)

- Small airways disease (scanning in inspiration und expiration to detect small airways disease using the air-trapping sign).

For the HR-chest inspiration/expiration technique (for small airways disease) the patient positioning should be in supine position with arms elevated over the head.

Scan parameters should include 0.6–1.0-mm collimation, a pitch of 1.25–1.5, 120 kV, 120 eff. mAs, reconstruction thickness of 1 mm at an increment of 3 mm, the kernel in high-resolution mode, and a rotation time of at least 0.5 s in the caudocranial scan direction. Contrast material is not necessary.

Lung Cancer Screening

- Screening examination for lung cancer (for populations with high risk for lung cancer, see text).

For lung cancer screening the patient positioning is supine, arms elevated over the head. Scanning with a low-dose technique is recommended to avoid higher radiation burden at the price of slight image degradation.

Scan parameters should include collimation from 0.6 mm (64 row) to 1.0 mm (4 row), pitch 1.25–1.5, 120 kV, 20 eff. mAs, reconstruction thickness of 1 mm (sharp kernel) and 3 mm (soft kernel) at an increment of 0.5 mm and 3 mm, respectively. A rotation time of at least 0.5 s in the caudocranial scan direction. Contrast material is not necessary.

Pediatric Routine Chest (Helical)

- Mediastinal and axillary lymph nodes.
- Tumors of the anterior, medial, and posterior mediastinum.
- Staging.
- Thoracic abnormalities.
- Abscesses.

For the examination of children, adaptation of the scanning parameters is essential. For the kV and mAs values please refer to the tables in Chap. 5.

Scan parameters should include collimation from 0.6 mm (64 row) to 2.5 mm (4 row), pitch 1.25–1.5, reconstruction thickness of 3 mm (soft kernel) at an increment of 2–3 mm. Rotation time of 0.5 s in the caudocranial scan direction. Contrast material: 2 mL/kg bodyweight, with an upper limit of 100 mL.

Scan Parameters

See Table 16.1.

Tips and Tricks

- For screening of lung nodules or inflammatory changes only, the low-dose protocol should be used.
- To confirm a nodule found on a chest radiograph, intravenous contrast administration is not mandatory.
- In pediatric patients, due to the short examination time, the bolus can be missed by errors in timing.

- Demarcation of the esophagus can be optimized by administering a barium suspension shortly before starting the scan.

Introduction

The lung is a very complex part of the body. Here, every imaging process deals with the problem of breathing, the transmitted movements of the heart, and that the great vessels induce movement of the lung. As a consequence, imaging must be fast, must allow differentiation of tissues with similar attenuation values and has to offer high resolution to detect small pathologies.

CT has dramatically altered the diagnostic approach to lung disease, because the images are free of superimposition of neighboring structures in the direction of the X-ray beam. In the late 1980s, high-resolution CT (HRCT) was added as a powerful tool for evaluation of diffuse lung disease. However, a complete acquisition of the whole chest could not be acquired with the HR mode due to limitations of the scanner and necessary breath-hold time of the patients.

A quantum leap in the development of CT scanners came with the introduction of multidetector row CT (MDCT) which provided the potential to combine a higher spatial resolution with a shorter acquisition time. Thus, for the first time it was possible to image the entire chest in one breath hold with a collimation of 1 mm, which meant scanning the whole lung volume in the HR mode. Using ECG triggering, the moving artifacts of the heart and the large vessels could be reduced or omitted.

Multidimensional imaging with near isotropic voxels and fewer artifacts is now possible with the latest scanners. Computer hardware and software have similarly improved such that a two- or three-dimensional image reconstruction (e.g., MIP, SSD, volume rendering, and virtual endoscopy) can be easily performed.

Table 16.1. List of common CT patterns and corresponding lung diseases

Parameters	4–8 slice scanners	10–16 slice scanners	32–64 slice scanners
Scanning parameters			
Tube voltage (kV)	120	120	120
Rotation time (s)	0.5	0.5	0.5
Tube current time product (mAs)	110–180[*]	110–180[*]	110–180[*]
Pitch corrected tube current time product (eff. mAs)	90–120[*]	90–120[*]	90–120[*]
Slice collimation (mm)	1/1.25	0.625/0.75	0.6/0.625
Norm. pitch	1.2–1.5 caudocranial direction	1.2–1.5 caudocranial direction	1.3–1.5 caudocranial direction
Reconstruction increment (mm)	5 For high resolution: 5[*]	5 For high resolution: 5[*]	5 For high resolution: 5[*]
Reconstruction thickness (mm)	5 For high resolution: 1–1.25 craniocaudal direction	5 For high resolution: 0.75–1 craniocaudal direction	5 For high resolution: 0.6–0.75 craniocaudal direction
Convolution kernel	High resolution/standard	High resolution/standard	High resolution/standard
Contrast material	If applicable	If applicable	If applicable
Volume (mL)	Monophasic	Monophasic	Monophasic
Injection speed (mL/s)	80	80	80
Saline flush (mL, mL/s)	3	3	3
Delay arterial (s)	30	30	30

[*] For parenchymal changes only (not applicable for metastasis or other nodular disease)

The Central Airways: Are Axial Slices not Enough?

Limitations of axial slices include the difficulty to visualize airways oriented obliquely to the axial plane, the inadequate display of complex three-dimensional relationships of the airways, underestimation of the craniocaudal extension of the disease, and limitation in the detection of subtle airway stenoses. Multiplanar and three-dimensional image reconstructions can help to overcome these limitations, but necessitate narrow collimations (1 or 2 mm). Beyond 3-mm collimation, the resulting stair-step ar-tifacts will degrade the image significantly. The use of overlapping reconstruction intervals is less important when very narrow collimation is used.

With 16- or 64-slice CT scanners, three-dimensional reconstructions can be created without the need for additional acquisitions, because the primary collimation is then 0.75 or 0.6 mm, respectively. For optimal visualization of anatomy and pathology in multiplanar and three-dimensional images, a standard or smoothing algorithm is preferable to an edge-enhancing or lung algorithm (Figs. 16.1–16.3).

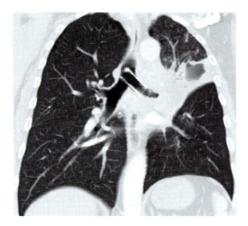

Fig. 16.1. Left side lung cancer. Palliation with stenting the left main bronchus. MPR. Note the stent dislocation into the distal tracheal lumen

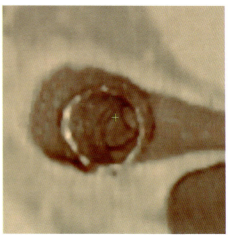

Fig. 16.3. Same patient as Fig. 16.1. Detailed view in virtual endoscopic technique. View from the trachea into the stent lumen

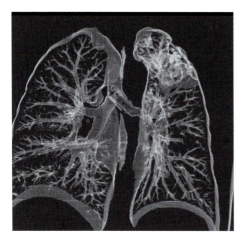

Fig. 16.2. Same patient as Fig. 16.1. Reconstruction with minIP. Note the dystelectasis in the left upper lobe

Airway imaging is performed routinely at deep inspiration. But to assess for excessive airway collapse, that is, to evaluate the degree of tracheobronchomalacia in patients with a large goiter preoperatively, we perform an additional sequence during dynamic exhalation. In this particular case, low-dose techniques (40 mAs or less) are sufficient for delineation of trachea dimensions.

Indications for multiplanar reformations:
- Airways stenoses and webs
- Complex airway diseases
- Extrinsic airway compression
- Tracheobronchomalacia
- Poststent placement

Lung Nodule Detection and Characterization

When you have a lung without a nodule, the slice thickness was too large!

Pulmonary nodules remain a diagnostic dilemma. They are often only incidentally detected or with a chest CT, performed to evaluate a nodule suspected at CR, more nodules could be identified. When any nodule found on CT images is operated on, the mortality becomes higher from surgery than from lung cancer. So, it is a great challenge to detect and to characterize the nodules, and to carefully recommend further evaluations after a nodule is identified (e.g., watch and wait, imaging with other modalities, biopsy, or surgery).

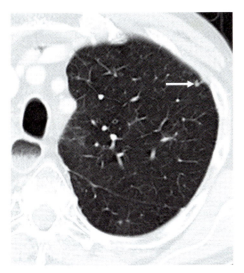 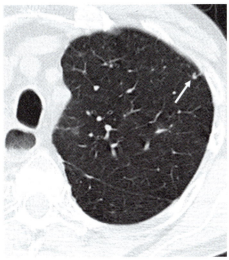

Fig. 16.4. Small subpleural lung nodule (*arrow*). Visualization with 120 kV and 120 mAs

Fig. 16.5. Small subpleural lung nodule (*arrow*). Visualization with 120 kV and 20 mAs. Please note the higher noise rate with 20 mAs, but the diagnosis can be made nonetheless

Attempts to differentiate nodules as benign versus malignant have relied on classifications focused on:

- Morphology
- Enhancement characteristics
- Densitometry
- Growth patterns

Multislice CT here offers some benefits to single row scanners in detection and characterization of lung nodules. On scans acquired with 8- to 12-mm collimation, which is typical for single-row CT scans used to scan the chest in a single breath hold, small lesions may be missed due to a partial volume effects. With 1-mm or thinner collimation, every nodule can be delineated and localized in a lung segment.

For the screening of high-risk populations for lung cancer, low-dose techniques (20 and 50 mA) are currently investigated. This reduces the radiation burden to 1/10 of the normal dose CT protocol. When comparing low-dose with diagnostic CT no decrease in recognition of small nodules could be found (Figs. 16.4 and 16.5).

For the large data sets that are produced, cine viewing or MIP facilitates differentiation of vessels from nodules.

Computer-aided diagnosis (CAD) may play a role to avoid false negative readings. Use of CAD as a second reader may not only decrease the number of missed nodules, but also improve clinical efficiency. Volume and morphologic analysis of nodules are also facilitated by computerized techniques. The follow-up of nodules and especially the detection of small size differences is fast and reliable for daily work (Figs. 16.6 and 16.7).

Morphologic patterns, which can help to differentiate a malignant from a benign intrapulmonary lesion, are:

- Margin contours (spiculated, lobulated, smooth)
- Feeding vessel sign
- Internal characteristics (pseudocavitation, air bronchograms)
- Halo sign
- Calcifications (benign: central, popcorn, solid, lamellated; malignant: stippled, eccentric)
- Fat

Utilizing nodules greater than 10 mm, Swenson et al. demonstrated in a multicenter

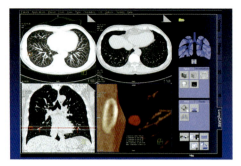

Fig. 16.6. Automatic nodule detection, segmentation and three-dimensional measuring. This allows for high quality follow-up examinations, where a nodule growth can be detected before the nodule has doubled its size (courtesy of P. Herzog, Munich)

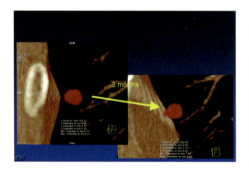

Fig. 16.7. Lung nodule in a three month follow-up. The volume of the lung node increases significantly from 163 to 260 mm³, but the diameter in the x- and y-axis increases only at 1.5 mm, which is not reliable to measure on axial images

study 98% sensitivity and 58% specificity for benignity using less than 15 HU as the maximal amount of enhancement from precontrast images. For smaller nodules, when respiratory motion is present or when the enhancement is heterogeneous due to partial necrosis, the value of enhancement for nodule characterization is substantially lower. However, multislice CT has facilitated characterization of small nodules by reducing partial volume effects. But it is important to keep in mind that every criterion is relative. Fat is a sign of benignity (lipoid pneumonia, hamartomas), but can be found in metastases from liposarcomas.

Entire calcification of a nodule is a sign of benignity (granuloma), but can be detected in mets from osteosarcomas.

The last important pattern is the growth rate, expressed as the term tumor volume doubling time (VDT). Radiographic studies have shown that lung cancers have a range between 20 and 400 days. That means stability on radiograph for two years implies benignity. Multislice CT offers the benefit of measuring nodule volume when nearly isotropic imaging is performed. Nodule volume quantification has the potential to detect smaller differences in nodule size at earlier intervals than simply relying on cross-sectional dimensions. Problems with this method are the reproducibility and partial volume effects.

Diffuse Lung Diseases

High-resolution CT (HRCT) is a sampling technique with large interspace gaps between the thinly collimated sections. Taking into account that diffuse interstitial lung disease involves multiple areas of the lung, this gap would not substantially degrade the diagnostic utility. Helical techniques using single-slice CT have not added benefit in most instances. Drawbacks of the above-mentioned HR scanning method are that familiar landmarks and the underlying normal lung (normal vascular, bronchial, and lobular) anatomy may not be well appreciated. If only HR scanning with gaps was performed, the lymph node evaluation and the nodule detection in the lung parenchyma were suboptimal. MDCT can fundamentally change the approach to diffuse lung disease. Scanning primarily with a thin collimation enables the evaluation of HR images when and where needed. Also, with reconstructed thicker images, the anatomic landmarks can be better visualized. With a 64-row scanner, for example, the acquisition of the entire lung with 1-mm reconstructed slice thickness takes fewer than 10 s, a time period in which even a dyspnoeic patient is able to hold his breath. Volumetric data sets obtained in the chest can be reconstructed with MPRs, offering that all zones of the lung can be evaluated simultaneously, from the apices through the bases, in either the coronal or sagittal direction. Variations in regional disease, including subtle variations in lung attenuation, will be better appreciated with this approach.

To diagnose small airways disease, the comparison of in- and expiratory thin collimated images is very helpful. The typical sign of small airways disease is the mosaic ventilation, which results from air trapping in affected lung zones and consecutive hyperinflation in correlation with the normal lung zones, where an increase in lung density can be found at expiration.

The best approach to diagnose diffuse lung disease is the recognition and analysis of the different patterns. The most important and common patterns will be listed in the following section.

- Nodule: round opacity, at least moderately well marginated and no greater than 3 cm (and usually less) in maximum diameter.
- Linear opacity: an elongated, thin line of soft-tissue attenuation.
- Septal thickening: abnormal widening of an interlobular septum or septa, usually caused by edema, cellular infiltration, or fibrosis. May be smooth, irregular, or nodular.
- Intralobular lines: fine linear opacities present in a lobule when the intralobular interstitium is thickened. When numerous, they may appear as a fine reticular pattern.
- Reticulation: innumerable, interlacing line shadows that suggest a mesh. A description term usually associated with interstitial lung disease. May be fine, intermediate, or coarse. Synonyma: reticular pattern.
- Cyst: a round, parenchymal space with a well-defined wall; usually air-containing when in the lung but without associated pulmonary emphysema (Figs. 16.8–16.10).
- Bulla: a round, focal air space, 1 cm or more in diameter, demarcated by a thin

wall; usually multiple or associated with other signs of pulmonary emphysema.
- Honeycombing: clustered cystic air spaces, usually of comparable diameters on the order of 0.3–1.0 cm, but as much as 2.5 cm, usually subpleural and characterized by well-defined walls, which are often thick.
- Ground-glass opacity: hazy increased attenuation of lung, but with preservation of bronchial and vascular margins; caused by partial filling of air spaces, interstitial thickening, partial collapse of alveoli, normal expiration, or increased capillary blood volume.
- Consolidation: homogeneous increase in pulmonary parenchymal attenuation that obscures the margins of vessels and airway walls. An air bronchogram may be present.
- Air trapping: decreased attenuation of pulmonary parenchyma, especially manifest as less than normal increase in attenuation during expiration. To be differentiated from the decrease attenuation of hypoperfusion (Fig. 16.11) secondary to locally increased pulmonary arterial resistance.

CT features of common lung diseases are listed in Table 16.2.

Pediatric Multidetector Chest CT: High-End Machine for Low-Size Patients?

Young patients will especially profit form shorter acquisition times in combination with higher resolution. Chest CT and CT angiography can be performed with doses of about 2 cc/kg bodyweight. Contrast can be injected either by the use of power injectors or by hand. The author recommends a manual injection if the angiocatheter is in peripheral portion of extremities, or when blood return is poor. To avoid scanning at the wrong time, we recommend a bolus tracking technology when possible. To reduce unnecessary radiation burden,

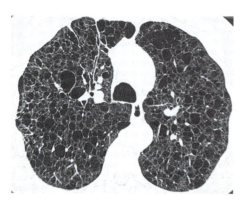

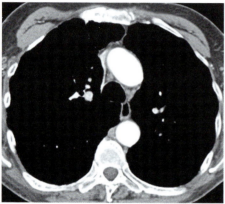

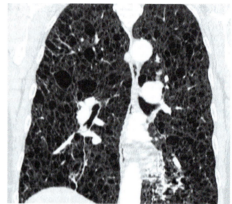

Fig. 16.8.–16.10. 1-mm high-resolution images and 6-mm images in soft-tissue kernel can be acquired with a single scan. Young female with lymphangioleiomyomatosis (LAM). The coronal MPR best visualizes the entire craniocaudal extension of the pathology

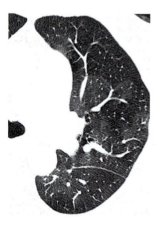

the milliampere and kilovolt values must be adjusted to age, bodyweight, and size. If just airway evaluation is indicated, then relatively low tube current and kilovoltage can be used (i.e., 80 to 100 kV[p], 20 to 40 mA). The indications for a chest CT in pediatric patients differs from the adults. Common indication in children are the evaluation of congenital abnormalities of the lung, mediastinum, and the heart (see Chap. 5), and as known from the adult group, evaluation of infection and complication of infections, and cancer detection and surveillance.

Fig. 16.11. HRCT. Patient with chronic pulmonary embolism. Note the mosaic pattern in the left lung, due to hypoperfusion in the low attenuation areas. In these lung segments, the vessel diameter is reduced

Table 16.2. List of parameters for 4-, 16-, and 64-row CT for different indication groups

Patterns	Common lung diseases[*]
Nodules	Sarcoidosis, HX, hypersensitivity pneumonitis, silicosis, metastatic cancer
Lines, thickened septa	Lung edema, lymphangitic carcinoma, infection (PCP, mycoplasma), drug reaction
Lines, intralobular or reticular	IPF, asbestosis, collagen vascular disease, pulmonary alveolar proteinosis
Lines, curvilinear, subpleural	Asbestosis, IPF, congestion in dependent lung
Lines, parenchymal bands	Asbestosis, scarring from pleural disease
Lung cysts	Distinguish from emphysema, HX, LAM, lymphoid interstitial pneumonitis
Honeycombing	Asbestosis, IPF, collagen vascular disease, sarcoidosis, hypersensitivity pneumonitis
Ground-glass opacity	BOOP, hypersensitivity pneumonitis, drug toxicity, DIP, pulmonary alveolar proteinosis, sarcoidosis
Consolidation	BOOP, eosinophilic pneumonia, alveolar cell carcinoma, lipoid pneumonia, pulmonary alveolar proteinosis, pulmonary embolism
Decreased lung attenuation	Constrictive bronchiolitis, panlobular emphysema, pulmonary embolism
Mosaic pattern	Constrictive bronchiolitis, pulmonary embolism, diseases causing ground-glass opacity

[*] Abbreviations: pulmonary histiocytosis X (HX), pneumocystis carinii pneumonia (PCP), idiopathic pulmonary fibrosis (IPF), lymphangioleiomyomatosis (LAM), bronchiolitis obliterans with organizing pneumonia (BOOP), desquamative interstitial pneumonia (DIP)

Literature
and Suggested Readings

- Arenas-Jimenez J, Alonso-Charterina S, Sanchez-Paya J, Fernandez-Latorre F, Gil-Sanchez S, Lloret-Llorens M (2000) Evaluation of CT findings for diagnosis of pleural effusions. Eur Radiol 10:681–690
- Austin JHM, Müller NL, Friedman PJ et al. (1996) Glossary of terms for CT of the lungs: recommendation of the nomenclature committee of the Fleischner Society. Radiology 200:327–331
- Boiselle P (ed) (2003) Multislice helical CT of the thorax. Radiol Clinic North Am 41(3):465–661
- Eibel R (2001) Primary chest film reading on coronal and sagittal MPRs. In: Reiser MF, Takahashi M, Modic M, Bruening R (eds) Multislice CT. Springer, Berlin Heidelberg New York, pp 155–164
- Eibel R, Tuengerthal S, Schoenberg SO (2003) The role of new imaging techniques in diagnosis and staging of malignant pleural mesothelioma. Curr Opin Oncol 15:131–138
- Fraser RS, Paré JA, Fraser RG, Paré PD (1994) Synopsis of diseases of the chest, 2nd edn. Saunders, Philadelphia
- McGuinness G, Naidich DP (2002) Multislice computed tomography of the chest. In: Silverman PM (ed) Multislice computed tomography. Lippincott Williams&Wilkins, Philadelphia, pp 117–167

17 MSCT Imaging of Pulmonary Embolism

A. Kuettner and A.F. Kopp

Indications

1. Atypical chest pain.
2. D-Dimer elevation.
3. Unclear dyspnoe.
4. Follow-up patients with known pulmonary embolism.
5. Screening for high-risk patients with known deep-vein thrombosis.

Patient Preparation

- Since this protocol may be used for patients in potentially life-threatening situations, no special preparation is needed. This protocol can also be used for critically ill patients.
- 20 or preferably 18 G i.v. access antecubitally. Also central i.v. catheters can be used if necessary. If a Shaldon catheter is present, it is the access of choice. Avoid the use of 20 or 22 G small-bore peripheral i.v. lines.
- Topogram/scan range: entire chest. Supine position (Fig. 17.1).
- Some centers prefer to additionally scan the abdomen, if a pulmonary embolism is detected. Thus, plan a conventional late-venous-phase abdominal scan incorporating the proximal deep femoral veins (mid-thigh) beforehand. This exam is only executed when a pulmonary embolism is detected. The advantage is that no additional CM is needed.

Scan Parameters

See Table 17.1.

Tips and Tricks

1. Make sure i.v. access is fully patent and all valves and lines are cleared, especially with ICU patients.
2. Execute one full table movement with all ICU patients to assure full clearance of all tubes and lines, especially all respiratory tubes.
3. Coronal reformats greatly facilitate the communication with referring clinicians who may not be as experienced in reviewing CT images as radiologists are.

Rationale for Scanning and History of Pulmonary Embolism Imaging

Pulmonary embolism (PE) is the cause of 10% of all deaths in hospital and is a contributing factor in another 10%. Many patients who have pulmonary embolism proven at autopsy did not have the diagnosis made ante mortem. Two recent studies show that the prevalence of pulmonary embolism among all patients who undergo CT scanning for reasons other than pulmonary embolism is about 1–2% [1,2].

The radiological diagnosis of pulmonary embolism is made using chest radiographs (CXR), ventilation perfusion lung scanning (VQ scans), or pulmonary angiography.

Chest X-ray is a nonspecific and relatively insensitive screening test. The classic plain-film sign of pulmonary embolism seen in less than 7% of cases, and in nearly half the cases when present, is not specific for pulmonary embolism. The main role of a chest X-ray has been to exclude other pa-

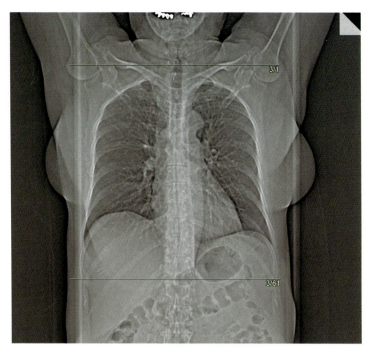

Fig. 17.1. Topogram. Arms above head. This is a standard protocol imaging the thorax only. Some centers prefer to plan an additional abdomen scan to look for DVT in case a PE is detected

thologies, such as pneumonia or an underlying neoplasm.

Nuclear scintigraphy or VQ lung scanning is a technique that provides reliable information about the probability of a pulmonary embolism only in combination with clinical information. If a VQ scan is read as high probability for pulmonary embolism in combination with high clinical suspicion, pulmonary embolism is indeed present in 96% of the cases. However, the problem remains that in clinical practice a considerable number of VQ scans are read as indeterminate [3,4].

Pulmonary angiography has been the gold standard for the evaluation of suspected pulmonary embolism. However, its use has been limited by a number of factors including the paucity of radiologists trained to do pulmonary angiography, the invasiveness of the procedure, its potential complications, and its increased risk in instable patients [5].

Multislice CT and PE Imaging

Already, the introduction of spiral CT with its considerably faster acquisition times as compared to sequential nonspiral CT brought considerable improvement especially to vascular imaging. Since 1992 studies have concluded that CT can depict thromboemboli in the second to fourth division pulmonary vessels [6]. By 1997, studies by Mayo concluded that "the sensitivity of spiral CT is greater than that of scintigraphy. Interobserver agreement is better with spiral CT" [7]. In the late 1990s some articles also addressed the comparison of conventional angiography and spiral CT angiography [8]. The results showed that CT had a 100% positive predictive value, with a prospective sensitivity of 91%. These encouraging results have been further improved by the introduction of multidetector CT (Fig. 17.2).

Table 17.1. Scan parameters

Parameters	4–8 slice scanners	10–16 slice scanners	32–64 slice scanners
Scanner settings			
Rotation time (ms)	500	370–500	330–420
Tube voltage (kV)	120	120	120
Tube current time product (mAs)	110	110	125
Pitch corrected tube current time product (eff. mAs)	120	120	140
Collimation (mm)	2.5	0.75	0.6
Norm. pitch	0.9	0.9	0.9
Reconstruction increment (mm)	3.0	0.8	0.4
Reconstr.-slice thickness (mm)	3.0	1.0	0.6
convolution kernel	standard	standard	standard
Specials	Bolus tracking	Bolus tracking	Bolus tracking
Scan range	Upper aperture to diaphragm	Upper aperture to diaphragm	Upper aperture to diaphragm
Scan direction	Craniocaudal	Craniocaudal	Craniocaudal
Contrast media application			
Concentration (mg iodine/mL)	350–400	350–400	350–400
Mono/Biphasic	Monophasic	Monophasic	Monophasic
Volume (mL)	120–150	80–120	60–120
Injection rate (mL/s)	3.5	3.5	3.5
Saline chaser (mL, mL/s)	30, 3.5	30, 3.5	30, 3.0
Delay (s)	Bolus tracking	Bolus tracking	Bolus tracking

The current generation of MDCT devices (up to 64 detectors) can obtain thin sections up to 0.5 mm with a resolution down to 0.4×0.4×0.4 mm and yet allow the study to be performed with a less than 10-s breath hold.

This may improve the diagnosis of pulmonary embolism and is especially important for determining the location and extent of the thrombus. Obviously, thin sections improve the depiction of small peripheral emboli. The high spatial resolution of sub-millimeter collimation data sets now allows evaluation of pulmonary vessels down to sixth-order branches and substantially increases the detection rate of segmental and subsegmental pulmonary emboli (Fig. 17.3) [9].

MDCT is especially useful for evaluating peripheral arteries that have an anatomic course parallel to the scan plane because these are the ones that tend to be most affected by volume averaging when thicker sections are used [10].

Many studies show that confidence in the evaluation of subsegmental arteries with thin-section MDCT by far exceeds the reproducibility of selective pulmonary angiography [5,11].

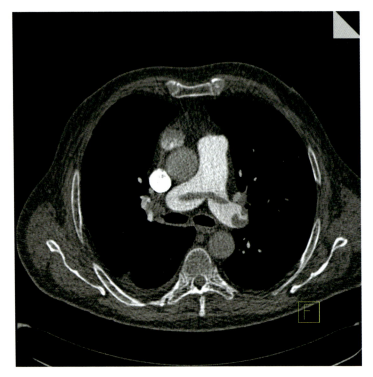

Fig. 17.2. Axial image of the pulmonary trunc. Note the large bilateral thrombus

New Clinical Implications

MDCT presents radiologists and clinicians a new challenge: the diagnosis of an isolated subsegmental embolus. In the past, such an isolated clot would often have gone unnoticed, especially in patients with no or minor symptoms. The improved detection of PE nodules has triggered a clinical debate about how to care for patients for which a diagnosis of isolated peripheral embolism has been established. The clinical importance of small peripheral emboli in subsegmental pulmonary arteries in the absence of a central embolus is uncertain. There is little disagreement about the fact that the presence of peripheral emboli may be an indicator of concurrent deep venous thrombosis (DVT), thus potentially heralding more severe embolic events [12]. The presence of some peripheral emboli may be of clinical importance in patients with cardiopulmonary restriction and in evaluating the development of chronic pulmonary hypertension in patients suffering from thromboembolic disease [13].

The main new clinical aspect is the high negative predictive value, which is almost 98% even when underlying pulmonary disease is present.

Clinical Diagnostic Algorithms

Current clinical algorithms for the exclusion of PE mainly rely on negative D-dimer tests. The sensitivity and negative predictive value of currently available test are between 90 and 100% and thus appropriately rule out the presence of PE. However, because of the lack of specificity of positive D-dimer tests and the fact that sensitivity does not always reach 100%, clinicians refuse to only rely on D-dimer testing.

If the presence of DVT can be established by ultrasound or fluoroscopy with patients suspected of having PE, some centers claim that no further workup of pulmonary cir-

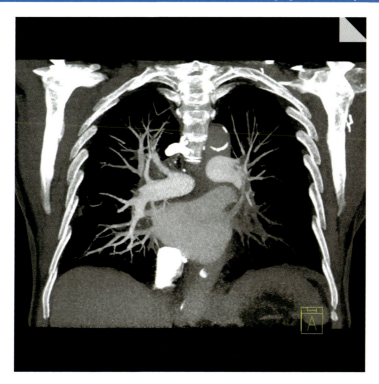

Fig. 17.3. MIP image of the thorax. The pulmonary embolism is almost completely obstructing the arteries of the left lower lobe

culation is required since the anticoagulant treatment regimen is the same for DVT and PE. Some centers, however, prefer to visually establish the presence of PE and thus perform a CT scan.

If no DVT can be established, CT angiography of the pulmonary vasculature is performed. If the result is positive, the patient is treated accordingly. If a good quality CT study does not reveal pulmonary embolism, the workup can be stopped at this point and other causes for the patient's symptoms should be considered [14].

In Fig. 17.4, a current clinical algorithm is described that uses MDCT as first-line imaging modality in combination with clinical symptoms and D-dimer testing.

Pulmonary Embolism in Pregnant Patients

Venous thromboembolism is a leading cause of maternal mortality and has been reported to occur in 0.5–3.0 of 1000 pregnancies. While the risk of thrombosis has usually been considered greatest during the third trimester and immediately postpartum, there is evidence that venous thromboembolism may occur with almost equal frequency in all trimesters. Established guidelines attempt to balance diagnostic efficacy and minimization of fetal exposure to ionizing radiation. Although ventilation–perfusion scanning is still considered the modality of first choice in pregnant women, recent studies were able to show that the mean fetal dose delivered with helical CT for a standard technique (120 kV, 100 mA, pitch 1) is less than that delivered with ventilation–perfusion scanning in all three trimesters [15].

The dose was less than 0.00006 Gy, well below the limit of 0.05 Gy that is considered safe for fetal exposure. Thus pregnancy should not preclude the use of CT for the diagnosis of PE. Also, accurate diagnosis is critical because there is substantial risk of

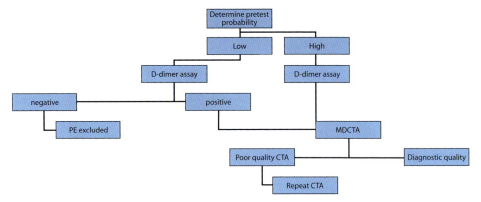

Fig. 17.4. Clinical management of patients with suspicion of PE. In lab tests, only D-dimer testing is used, CT is the primary imaging modality

morbidity to both mother and fetus from potentially unnecessary treatment. Thus to rule out PE is important, especially during pregnancy.

Scanning Technique

The use of MDCT as a diagnostic instrument for pulmonary thromboembolism may create inconclusive exams if contrast in the pulmonary artery is inadequate. The new scanner generations enable acquisition during the maximal phase of enhancement. Although this reduces the total dose of contrast material necessary, the acquisition speed may also result in incorrect CM timing.

Many technical devices have been introduced to obtain accurate timing of the bolus injection. The most commonly employed are a test bolus and automated bolus triggering associated with a mandatory saline flush after the bolus injection in order to reduce streak density artifacts in the vena cava and to optimize the use of the contrast material. Most injection protocols are adapted in order to reach the maximum iodine concentration in the shortest time possible. This can be obtained using a higher injection rate. However, increase of the injection flow rate to above 6 mL/s is not practical for peripheral venous injection or for most central i.v. lines. Instead, the concentration of iodine can be increased to values of 350–400 mg I/mL without the side effects of a resulting higher viscosity. To visualize the entire thorax, 60–80 mL of CM are sufficient to obtain well-opacified images. To rule out significant thrombosis in deep femoral/iliac veins the amount may be increased to 100–120 mL CM. The use of automated bolus detection currently seems to be the most practical approach (ROI in pulmonary trunc, level: 100–120 HU). It is quick and reliable.

Since MDCT is able to detect emboli even in sixth-order branches, motion artifacts due to the patient's respiration or transmitted cardiac motion may distort image quality. The short acquisition time enables even dyspnoeic patients to maintain a thorough breath hold. Retrospective ECG-gated acquisition techniques may be applied to effectively reduce transmitted pulsation artifacts. However no study has yet proven its clinical superiority over conventional scanning techniques especially when taking the considerably higher radiation dose into consideration.

References

1. Gosselin MV, Rubin GD, Leung AN, Huang J, Rizk NW (1998) Unsuspected pulmonary embolism: prospective detection on routine helical CT scans. Radiology 208(1):209–215

2. Winston CB, Wechsler RJ, Salazar AM, Kurtz AB, Spirn PW (1996) Incidental pulmonary emboli detected at helical CT: effect on patient care. Radiology 201(1):23–27

3. Bajc M, Albrechtsson U, Olsson CG, Olsson B, Jonson B (2002) Comparison of ventilation/perfusion scintigraphy and helical CT for diagnosis of pulmonary embolism; strategy using clinical data and ancillary findings. Clin Physiol Funct Imaging 22(6):392–397

4. Blachere H, Latrabe V, Montaudon M, Valli N, Couffinhal T, Raherisson C, Leccia F, Laurent F (2000) Pulmonary embolism revealed on helical CT angiography: comparison with ventilation-perfusion radionuclide lung scanning. AJR Am J Roentgenol 174(4):1041–1047

5. Diffin DC, Leyendecker JR, Johnson SP, Zucker RJ, Grebe PJ (1998) Effect of anatomic distribution of pulmonary emboli on interobserver agreement in the interpretation of pulmonary angiography. AJR Am J Roentgenol 171(4):1085–1089

6. Remy-Jardin M, Remy J, Wattinne L, Giraud F (1992) Central pulmonary thromboembolism: diagnosis with spiral volumetric CT with the single-breath-hold technique--comparison with pulmonary angiography. Radiology 185(2):381–387

7. Mayo JR, Remy-Jardin M, Muller NL, Remy J, Worsley DF, Hossein-Foucher C, Kwong JS, Brown MJ (1997) Pulmonary embolism: prospective comparison of spiral CT with ventilation-perfusion scintigraphy. Radiology 205(2):447–452

8. Remy-Jardin M, Remy J, Deschildre F, Artaud D, Beregi JP, Hossein-Foucher C, Marchandise X, Duhamel A (1996) Diagnosis of pulmonary embolism with spiral CT: comparison with pulmonary angiography and scintigraphy. Radiology 200(3):699–706

9. Ghaye B, Szapiro D, Mastora I, Delannoy V, Duhamel A, Remy J, Remy-Jardin M (2001) Peripheral pulmonary arteries: how far in the lung does multi-detector row spiral CT allow analysis? Radiology 219(3):629–636

10. Schoepf UJ, Holzknecht N, Helmberger TK, Crispin A, Hong C, Becker CR, Reiser MF (2002) Subsegmental pulmonary emboli: improved detection with thin-collimation multi-detector row spiral CT. Radiology 222(2):483–490

11. Stein PD, Henry JW, Gottschalk A (1999) Reassessment of pulmonary angiography for the diagnosis of pulmonary embolism: relation of interpreter agreement to the order of the involved pulmonary arterial branch. Radiology 210(3):689–691

12. Patriquin L, Khorasani R, Polak JF (1998) Correlation of diagnostic imaging and subsequent autopsy findings in patients with pulmonary embolism. AJR Am J Roentgenol 171(2):347–349

13. Goodman LR, Lipchik RJ, Kuzo RS, Liu Y, McAuliffe TL, O'Brien DJ (2000) Subsequent pulmonary embolism: risk after a negative helical CT pulmonary angiogram--prospective comparison with scintigraphy. Radiology 215(2):535–542

14. Schoepf UJ, Costello P (2003) Multidetector-row CT imaging of pulmonary embolism. Semin Roentgenol 38(2):106–114

15. Winer-Muram HT, Boone JM, Brown HL, Jennings SG, Mabie WC, Lombardo GT (2002) Pulmonary embolism in pregnant patients: fetal radiation dose with helical CT Radiology 224(2):487–492

18 Mediastinum, Pleura, and Chest Wall

R. Eibel

Indications

- Acute mediastinitis.
- Chronic sclerosing mediastinitis.
- Tumors of the mediastinum: thymic lesions (thymic hyperplasia, thymolipoma, thymic cysts, thymoma, thymic neuroendocrine neoplasms, thymic carcinoma, thymic lymphoma, Germ cell neoplasms (teratoma, seminoma, endodermal sinus tumor, choriocarcinoma), tumors of thyroid and parathyroid tissue, tumors of adipose tissue (lipoma, lipomatosis), tumors of vascular tissue (hemangioma, angiosarcoma, hemangiopericytoma, lymphangioma).
- Lymph node enlargement (primary mediastinal lymphoma, angiofollicular lymph node hyperplasia).
- Masses situated in the anterior cardiophrenic angle (pleuropericardial fat, mesothelial cysts, hernia through the foramen of Morgagni, enlargement of diaphragmatic lymph nodes).
- Dilatation of the main pulmonary artery, of the major mediastinal veins, of the aorta, or of its branches (including aortic tears, dissections).
- Tumors and tumor-like conditions of neural tissue (tumors arising from peripheral nerves, from sympathetic ganglia and aorticosympathetic paraganglioma, and from meningocele and meningomyelocele).
- Posterior mediastinal cysts (gastroenteric cysts, esophageal cysts, thoracic duct cyst).
- Diseases of the esophagus (neoplasms, diverticula, megaesophagus).
- Tracheoesophageal and bronchoesophageal fistulae.
- Mediastinal masses due to transdiaphragmatic herniation of abdominal contents.
- Pleural plaque.
- Diffuse pleural thickening.
- Pleural tumor.
- Diaphragmatic injuries.

Scan Parameters

See Table 18.1.

Tips and Tricks

See text below.

Introduction

This chapter will focus on the mediastinum and chest wall including thoracic trauma and the pleura.

The mediastinum contains central cardiovascular and tracheobronchial structures, the esophagus, nerves, and lymph nodes. The most common is an anatomic scheme in which the mediastinum is divided into anterior, middle, and posterior compartments. Furthermore, this division of the mediastinum corresponds to easily recognizable regions as seen on the lateral chest radiograph.

The pleura is a serosal membrane that envelopes the lung and lines the costal surface, diaphragm, and mediastinum. It is composed of two layers, the visceral and the parietal pleura, which join at the hilum. The normal costal, diaphragmatic, and mediastinal pleura is not visible on plain film

Table 18.1. List of parameters for 4-, 16-, and 64-row CTs for different indication groups

Parameters	4–8 slice scanners	10–16 slice scanners	32–64 slice scanners
Scanning parameters			
Tube voltage (kV)	120	120	120
Rotation time (s)	0.5	0.5	0.33–0.5
Tube current time product (mAs)	120–225	120–225	120–225
Pitch corrected Tube current time product (eff. mAs)	100–150	100–150	100–150
Slice Collimation (mm)	1/1.25 or 2.5 for optimized scan time	0.625/0.75 or 1.25/1.5 for optimized scan time	0.6/0.625
Norm. pitch	1.2–1.5	1.2–1.5	1.2–1.5
Reconstruction increment (mm)	5 For recons 1.0	5 For recons 0.6	5 For recons 0.5
Reconstruction thickness (mm)	5[*] For recons 1.5–2.5	5[*] For recons 0.75–1	5[*] For recons 0.6–1
Convolution kernel	Standard[**]	Standard[**]	Standard[**]
Contrast material	Yes	Yes	Yes
Volume (mL)	100	80	80
Injection speed (mL/s)	3	3	3
Saline flush (mL, mL/s)			
Delay arterial (s)	30	40	40

[*] For the evaluation of chest wall and pleural diseases, especially for detection of small pleural calcifications, thin slices (2–3 mm) are necessary.

[**] For the workup of cases in which the combined investigation of lung parenchyma and mediastinal and hilar soft tissue is necessary, the Combi Thorax protocol is ideal. This protocol should be used for the combined evaluation of HR lung and soft-tissue mediastinum. It is also recommended for delineation of pleural disease, because of the possibility to reconstruct thin slice, where pleural abnormalities are found on thicker slices. Demarcation of the esophagus can be optimized by giving a barium suspension shortly before starting the scan.

Scan parameters (Combi Thorax) should include 0.6 mm (64 row) to 2.5 mm (4 row) collimation, pitch 1.25–1.5, 120 kV, 120 eff. mAs, reconstruction thickness of 1 mm (sharp kernel) and 5 mm (soft kernel) at an increment of 0.5 mm and 3 mm, respectively. A rotation time of at least 0.5 s in the caudocranial scan direction. Contrast material is recommended in a dose of 80–90 mL and at a flow rate of 3 mL/s.

or CT. The intercostal stripe, which can be detected at HRCT represents a combination of the two pleural layers, the endothoracic fascia, and the innermost intercostal muscle. To detect real pleural thickening, it is recommended to look for soft tissue density between the inner rib and the lung (Fig. 18.5).

The symmetry of the chest cage and the axillae allow, in most cases, easy detection and characterization of abnormalities in CT, including pathological enlarged lymph

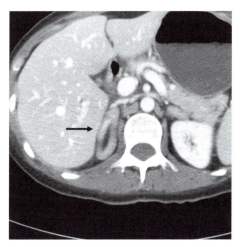

Fig. 18.1. Patient with Cushing syndrome. Ap-dominal CT delineated hyperplasia of both adrenal glands (*arrow* indicates right adrenal gland)

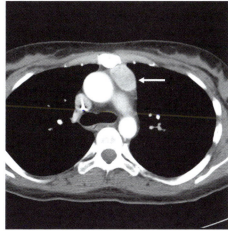

Fig. 18.2. In chest CT, a soft tissue mass in the anterior mediastinum was found (*arrow*). Histology: thymic carcinoid

nodes. The first rib can be readily identified as it lies adjacent to the medial end of the clavicle at the level of the sternoclacicular joint. The second, third, and fourth ribs can usually be identified at the same level by counting posteriorly along the rib cage. By proceeding sequentially caudally, each next vertebra and corresponding rib can be identified. Using coronal or sagittal reformations can overcome this problem by visualization of the entire spine in one image.

The Mediastinum

The good news is that primary diseases of the mediastinum are rare in comparison to the other thoracic diseases. The bad news is that by using plain film and physical examinations a lot of mediastinal pathologies are not or infrequently detected and thus even a suspicion of a mass requires a CT.

Acute mediastinitis is a severe disease resulting from, in the majority of patients, esophageal perforation by a primary carcinoma, an impacted foreign body, or diagnostic or therapeutic instrumentation. After severe vomiting (Boerhaave's syndrome), spontaneous perforation can develop. The "typical" finding here on plain film is a widening of the mediastinum. Air collections (pneumomediastinum) can raise the suspicion of esophageal perforation. With CT the sensitivity to detect free air or the primary cause of mediastinitis is much higher than with plain film. Intravenous contrast is mandatory to visualize abscess formation. It can help to detect an esophageal defect when the patient swallows diluted contrast material directly prior to the scan. Chronic sclerosing mediastinitis is a rare condition, characterized by chronic inflammation and fibrosis of mediastinal soft tissue. CT detects a mediastinal or hilar mass, calcifications in the mass or adjacent lymph nodes, and tracheobronchial tree narrowing.

Table 18.2 gives an overview of the mediastinal tumors and their typical locations.

For a short overview, the CT criteria are summarized here for the more common of the above-mentioned masses.

- Thymic hyperplasia: enlargement of the entire organ with preservation of organ contours.
- Thymolipoma: fat attenuation values, very soft tissue, slumps toward diaphragm.
- Thymic cysts: low-density fluid (0–10 HU), small wall calcification is possible.

Table 18.2. Most common mediastinal tumor entities and their typical locations

Location	Tumor
Anterior mediastinum	• Thymic lesions (thymic hyperplasia, thymolipoma, thymic cysts, thymoma, thymic neuroendocrine neoplasms (Figs. 18.1 and 18.2), thymic carcinoma, thymic lymphoma (Fig. 18.3) • Germ cell neoplasms (teratoma, seminoma, endodermal sinus tumor, choriocarcinoma) • Tumors of thyroid and parathyroid tissue • Tumors of adipose tissue (lipoma, lipomatosis) • Tumors of vascular tissue (hemangioma, angiosarcoma, hemangiopericytoma, lymphangioma) • Tumors of muscle • Fibrous and fibrohistiocytic tumors
Middle mediastinum	• Lymph node enlargement (primary mediastinal lymphoma, angiofollicular lymph node hyperplasia) • Aorticopulmonary paraganglioma • Masses situated in the anterior cardiophrenic angle (pleuropericardial fat, mesothelial cysts, hernia through the foramen of Morgagni, enlargement of diaphragmatic lymph nodes) • Dilatation of the main pulmonary artery • Dilatation of the major mediastinal veins • Dilatation of the aorta or its branches • Tumors and tumor-like conditions of neural tissue (Tumors arising from peripheral nerves, from sympathetic ganglia and aorticosympathetic paraganglioma, meningocele and meningomyelocele)
Posterior mediastinum	• Posterior mediastinal cysts (Gastroenteric cysts, Esophageal cysts, Thoracic duct cyst) • Diseases of the esophagus (Neoplasms, Diverticula, Megaesophagus) • Tracheoesophageal and bronchoesophageal fistulae • Mediastinal masses due to transdiaphragmatic herniation of abdominal contents • Diseases of thoracic spine (Neoplasms, Infectious spondylitis, Fracture with hematoma formation) • Extramedullary hematopoises

- Thymoma: homogenous soft tissue with smooth borders and homogenous enhancement, sometimes calcifications.
- Thymic neuroendocrine neoplasms: homogeneous, lobulated, rare calcifications.
- Thymic carcinoma: heterogeneous attenuation, irregular interface with lung, metastases. Sometimes CT fails in predicting malignancy, if no direct signs (invasion, metastases) are visible.
- Teratoma: uni- or multicystic, fat and calcifications. Cave: If larger and signs of invasion are visible: malignant transformation.
- Seminoma: lobulated noncalcified mass, undistinguishable from other malignant germ cell tumors.
- Lipomatosis: smooth and symmetric mediastinal widening with fat attenuation values.
- Lymphangioma: the cystic variation in children (cystic hygroma) and the well-defined variety of adults with low attenuation values, tumor molds to the mediastinal contours.

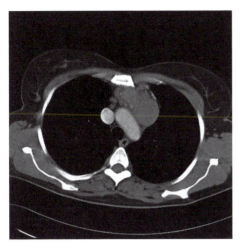

Fig. 18.3. M-Hodgkin. Large mass in the anterior mediastinum

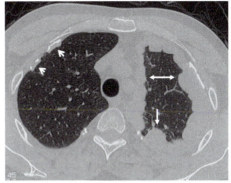

Fig. 18.4. HRCT. Malignant pleural mesothelioma at the left side (*long arrows*) and calcified pleural plaque at the right lateral pleural (*short arrows*)

- Lymphoma: asymmetric lymph node enlargement, but not unilateral. Calcifications after radiation and occasionally after chemotherapy. Hodgkin's lymphoma can also present as an anterior mediastinal mass usually caused by primary involvement of the thymus rather than by enlarged lymph nodes. Non-Hodgkin's lymphomas are seen with extranodal spread more often.
- Schwannoma: round or oval paravertebral mass with mixed attenuation, dumbbell configuration, when originating in a nerve root.
- Ganglioneuroma: homogeneous lesion in the paravertebral zone with an elongated, flattened configuration with a broad base toward the mediastinum.
- Paraganglioma: indistinguishable from the other neurogenic neoplasms.
- Gastroenteric cyst (neurenteric cyst): homogeneous (fluid content), sharply defined mass in the paravertebral location. Contains gas, if a communication with the esophagus exists.

Look carefully for signs of local invasion and metastatic spread. Homogeneous soft tissue attenuation and depiction of calcification are not pathognomonic for benignity.

Pleural Disease: Effusion and More

With CT, four types of pleural disease can be differentiated: pleural plaques, diffuse pleural thickening, pleural tumors and pleural effusions. From the etiologic, diagnostic, therapeutic, and prognostic points of view it is necessary to differentiate these entities.

A pleural plaque is a marker of asbestos exposure (Fig. 18.4). It represents a deposition of hyalinized collagen fibers in the parietal pleura, most commonly found along the sixth through ninth ribs and along the diaphragm. With CT it can be clearly separated from the extrapleural fat and the endothoracic fascia. Calcifications are identified by chest X-ray in 20% of the detected pleural plaques, on CT scanning in 50%, and at autoptic examination in 80%. Sometimes these plaques can look like "tabloids" or have a nodular configuration with impingement of the adjacent lung parenchyma.

Diffuse pleural thickening on the other hand is a nonspecific response of the pleura to a number of agents, not a specific marker of asbestos exposure (Fig. 18.5). Inflammation, trauma, neoplasia, embolism, and radiation can each result in diffuse pleural thickening. There is an involvement of the parietal and visceral pleura. After initial obliteration of the costophrenic sulci devel-

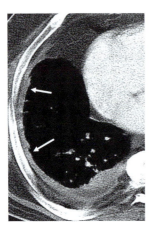

Fig. 18.5. Diffuse pleural thickening (*arrows*)

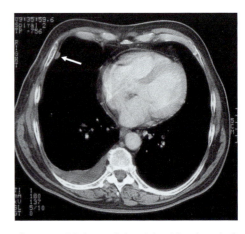

Fig. 18.6. Etiology of the right side pleural effusion? Note the ventro-lateral pleural plaque (courtesy of S. Tuengerthal, Heidelberg)

opment of pleural retraction and cicatrisation is possible, sometimes encircling the lung surface and involving the mediastinal pleura. CT criteria include an extent of more than 8 cm in the craniocaudal direction, 5 cm in cross section, and a thickness of more than 3 mm.

A pleural tumor is defined as a pleural nodule more than 30 mm in diameter. The majority of pleural tumors are malignant and most are metastatic diseases (primary pleural membrane tumors, pleural invasion by primary bronchogenic carcinoma, subpleural tumors like lymphoma, hematogenous dissemination to the pleura and direct pleural seeding).

CT findings indicating malignant pleural disease instead of benign disease include mediastinal pleural involvement, pleural nodularity, and pleural thickening of more than 1 cm each. They have a high specificity; with the exception of pleural thickening more than 1-cm. Detection of subpleural soft tissue hypertrophy in fat tissue is an important CT finding for benign disease and is present in half of the benign cases. Signs of invasion of mediastinal or osseous structures, transdiaphragmatic growth, and metastases to lymph nodes and distant organs by pleural disease are clear findings of malignant disease.

A drawback of CT is the sensitivity and specificity of a correct lymph node staging.

Although distant metastases are uncommon, intrathoracic disease, particularly to regional lymph nodes, is reported in 34 to 50% of patients. Therefore biopsy is recommended for a definite diagnosis.

Pleural effusion is one of the most common pleural abnormalities, and can occur without other pathologies in the thorax. But because an effusion is not a physiologic variant, the underlying cause must always be evaluated. Specific causes are infection (bacteria, fungi, viruses and parasites), connective tissue diseases (systemic lupus erythematosus, rheumatoid disease), asbestosis (Fig. 18.6), drugs, neoplasms (lung cancer, lymphoma, leukemia, multiple myeloma, metastases), thromboembolism, cardiac decompensation, and trauma. A variety of intraabdominal and pelvic disorders are also associated with pleural effusion (such as pancreatitis, sequela of abdominal surgery, subphrenic abscess, Meigs–Salmon syndrome, dialysis, hydronephrosis and urinothorax, nephritic syndrome, cirrhosis, acute glomerulonephritis and uremic pleuritis). CT can be very helpful in diagnosing the etiology of pleural fluid. But how safe is CT to distinguish between transudate and exudate? A study form Arenas-Jiménez et al. showed that the delineation of pleural nodules, nodular pleural thickening, and extrapleural fat of increased density only appeared in exudates. Differentiation between empyemas and parapneumonic effusions cannot be established on the basis of CT findings, but localization, thickening of any pleural surface, and increased density of extrapleural fat are more frequently encountered in empyemas.

Thoracic Trauma: One-Stop Shopping?

Some years ago, severely ill trauma patients received plain film investigations of the skeleton, the chest, and abdomen. In correlation with ultrasound findings and physical examination, a CT was performed. Multislice CT has now dramatically changed the approach to the severely injured individual. CT has a higher sensitivity and specificity for detection and characterization of thoracic injuries, especially those of the heart, pericardium and the great vessels, the lungs, mediastinum and diaphragm, the thoracic spine, sternum, and ribs. Whole-body scanning in 1 min has become reality, and using a 16-row scanner, the thorax can be acquired in about 10 s. After the patient leaves the CT room, reconstructions in the lung, soft, and bone tissue kernel can be performed, adapting to the different regions of interest. Even more complex reformations (MPR, volumetric methods) can be calculated in retrospect, and the patient avoids delay in treatment of other injuries. It is important to implement a generally accepted algorithm for the optimal use of MDCT in the emergency situation in the near future. Despite unknown renal status (elevation of creatinine, perhaps), intravenous contrast is recommended in nearly every case.

Pneumothorax and pneumomediastinum are serious conditions, because under assisting ventilation even a small pneumothorax may rapidly progress to a tension-type pneumothorax and subsequent cardiovascular compromise. The plain film often fails in delineating these lesions at early stages. As a consequence, after any significant chest trauma, CT with intravenous contrast is highly recommended. Typical lung injuries are contusion, laceration,

and tears or ruptures of the bronchi and trachea. Again, multiplanar reformations can help to localize the lesions. Especially because most of the trachea tears are horizontally orientated, they may be missed in axial scans, but can be found in sagittal or coronal reformations when previously scanning with a thin collimation (4×1 mm, 16×0.75 mm, and 64×0.6 mm).

The sensitivity of detecting diaphragmatic injuries with plain film is low (46%). With MDCT the sensitivity can be elevated up to 71%. Again the sagittal and coronal reformation can make the diagnosis easier, because defects of the diaphragm and herniations can be appreciated in one slice.

High acceleration/deceleration traumas play an increasing role in the emergency room. Motor vehicle accidents lead to many more vascular and cardiac injuries compared to 20 years ago. With plain films, the diagnosis of aortic tears can be made indirectly, by widening of the mediastinum, unsharpness of the aortic knob, and the delineation of pleural effusion. CT is the gold standard in the emergency situation for evaluation of the heart and the great vessels, because the direct signs of aortic injury are both more accurate than indirect signs and show higher interobserver agreement. Dissections can be found without performing a more invasive angiography or transesophageal endoscopy. In this sense, plain films have no value for diagnosis.

In the hospital of the author, whole-body CT is beginning to replace plain films of the chest and spine in critically ill trauma victims. MDCT allows for thinner collimation without sacrificing speed, and the high spatial resolution is the basis for superb 2D and 3D reformations that give helpful additional information to the referring physician.

The Chest Wall

Abnormalities of the ribs can be divided into a congenital and an acquired group. Congenital anomalies are rib fusions and various types of bifid ribs, which are generally asymptomatic. Additional cervical ribs may result in clinical symptoms, when they compress subclavian vessels or the brachial plexus. Erosion and inferior notching of ribs can have a lot of causes, like aortic obstruction, superior vena cava obstruction, arteriovenous fistula, intercostals neurinoma or hyperparathyroidism. These osseous finding are easily detectable on plain films. CT is useful to visualize the cause of the acquired rib alterations in addition to other findings (history of the patient, laboratory findings, ultrasound, etc.).

Indications for CT are neoplasms and nonneoplastic tumors of the chest wall and trauma conditions. In general, benign and malignant primary neoplasms that originate in the chest wall are uncommon. In adults, the most common benign tumor of the chest wall is lipoma; the most common malignant neoplasms are fibrosarcoma and malignant fibrohistiocytoma. In children, the most frequent malignant tumors are primitive neuroectodermal tumor, rhabdomyosarcoma, and extraosseous Ewing's sarcoma. When looking at the bony structures, most of the neoplasms of the thoracic skeleton occur in the ribs and are metastases. The most common primary malignant tumor of the thoracic skeleton is chondrosarcoma. Osteogenic sarcoma, malignant fibrohistiocytoma, hemangiopericytoma, and fibrosarcoma are less frequent. The most common benign type is osteochondroma, followed by enchondroma and bone islands. Myeloma is the most frequent malignant neoplasms of reticuloendothelial

origin. CT and especially the multiplanar reformations can assist in delineating the pathological process and its anatomic relationships, but in most of the cases a pathologic correlation is necessary.

Literature
and Suggested Readings

- Arenas-Jiménez J, Alonso-Charterina S, Sanchez-Paya J, Fernandez-Latorre F, Gil-Sanchez S, Lloret-Llorens M (2000) Evaluation of CT findings for diagnosis of pleural effusions. Eur Radiol 10:681–690
- Austin JHM, Müller NL, Friedman PJ et al. (1996) Glossary of terms for CT of the lungs: Recommendation of the nomenclature committee of the Fleischner Society. Radiology 200:327–331
- Boiselle Ph (ed) (2003) Multislice helical CT of the thorax. Radiologic Clinics of North America 41(3):465–661
- Eibel R (2001) Primary chest film reading on coronal and sagittal MPRs. In: Reiser MF, Takahashi M, Modic M, Bruening R (eds) Multislice CT. Springer, Berlin Heidelberg New York, pp 155–164
- Eibel R, Tuengerthal S, Schoenberg SO (2003) The role of new imaging techniques in diagnosis and staging of malignant pleural mesothelioma. Curr Opin Oncol 15:131–138
- Fraser RS, Paré JA, Fraser RG, Paré PD (1994) Synopsis of diseases of the chest, 2nd edn. Saunders, Philadelphia
- McGuinness G, Naidich DP (2002) Multislice computed tomography of the chest. In: Silverman PM (ed) Multislice computed tomography. Lippincott Williams&Wilkins, Philadelphia, pp 117–167

19 Thoracic Aorta

A. Kuettner

Indications

- Assessment of aortic diameter in patients with suspected aortic dilatation.
- Preoperative planning scan.
- Suspected aortic dissection and/or follow-up.
- Suspected aortic rupture.
- Follow-up after aortic valve replacement with or without conduit implantation.
- Follow-up after ascending aorta replacement.

Patient Preparation

- 20 or 18 G i.v. access antecubitally, supine position.
- Topogram/scan range: entire chest/diaphragm to mid-supraaortic branches (Fig. 19.1).
- Placement of ecg-leads (if gated scan is necessary).
- If the coronary arteries are of interest (e.g, before ascending aorta replacement), a beta-blocker regimen analogous to the coronaries is recommended (see Chap. 21).

Scan Parameters

See Table 19.1.

Tips and Tricks

- Make sure i.v. access is fully patent.
- For good vessel opacification use contrast media containing >350 mg iodine/mL).

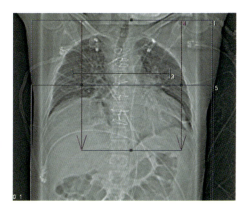

Fig. 19.1. Topogram. Arms above the head. The ecg-gated scan range should encompass the suspected anatomical site of a given suspected pathology (e.g., aortic aneurysm). If possible, scan the entire chest with the diaphragm as lower limit and the supraaortic branches as upper limit. If a second nongated thorax spiral scan is required, it should be executed in the opposite scan direction (flying-thorax) with no additional contrast applied

- If a gated spiral is followed by an ungated spiral scan, the first scan should be executed craniocaudally and the second caudocranially to avoid any delay between scans. By doing so, no additional CM is needed for the second spiral ("flying thorax").

Anatomical and Technical Considerations

Since helical single slice CT scanners became available, the assessment of the aortic arch using computed tomography has been established as the modality of choice for most

Table 19.1. Scan parameters

Parameters	4–8 slice scanners	10–16 slice scanners	32–64 slice scanners
Scanner settings			
Tube voltage (kV)	120	120	120
Tube current time product (mAs)	110	160	170
Pitch corrected tube current time product (eff. mAs)	300	650	850
Collimation (mm)	2.5	0.75	0.6
Norm. pitch	0.375	0.25	0.2
Reconstr.-slice thickness (mm)	3.0	1.0	0.6
convolution kernel	standard	standard	standard
Specials	Retrospective ECG-gating	Retrospective ECG-gating	Retrospective ECG-gating
	ECG-pulsing for HR<60	ECG-pulsing for HR<70	ECG-pulsing for HR<80
Scan range	Base of heart to beginning of aortic arch	Base of heart to beginning of aortic arch	Base of heart to beginning of aortic arch
Scan direction	Caudocranial	Caudocranial	Caudocranial
Contrast media application			
Concentration (mg iodine/mL)	350–400	350–400	350–400
Mono/Biphasic	Biphasic	Biphasic	Monophasic
Volume (mL)	150	120	100
Injection rate (mL/s)	4.0, 2.5	4.0, 2.5	5.0
Saline chaser (mL, mL/s)	30, 2.5	30, 2.5	60, 5.0
Delay (s)	Test bolus	Test bolus	Test bolus or bolus tracking

pathologies [1]. With the introduction of multislice systems the scanning techniques were gradually refined [2–5], but still there are pitfalls to be taken into account when interpreting CT scans [6]. From a CT imaging perspective, the thoracic aortic arch can be divided into segments considerably affected by cardiac motion such as the proximal ascending aorta. All other segments such as the large supraaortic branches, the brachiocephalic trunk, the left common carotid artery and the left subclavian artery as well as the small intercostal and spinal branches are commonly not affected by cardiac motion [7]. All cardiac-motion affected segments can be scanned using ecg-gated techniques [7,8]; all other structures can be scanned using conventional nongated CT protocols. However, ecg-gated protocols use a considerably higher dose level (9–10 mSv vs. 3–4 mSv) than nongated protocols, thus choosing the appropriate scan protocol depends not only on the anatomic structure in questions, but the effective dose needed for a particular scan protocol should be taken into account [8].

With the introduction of scanners acquiring up to 64 slices per rotation, the entire chest may be scanned using ecg-gated techniques (Fig. 19.2). For all previ-

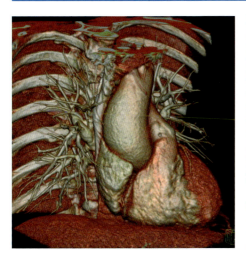

Fig. 19.2. 3D volume-rendered image of a 64-slice scan. Large ascending aorta aneurysm displayed with excellent image quality with no motion artifacts present

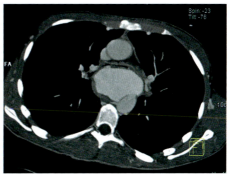

Fig. 19.3. Axial image of a ruptured descending aorta: 22-year-old patient with progressive dysphagia and progressive dyspnea. Initial diagnosis made with a nongated helical single-slice scanner was aortic aneurysm of the descending aorta. Note the site of rupture as well as the large pseudo-aneurysm. The trachea, as well as the esophagus, are severely compressed accounting for the patient's symptoms

ous scanner generations up to 16 slices, the scan range is limited, so that the entire chest may not be covered within a reasonable breath hold time and only regions with suspected motion artifacts may be scanned using ecg-gating. Regardless of scanner types, if a particular pathology is known, the scan range should be set accordingly. If a pathology is suspected, but the exact location is unknown (e.g., aortic dissection), the entire ascending aorta should be taken into the ecg-gated scan range. Since a complete scan of the entire chest is most often required to answer all medical questions, a second scan of the chest using a nongated protocol should be performed. If both scans have opposite scan directions, no additional contrast media is required for the second spiral since adequate opacification still remains from the first scan (flying thorax technique: first scan craniocaudal, second scan caudocranial or vice versa).

Image Reconstruction

For ecg-gated image reconstruction, standard built-in preset reconstruction algorithms used for cardiac imaging and provided by each manufacturer can be also used for aortic imaging. Generally, the reconstruction window is set to start at 60% RR-interval. If significant motion artifacts, an additional test-series reconstructing single slices in 5% steps at a given z-position is recommended, ranging from 0 to 95% relative to the RR-interval. The time point with the least motion artifacts is then chosen to reconstruct the entire stack of images of the MDCTA scan. Typically, a slice thickness of image thickness 0.6–1 mm with a reconstruction increment of 0.4–0.8 mm and a medium smooth reconstruction kernel is used. The second flying thorax can be reconstructed using 1-mm slices with an increment of 0.8 mm; the kernel can be medium smooth.

Visualization Techniques

For the assessment of the aortic arch, axial image interpretation is still the most commonly used and most efficient way of quickly assessing the aorta (see Fig. 19.3). Maximum intensity projections (MIPs) or double oblique multiplanar reformats (MPR) in parallel alignment to the aortic arch are also a very convenient and efficient way to visualize and diagnose the entire aorta (see

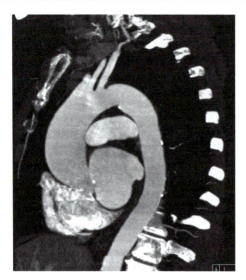

Fig. 19.4. Curved MIP of the same patient as in Fig. 19.2. In one single image, all relevant anatomical information for a potential surgical intervention is provided: maximum diameter, distance from the sternum, absent affection of the supracoronary branches, and diameter of the aorta on the level of the aortic bulb

Fig. 19.4). Curved MIP projections, projecting the vessel in a single plane are helpful for the assessment of any vascular diameters. VRT images may be helpful for the purpose of better anatomic orientation (see Figs. 19.2 and 19.5), but should not be used for detailed diagnosing.

References

1. Rubin GD (1997) Helical CT angiography of the thoracic aorta. J Thorac Imaging 12:128–149
2. Alkadhi H, Wildermuth S, Desbiolles L et al. (2004) Vascular emergencies of the thorax after blunt and iatrogenic trauma: multi-detector row CT and three-dimensional imaging. Radiographics 24:1239–1255
3. Castaner E, Andreu M, Gallardo X et al. (2003) CT in nontraumatic acute thoracic aortic disease: typical and atypical features and complications. Radiographics 23:S93–110
4. Kapoor V, Ferris JV, Fuhrman CR (2004) Intimomedial rupture: a new CT finding to distinguish true from false lumen in aortic dissection. AJR Am J Roentgenol 183:109–112
5. Khan IA, Nair CK (2002) Clinical, diagnostic, and management perspectives of aortic dissection. Chest 122:311–328
6. Batra P, Bigoni B, Manning J et al. (2000) Pitfalls in the diagnosis of thoracic aortic dissection at CT angiography. Radiographics 20:309–320
7. Roos JE, Willmann JK, Weishaupt D et al. (2002) Thoracic aorta: motion artifact reduction with retrospective and prospective electrocardiography-assisted multi-detector row CT. Radiology 222:271–277
8. Hofmann LK, Zou KH, Costello P et al. (2004) Electrocardiographically gated 16-section CT of the thorax: cardiac motion suppression. Radiology 233:927–933

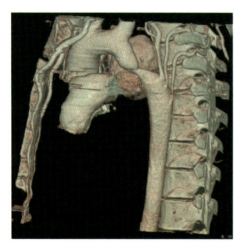

Fig. 19.5. 3D VRT image of the same aorta as in Fig. 19.3. The site of rupture is proximal to an unknown congenital aortic coarctation. This image is an excellent anatomical overview to demonstrate the anatomical relationship between the pseudo-aneurysm and the coarctation

20 Calcium Screening

R. Fischbach

Indications

- Suspected coronary artery disease.
- Differential diagnosis of symptomatic patients with atypical chest pain.
- Risk stratification in asymptomatic individuals with an intermediate to high risk for a future myocardial event.
- Follow-up of patients with coronary atherosclerosis and lipid lowering therapy.

Patient Preparation

No special preparation.

Patient Positioning

Supine, arms elevated, ECG leads attached, table height should position the heart in the isocenter of the gantry.

Scan Range

One centimeter below the tracheal bifurcation to diaphragm. Scan range must include the entire cardiac volume (Fig. 20.1).

Scan Parameters

See Tables 20.1 and 20.2.

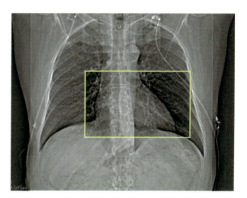

Fig. 20.1. Scan range for calcium scanning. The scan volume should include the entire heart from the mid level of the pulmonary artery (approx. 1 cm below the tracheal bifurcation) down to the diaphragm

Tips and Tricks

Motion-free images are crucial for exact and reproducible scoring results.

- In sequential scanning, usually a scan start at 60% of the RR interval works best. The scan window can be tested by using a single section test scan at the mid level of the right coronary artery. If the right coronary artery does not show motion artifacts, other vessels will also usually be motion free.
- In spiral scanning, the image reconstruction window should be set to 60% of the RR interval. If motion artifacts are present, a different reconstruction window can be selected to minimize motion artifacts.

Table 20.1. Calcium quantification, sequential scan technique

Parameters	4–8 slice scanners	10–16 slice scanners	32–64 slice scanners
Tube voltage (kV)	120	120	120
Tube current (mAs)	100	100	100
Collimation (mm)	2.5	1.5	0.6
Table feed (mm)	10	18	18
Rotation time (ms)	500	420	330
Reconstr.-slice thickness (mm)	2.5	3	3
Reconstruction increment (mm)	2.5	3	3
convolution kernel	standard	standard	standard
Specials	ECG triggering, 60% RR interval		
Scan range	Carina-diaphragm		
Scan direction	Craniocaudal		
Field of view (cm)	22		
Contrast media application	NA		

Table 20.2. Calcium quantification, spiral scan technique

Parameters	4–8 slice scanners	10–16 slice scanners	32–64 slice scanners
Tube voltage (kV)	120	120	120
Tube current time product (mAs)	40	30	20
Pitch corrected tube current time product (eff. mAs)	100	100	100
Collimation (mm)	2.5	1.5	1.2
Normalized pitch	0.365	0.283	0.20
Table feed (mm)	3.7	6.8	4.8
Rotation time (ms)	500	420–330	330
Reconstr.-slice thickness (mm)	3	3	3
Reconstruction increment (mm)	1.5	1.5	1.5
convolution kernel	standard	standard	standard
Specials	ECG gating, 60% RR interval		
Scan range	Carina-diaphragm		
Scan direction	Craniocaudal		
Field of view (cm)	22		
Contrast media application	NA		

- In patients with a high heart rate a systolic reconstruction window (25–30% RR) may yield better results.
- Oral premedication with a beta blocker may be considered in patients with a heart rate above 70 beats/min when using a scanner with rotation times >370 ms.
- Overlapping image reconstruction improves the measurement reproducibility and increases sensitivity for small calcifications.
- Lung windows should be inspected when reading the study, since patients at risk for coronary heart disease have an increased risk for bronchogenic carcinoma.

Anatomy

The right coronary artery (RCA) arises from the sinus of Valsalva and follows the right atrioventricular groove to the inferior surface of the heart. At the cardiac crux it bifurcates into the posterior descending and posterolateral branches. The left coronary artery arises approximately 1 cm above the level of the RCA and divides into the left anterior descending (LAD) branch and left circumflex (LCx) branch. The LAD follows the anterior interventricular groove to the cardiac apex while the LCx lies in the left atrioventricular groove.

Medical Indications

Symptomatic Patients Suspected of Having Coronary Heart Disease

A negative coronary calcium scan almost rules out obstructive coronary artery disease in symptomatic patients. A negative predictive value of 98% has been reported in patients with acute chest pain and nonspecific ECG [1]. In patients with an equivocal stress test, identification of coronary artery calcification may be helpful, since coronary artery calcification correlates with the presence of a significant stenosis. Coronary calcifications are found in individuals with obstructive coronary heart disease with a sensitivity ranging from 90–100% and a specificity of 45–76%.

Asymptomatic Individuals with Increased Coronary Risk

Since coronary artery calcification is a surrogate marker for coronary atherosclerotic plaque, it is diagnostic of coronary atherosclerosis. The amount of coronary calcium correlates with the total coronary plaque burden and can be seen as a measure of life-long risk-factor exposure of the arterial wall and an individual's response to such risk-factor exposure. Coronary artery calcification may be present long before clinical manifestation of coronary heart disease (CHD) and may therefore help to identify patients at risk for a future myocardial event, who could potentially benefit from early preventive efforts.

Patients with Coronary Atherosclerosis and Lipid Lowering Therapy

Recent studies have shown the ability of calcium quantification to monitor the progression of coronary calcification and to document the effect of risk factor modification and medical treatment. In 66 patients with coronary calcifications, the observed increase in coronary calcium volume score was 25% without treatment and decreased to 8.8% with statin treatment [2]. Progression of coronary calcification despite lipid-lowering therapy seems to be associated with a significantly increased myocardial risk.

Incidence, Risk Factors

Coronary heart disease remains the major cause of mortality and morbidity in the industrialized nations and accounts for 54% of all cardiovascular deaths and 22% of all deaths in the United States [3]. Sudden coronary death or nonfatal myocardial infarction is the first manifestation of disease in up to 50% of CHD victims. CHD typically manifests in middle-age or older and predominantly in male individuals. Well-recognized risk factors are tobacco smoking, high LDL cholesterol levels, low HDL cholesterol levels, diabetes mellitus, arterial hypertension, and a family history of premature myocardial infarction. Algorithms or scoring systems derived from large prospective epidemiological studies like the Framingham Study in the United States and the Prospective Cardiovascular Münster (PROCAM) Study in Europe can be used to calculate a person's global risk of CHD. A calculated risk greater than 20% in 10 years is considered as high and international expert guidelines recommend initiating treatment of hypertension and hypercholesterolemia in these individuals. Since one third of all coronary events occur in persons with an intermediate risk category (10-year risk 10–20%), there is also considerable need to improve the sensitivity and specificity of coronary risk prediction in this group [4,5].

Staging

Calcifications of the coronary arteries are quantified using either the traditional calcium score (Agatston score), a volume score, or calibrated calcium mass. A threshold of 130 Hounsfield units (HU) is set to identify calcifications. The Agatston score has an inferior reproducibility compared to volume or mass scores and its use with MSCT has been criticized, since it had been designed for a special scan protocol and modality (electron beam CT, EBCT). Calcium mass quantification is independent of scanner hardware and image acquisition parameters when using appropriate scanner calibration as is recommended [6,7].

The report should include the number of calcified vessels, Agatston score, calcium volume score, and calibrated calcium mass. Empirical guidelines for clinical interpretation of calcium scores based on EBCT results have been suggested (Table 20.3).

Since a high calcium score indicates a significant plaque burden, absolute values will provide a certain orientation, when assessing a calcium scan. The prevalence of coronary artery calcification increases with age and shows significant differences between men and women. Therefore, interpretation of calcium scores should also consider the expected normal range. A score above the 75th percentile for age and gender represents a significantly increased risk for future myocardial infarction.

The calcium score or calcium mass seems to be an independent predictor of myocardial events and can provide additional information to that obtained by clinical risk assessment. Calcium score results can be used to test whether and to what extent risk factor exposure has led to expression of coronary atherosclerotic lesions. This information may put an individual in a lower or higher clinical risk group [8].

CT Characteristics

Calcifications are easily recognized in CT due to the high attenuation differences with the surrounding epimyocardial fat. Ostial lesions at the aorta are not included in the calcium measurement. Calcifications of the mitral valve annulus can be confused with calcifications of the LCx. These calcifications are surrounded by myocardium.

Differential Indication

CT is the only modality to reliably quantify coronary artery calcifications. It has a much higher sensitivity than fluoroscopy. Electron beam CT was used for calcium quantification prior to the introduction of MSCT. Initial experience shows good correlation of EBCT measurement and prospectively triggered MDCT [9,10]. EBCT is not widely available, has a slightly better temporal resolution than current generation MSCT systems, but suffers from dose limitations leading to increased image noise.

Table 20.3. Guidelines for coronary calcium score interpretation (adapted from Rumberger JA et al. [11])

Agatston score	Atherosclerotic plaque burden	Probability of significant CAD	Implications for cardiovascular risk	Recommendations
0	No plaque	Very unlikely, <5%	Very low	Reassure patient. Discuss general guidelines for primary prevention of CV diseases.
1–10	Minimal	Very unlikely, <10%	Low	Discuss general guidelines for primary prevention of CV diseases.
11–100	Mild	Mild or minimal coronary stenoses likely	Moderate	Counsel about risk factor modification, strict adherence with primary prevention goals. Daily ASA.
101–400	Moderate	Nonobstructive CAD highly likely, obstructive disease possible	Moderately high	Institute risk factor modification and secondary prevention goals. Consider exercise testing. Daily ASA.
>400	Extensive	High likelihood (>90%) of at least one significant coronary stenosis	High	Institute very aggressive risk factor modification. Consider exercise or pharmacologic nuclear stress testing. Daily ASA.

References

1. McLaughlin VV, Balogh T, Rich S (1999) Utility of electron beam computed tomography to stratify patients presenting to the emergency room with chest pain. Am J Cardiol 84:327–328

2. Achenbach S, Ropers D, Pohle K, Leber A, Thilo C, Knez A, Menendez T, Maeffert R, Kusus M, Regenfus M, Bickel A, Haberl R, Steinbeck G, Moshage W, Daniel WG (2002) Influence of lipid-lowering therapy on the progression of coronary artery calcification: a prospective evaluation. Circulation 106:1077–1082

3. American Heart Association (2002) Heart disease and stroke statistics – 2003 update. American Heart Association, Dallas, TX

4. Schmermund A, Erbel R (2001) New concepts of primary prevention require rethinking. Med Klin 96:261–269

5. Taylor AJ, Burke AP, O'Malley PG, Farb A, Malcom GT, Smialek J, Virmani R (2000) A comparison of the Framingham risk index, coronary artery calcification, and culprit plaque morphology in sudden cardiac death. Circulation 101:1243–1248

6. Hong C, Becker CR, Schoepf UJ, Ohnesorge B, Bruening R, Reiser MF (2002) Coronary artery calcium: absolute quantification in nonenhanced and contrast-enhanced multi-detector row CT studies. Radiology 223:474–480

7. Ulzheimer S, Kalender WA (2003) Assessment of calcium scoring performance in cardiac computed tomography. Eur Radiol 13:484–497

8. Greenland P, LaBree L, Azen SP, Doherty TM, Detrano RC (2004) Coronary artery calcium score combined with Framingham score for risk prediction in asymptomatic individuals. JAMA 291:210–215

9. Becker CR, Kleffel T, Crispin A, Knez A, Young J, Schoepf UJ, Haberl R, Reiser MF (2001) Coronary artery calcium measurement: agreement of multirow detector and electron beam CT. AJR Am J Roentgenol 176:1295–1298

10. Stanford W, Thompson BH, Burns TL, Heery SD, Burr MC (2004) Coronary artery calcium quantification at multi-detector row helical CT versus electron-beam CT. Radiology 230:397–402

11. Rumberger JA et al. (1999) Mayo Clin Proc 74:243–252

21 Coronary Imaging

A. Kuettner

Indications

As coronary CTA is a new modality, no definitive clinically proven indication exists at present. It is only agreed that for the assessment of suspected coronary artery anomaly, coronary CTA is the modality of choice [1]. There is also rising evidence that the method has a high negative predictive value and is able to rule out significant coronary artery stenosis [2,3]. For all other possible uses of coronary CTA, including plaque assessment and follow-up, no hard indication currently exists.

1. Assessment of suspected coronary artery anomaly.
2. To rule out significant coronary artery stenosis in patients with low to medium risk for coronary artery disease with atypical symptoms and/or nondeterminative stress-ecg, echocardiography, or myocardial szintigraphy.
3. Follow-up after coronary intervention to rule out restenosis.
4. Follow-up patients with hemodynamically nonsignificant atherosclerotic wall changes and plaque to determine progression or regression of plaque burden with or without medical therapy.
5. Assessments of left ventricular and left atrial thrombi, if other modalities (echo or MRI) are not available or yield no definite diagnosis.

Contraindications

1. Patients with known severe coronary calcifications.

2. Patients with known diffuse multivessel disease.

Patient Preparation

- β-blockage prior to the scan is strongly recommended if clinically possible. Target heart rate 50–60 bpm; method: 50–100 mg metoprololtartrate 30–60 min prior to the scan. Use 100 mg when possible, reduce to 50 mg when the patient already receives a concomitant β-blocker and has a heart rate that is not <65 bpm, for small patients, and in general for patients with heart rates of 60–65 bpm. No β-blocker should be given when general contraindication for β-blocker is present or for heart rates <55 bpm.
- 20 or 18 G i.v. access antecubitally, supine position.
- Topogram/scan range: entire chest/base of heart to carina (Fig. 21.1).
- Placement of ecg-leads.
- Immediately prior to the scan application of 0.8 mg nitroglycerin orally, or alternatively 2.5 mg of isosorbide dinitrate (coronary dilatiation).

Scan Parameters

See Table 21.1.

Tips and Tricks

1. Make sure i.v. access is fully patent.
2. Attach ecg-leads after patient has lifted his/her arms above the head to avoid

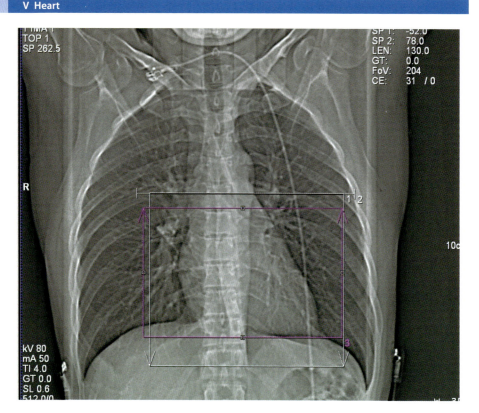

Fig. 21.1. Topogram. Arms above the head. The calcium scoring scan prior to the scan can be used as an additional localizer for the contrast-enhanced spiral, which is usually smaller than the nonenhanced scan. The carina is the upper border, while the base of the heart is the lower border

dislocation and use the "rules" of each manufacturer for positioning (not a "normal" diagnostic ecg).

3. Have the patient start to hold their breath about 5 s prior to the scan (Valsalva maneuver will lead to a decrease of the heart rate).

Rationale for Scanning

Coronary artery disease (CAD) constitutes a major clinically relevant disease in the western industrialized world causing 600,000 deaths annually [4]. The current gold standard to assess the morphological severity of CAD is conventional invasive coronary angiography. In 1999, more than 1.83 million conventional angiographic examinations were performed in the US, of which two thirds were of diagnostic nature only, with no associated intervention [5]. In Europe, similar numbers are available. In Germany alone, the total number of coronary catheter angiography (CCA) rose by 45% from 409,000 in 1995 to more than 594,000 annual procedures in the year 2000 [6]. The fraction of interventional procedures are constantly low at about 30%, which is comparable to US statistics (AHA). Although coronary angiography has become a safe procedure with only a small associated risk, the inconvenience for the patient, as well as the economic burden, have fuelled the quest to find an alternative, noninvasive method to visualize and assess coronary plaque burden.

Table 21.1. Scan parameters

Parameters	4–8 slice scanners	10–16 slice scanners	32–64 slice scanners
Scanner settings			
Tube voltage (kV)	120	120	120
Rotation time (s)	0.5	0.375–0.5	0.33–0.4
Tube current time product (mAs)	150	140–160	150–180
Pitch corrected tube current time product (eff. mAs)	400	550–650	750–900
Collimation (mm)	1.00/1.25	0.625/0.75	0.6/0.625
Norm. pitch	0.375*	0.25*	0.2*
Recon. increment	1	0.8	0.4–0.6
Reconstr.-slice thickness (mm)	1.25	1.0	0.6–0.75
convolution kernel	standard/high res	standard/high res	standard/high res
Specials	Retrospective ECG-gating	Retrospective ECG-gating	Retrospective ECG-gating
	ECG-pulsing for HR<60	ECG-pulsing for HR<70	ECG-pulsing for HR<80
Scan range	Base of heart to carina	Base of heart to carina	Base of heart to Carina
Scan direction	Caudocranial	Caudocranial	Caudocranial
Contrast media application			
Concentration (mg iodine/mL)	350–400	350–400	350–400
Mono/Biphasic	Biphasic	Biphasic	Monophasic
Volume (mL)	120–150	80–100	60–80
Injection rate (mL/s)	4.0, 2.5	4.0, 2.5	5.0
Saline chaser (mL, mL/s)	30, 2.5	30, 2.5	60, 5.0
Delay (s)	Test bolus	Test bolus	Test bolus or bolus tracking

Anatomy

When assessing the heart the following structures should be viewed for diagnosis (Fig. 21.2):

- Right coronary artery (RCA), having four segments: proximal (1), middle (2), distal (3), and posterior descending branch (4).
- Left main coronary artery (5).
- Left anterior descending artery (LAD) subdivided into five segments: proximal (6), middle (7), distal (8), first diagonal (9), and second diagonal branch (10)
- Circumflex artery (RCX) having three segments: proximal (11), distal (12), and first marginal branch (13).
- All cardiac chambers.
- Mitral and aortic valve.

Scanning

After preparing the patient (see above) a calcium scan is routinely performed before the

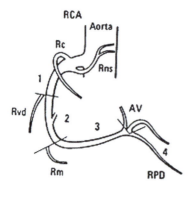

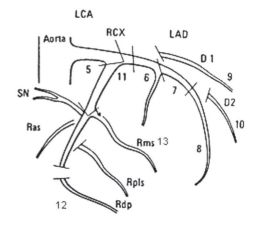

AHA Coronary segments modified

Fig. 21.2. Schematic coronary tree, modified from the AHA classification, with a total of 13 coronary segments used at our institution to report coronary lesions. Since the distal RCX has a considerable interindividual variance, all branches distal to the first marginal branch are distal segments

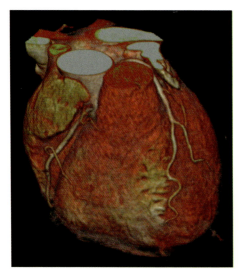

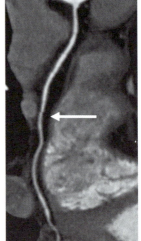

Fig. 21.3. 3D volume-rendered image. Can be used for global orientation and presentation of diagnosis (normal finding). These images should not be used for reading

Fig. 21.4. Curved MPR of a right coronary artery, no stenosis present. This postprocessing type can be used for demonstration of diagnosis for a single coronary artery. Can also be used for cautious reading, note that motion artifacts (*arrow*) may look like a coronary stenosis

contrast-enhanced scan (for the scan protocol, see Chap. 20). If the calcifications are significant, a contrast-enhanced scan may not bring any further information since the coronary lumen may be obscured by calcifications. This effect is especially important when using 4-slice scanners. The threshold for a diagnostic contrast enhanced scan may be as low as 335 Agatston Score. When us-

ing a 16-slice scanner the threshold may rise to 1000 Agatston [7,8]. If calcifications are detected exceeding these limits, the exam should be terminated before contrast-enhanced scanning and the patient referred to conventional coronary angiography. For >16-slice-scanners there are no calcium limits established at present.

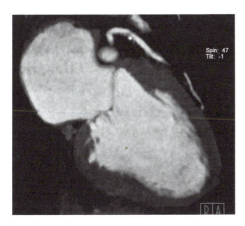

Fig. 21.5. Double oblique MIP (4–6 mm) used for primary reading. Since the entire coronary vessel can not be visualized, one has to interactively scroll through the stack of images. Medium-grade stenosis at proximal LAD (*arrow*)

If the calcium score does not exceed the limits stated above, the CTA scan is performed.

Postprocessing and Image Interpretation

For image reconstruction, a preset reconstruction algorithm provided by each manufacturer can be used. Generally, the reconstruction window is set to start at 60% RR interval. If coronary segments show motion artifacts, an additional test-series reconstructing single slices in 5% steps at a given z-position is recommended, ranging from 0 to 95% relative to the RR interval. The time point with the least motion artifacts is then chosen to reconstruct the entire stack of

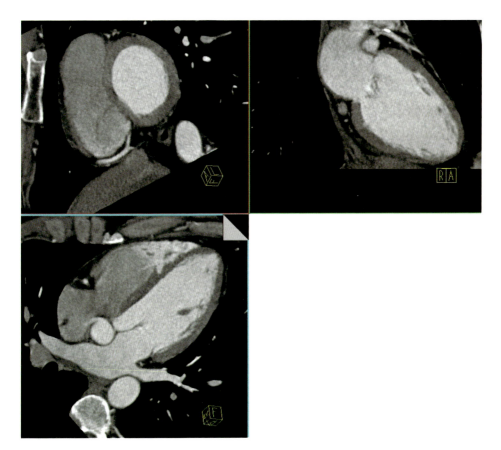

Fig. 21.6. Double oblique MIP as four-chamber view, long-axis view, and short axis view (4–6 mm). Scrolling through the image stack in this direction serves as assessment for general cardiac noncoronary morphology, such as valves, myocardium, or the presence of intracavital thrombi

images of the MDCT scan. Typically a slice thickness of 0.6–1 mm with an increment of 0.4–0.8 mm and a medium-smooth reconstruction kernel is used. Most vendors recommend specifically adapted cardiac kernels that should be used.

Generally, advanced postprocessing techniques such as 3D volume rendering and curved maximum intensity projections (curved MIPs) are too time-consuming and often of limited use for the physician reading cardiac images (Figs. 21.3 and 21.4). Image-interpretation techniques, such as double-oblique MIPs or MPRs (reconstructed thickness with overlap 2–6 mm), yield fully diagnostic results. It is recommended that each coronary segment should be evaluated interactively by scrolling through the dataset in an adapted right anterior oblique (RAO) viewing angle for the LAD and a left anterior oblique (LAO) viewing angle for the RCA and RCX. If a suspected lesion is detected, the degree of stenosis should be established in at least two orthogonal viewing angles to account for potentially eccentric lesions (Fig. 21.5).

After having assessed the coronaries, the left atrium and ventricle should be assessed. The best visualization technique is a standard MPR in short and long axis view as well as the four-chamber view. The presence of intracavital thrombi, as well as the assessment of the myocardium regarding signs of hypertrophy, presence of scar tissue, or presence of aneurysms should be performed (Fig. 21.6).

The right atrium and ventricle is usually difficult to assess using CT imaging due to the contrast media influx artifacts. Only enlarged right cavities or obvious masses should be reported.

Since the tricuspid valve is virtually never and the pulmonary valve rarely visualized, only the aortic and mitral valve should be assessed. Calcifications of either valve indicate that there is a higher likelihood of valve stenosis or insufficiency present. Exact determination of valve functionality is not clinically feasible at present.

References

1. Sandstede J (2004) Working group on cardiac imaging. German Roentgen Society
2. Martuscelli E, Romagnoli A, D'Eliseo A et al. (2004) Accuracy of thin-slice computed tomography in the detection of coronary stenoses. Eur Heart J 25:1043–1048
3. Mollet NR, Cademartiri F, Nieman K et al. (2004) Multislice spiral computed tomography coronary angiography in patients with stable angina pectoris. J Am Coll Cardiol 43:2265–2270
4. Wielopolski PA, van Geuns RJ, de Feyter PJ et al. (2004) Coronary arteries. Eur Radiol 10:12–35
5. Schoepf UJ, Becker CR, Ohnesorge BM et al. (2004) CT of coronary artery disease. Radiology 232:18–37
6. Mannebach H, Hamm C, Horstkotte D (2002) 18th report of the statistics of heart catheter laboratories in Germany. Results of a combined survey by the Committee of Clinical Cardiology and the Interventional Cardiology and Angiology Working Group (for ESC) of the German Society of Cardiology-Heart- and Cardiovascular Research 2001. Z Kardiol 91:727–729
7. Kuettner A, Kopp AF, Schroeder S et al. (2004) Diagnostic accuracy of multidetector computed tomography coronary angiography in patients with angiographically proven coronary artery disease. J Am Coll Cardiol 43:831–839
8. Kuettner A, Trabold T, Schroeder S et al. (2004) Noninvasive detection of coronary lesions using 16-detector multislice spiral computed tomography technology: initial clinical results. J Am Coll Cardiol 44:1230–1237

22 Functional Cardiac Imaging

A. H. Mahnken, M. Heuschmid, and A. Kuettner

Indications

To date, there is no evidence-based indication to assess cardiac function using retrospectively electrocardiogram-gated (ECG-gated) multislice spiral computed tomography (MSCT) imaging as a standalone exam. Thus all functional imaging and evaluation is taken from exams assessing cardiac and coronary morphology. These exams enable assessment of cardiac function as follows:

1. Determination of global left ventricular function:
   End-diastolic volume (EDV)
   End-systolic volume (ESV)
   Stroke volume (SV)
   Ejection fraction (EF)
   Cardiac output (CO)
   Peak filling rate (PFR)
   Peak ejection rate (PER)
   Time to PER (TPER)
   Time from end-systole to PFR (TPFR)
   Myocardial mass
2. Regional wall motion analysis

Patient Preparation

- For functional assessment, no β-blockage is in principle necessary. However, since β-blockage prior to the scan is recommended for coronary analysis, and since functional assessment is always part of a comprehensive cardiac assessment, most patients will be β-blocked prior to the scan. Thus, one has to be aware of potentially altered cardiac functional data when using CT.
- 20 or 18 G i.v. access antecubitally, supine position.

- Topogram/scan range: entire chest/base of heart to carina (Fig. 22.1).
- Placement of ECG-leads.

Tips and Tricks

1. Make sure i.v.-access is fully patent.
2. Attach ECG-leads after patient has lifted his/her arms above the head to avoid dislocation and use the "rules" of each manufacturer for positioning (not a "normal" diagnostic ECG).
3. Have the patient start to hold their breath about 5 s prior to scan (Valsalva maneuver will lead to decrease of heart rate).
4. It is not necessary to disable the ECG-dependent dose modulation to obtain better image quality in systole; the image quality is fully diagnostic to assess regional wall movement.

Rationale for Scanning

For an efficient management of patients with cardiac disease, whether it be coronary artery disease (CAD), dilative cardiomyopathy, valve disorders, or congenital heart disease, a comprehensive, noninvasive examination is desirable, assessing both, coronary morphology as well as left ventricular (LV) function. Recently, retrospectively ECG-gated MSCT proved its ability to acquire thin section coronary angiograms, providing a good sensitivity and specificity for the detection of coronary artery stenosis [1]. Assessment of LV volumes also proved feasible [2]. So far, evaluation of the LV-function was limited due to a tem-

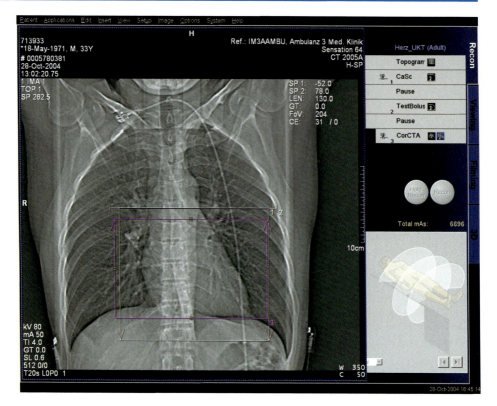

Fig. 22.1. Topogram. Arms above the head. The topogram is identical to that of a gated cardiac scan; no modifications are needed. The carina is the upper border, the heart's base is the lower border

poral resolution restricted to 125–250 ms for 4-slice systems and 94–188 ms for 16-slice systems. Currently available systems with 64-slices have a temporal resolution up to 85–165 ms. Although global LV-function could already be assessed with good correlation to biplane ventriculography, echocardiography, and magnetic resonance imaging (MRI) for 4-slice systems [3,4,5], the latter is still superior when compared with 4-slice CT, calling for improved temporal resolution and shorter scan times for MSCT systems, such as 16- or 64-slice systems. However, there are only few studies assessing regional wall-motion analysis from MSCT data, showing that MSCT wall-motion analysis is limited by the temporal resolution [6].

Anatomy

When assessing functional aspects of the heart, the following structures should be viewed for diagnosis (Fig. 22.2):

1. Left atrium and ventricle.
2. Right atrium and ventricle (size and shape only).
3. Possible intracavital masses (e.g., thrombi).
4. Mitral and aortic valve leaflets.
5. Mitral and aortic valve anulus.

To report findings concerning the left ventricle, the AHA segment model can be used as a widely accepted gold standard (Fig. 22.2). However, when communicating with referring physicians the strict number-

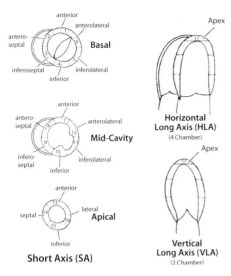

Apex

Horizontal
Long Axis (HLA)
(4 Chamber)

Apex

Vertical
Long Axis (VLA)
(2 Chamber)

Fig. 22.2. Left ventricular segmentation model according to the AHA classification bases on short axis views. There are 17 different segments, one ring of six segments at a basal short axis view, six segments at a mid ventricular short axis view and four segments apically. The apex itself is considered the 17th segment

ing is often replaced by anatomical description such as, e.g., "inferolateral" instead of "segment 5 and 11."

Scanning

For functional assessment, no other special scanning parameters are required than those of a regular cardiac scan for coronaries and/or bypasses.

Functional parameter assessment is always complementary information taken from morphological studies. Thus ECG-dependent dose modulation techniques should be applied whenever possible. Since β-blockers are important to improve image quality in coronary MSCT angiography, their potential benefit on image quality has to be weighted higher than subsequent alterations of functional parameters.

Postprocessing and Image Interpretation

For quantitative assessment of left ventricular function only the end-systolic and end-diastolic phase is needed for image reconstruction whereas for semi-quantitative assessment of regional wall-motion abnormalities, about 20 datasets throughout the cardiac cycle are required. They may either be complete datasets of the entire volume or different sections such as short or long axis views (see Fig. 22.3). Generally, most workstations handle complete volume datasets up to 10 different cycles, whereas for defined views, up to 25 different time points in the RR-cycle can be analyzed. Thus for all practical purposes, the authors recommend reconstructing two complete datasets in end-systolic and end-diastolic phase for assessment of quantitative functional parameters. For semiquantitative wall-motion analysis, 20–25 cycles in the RR interval in the short axis as well as the two-, three-, and four-chamber view should be reconstructed.

To determine end-systole and end-diastole, a mid-left ventricular axial test series can be performed at 4–5% steps throughout the RR interval, yielding an accurate determination of both phases. Alternatively, assessment of short axis views from 20–25 phases allows a more precise determination of end-systole and end-diastole. However, this technique is much more time consuming.

Since most algorithms use a modified Simpson rule, 8–12 double oblique MIPs or MPRs are reconstructed along the ventricular axes with a slice thickness of ≤8 mm without interslice gaps. One set of images is calculated for end-systole and diastole. The first image should encompass the apex; the last image should visualize at least 50% of the myocardial circumference (Fig. 22.4). The most frequent cause for inaccurate results is the variance of the basal image. Mostly, the papillary muscles are considered to be part of the ventricular blood pool. Depending on the workstation used,

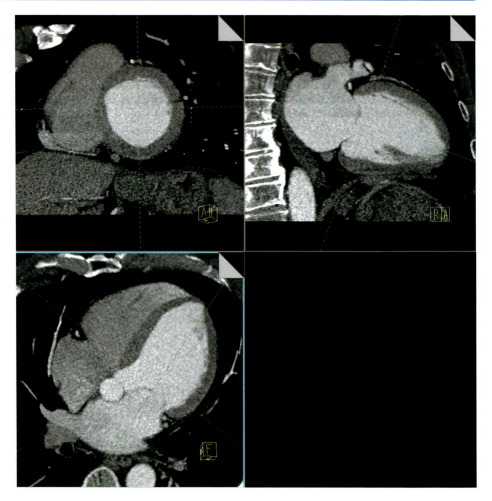

Fig. 22.3. For easy assessment three planes perpendicular to each other are most suited: short axis, two-chamber view, and four-chamber view. To clarify this simple principle, all orientation lines have been left in the images. The *green line* is parallel to the septum, the *blue line* through the mid-mitral valve through the apex, and the *red line* is orthogonal to the *green* and *blue line*

the epi- and endocardial border is more or less automatically detected with manual corrections needed. All quantitative parameters are automatically computed and derived from the measurements.

For semiquantitative wall-motion analysis, the acquired image series are viewed in cine mode. By observing the movement of the left ventricular wall, four different motion patterns can be described.

1. Normal, timely, and inward-directed wall motion of left ventricular wall with adequate wall thickening is described

as normokinesis. Only fully contractile, nonischemic myocardial segments are considered to be normokinetic. CAVE: The analysis is performed under resting conditions, thus partly ischemic wall segments may appear normokinetic at rest and hypokinetic under stress conditions. This borderline ischemia will be missed using cardiac MSCT.

2. Regional inward wall motion that is either smaller in amplitude or not timely synchronized with the other wall segments with visibly impaired wall thickening is called hypokinesis. Ischemic

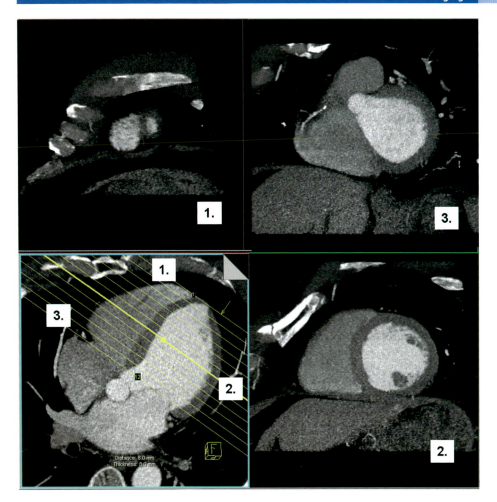

Fig. 22.4. Reconstruction principle for quantitative assessment of the LV-function. Since most algorithms use a modified Simpson rule, 8–12 double oblique short axis MIPs or MPRs are calculated. Identically orientated sets of images are calculated for end-systole and end-diastole. The first image encompasses the apex (1), the last image (3) should visualize at least 50% of the myocardial circumference

segments/small myocardial infarctions may display this behavior.

3. Regional wall sections that do not move at all through the cardiac cycle or only display passive movement ("dragged along" by other wall segments) and/or show no signs of wall thickening are described as akinetic segments. Myocardium that is either scarred or significantly ischemic may display this movement pattern. The underlying cause is most likely a severe coronary stenosis or a consequence of a myocardial infarction.

4. Regionally thinned wall sections that perform an outward bound wall movement in systole are described as dyskinetic segments. Only large areas with a thinned and severely scarred wall due to significant myocardial infarction display this moving pattern (e.g., aneurysms).

If a wall-motion abnormality is detected, it should be correlated with the coronary anatomy and its supply territories to discriminate a possible target vessel (see Fig. 22.5).

Coronary Artery Territories

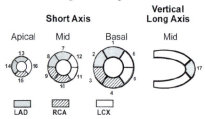

Fig. 22.5. Left ventricular myocardial territories as supplied by the three different coronary arteries. This territorial supply is valid for most anatomical variants, but it may vary for left or right dominant coronary artery tree anatomy

For a complete diagnosis, the presence of intracavital thrombi, as well as the assessment of the myocardium regarding signs of LV-hypertrophy should be performed.

The right atrium and ventricle is difficult to assess using CT imaging. However, enlarged right cavities or obvious masses should be reported. To rule out or diagnose small right atrial thrombi is virtually impossible, since contrasted blood from the upper vena cava mixes with noncontrasted blood in the right atrium/ventricle, causing the presence of multiple hypo- and hyperdense areas in which hypodense thrombi may be masked or artificially created.

Since the tricuspid valve is also virtually never and the pulmonary valve rarely visualized only the aortic and mitral valve can be routinely assessed. Calcifications of either valve indicate that there is a higher likelihood of valve stenosis. Large ascending aortic aneurisms may indicate the presence of an aortic valve insufficiency. However, exact determination of valve functionality is not clinically feasible at present. If a dysmorphic valve is diagnosed for the first time using MSCT, a complementary exam such as echocardiography or cardiac MRI is indicated.

References

1 Ropers D, Baum U, Pohle K, Anders K, Ulzheimer S, Ohnesorge B, Schlundt C, Bautz W, Daniel WG, Achenbach S (2003) Detection of coronary artery stenoses with thin-slice multi-detector row spiral computed tomography and multiplanar reconstruction. Circulation 107:664–666
2 Juergens KU, Grude M, Fallenberg EM, Opitz C, Wichter T, Heindel W, Fischbach R (2002) Using ECG-gated multidetector CT to evaluate global left ventricular myocardial function in patients with coronary artery disease. AJR Am J Roentgenol 179:1545–1550
3 Heuschmid M, Kuttner A, Schroder S, Trebar B, Burgstahler C, Mahnken A, Niethammer M, Trabold T, Kopp AF, Claussen CD (2003) Left ventricular functional parameters using ECG-gated multidetector spiral CT in comparison with invasive ventriculography. Rofo 175:1349–1354, in German
4 Mahnken AH, Koos R, Katoh M, Spuentrup E, Busch P, Wildberger JE, Kuhl HP, Gunther RW (2005) Sixteen-slice spiral CT versus MR imaging for the assessment of left ventricular function in acute myocardial infarction. Eur Radiol 15(4):714–20
5 Dirksen MS, Bax JJ, de Roos A, Jukema JW, van der Geest RJ, Geleijns K, Boersma E, van der Wall EE, Lamb HJ (2002) Usefulness of dynamic multislice computed tomography of left ventricular function in unstable angina pectoris and comparison with echocardiography. Am J Cardiol 90:1157–1160
6 Mahnken AH, Spuentrup E, Niethammer M, Buecker A, Boese J, Wildberger JE, Flohr T, Sinha AM, Krombach GA, Gunther RW (2003) Quantitative and qualitative assessment of left ventricular volume with ECG-gated multislice spiral CT: value of different image reconstruction algorithms in comparison to MRI. Acta Radiol 44:604–611

23 Bypass Imaging

A. Kuettner

Indications

1. Long term follow-up of arterial or venous coronary bypass grafts.
2. Assessment of bypass graft patency in the acute postoperative phase.

Patient Preparation

- Since most bypass patients receive a β-blocker as concomitant drug, an additional β-blockage prior to the scan may not be necessary. The target heart rate is 50–60 bpm, analogous to the cardiac scan. Method: 50 mg metoprololtartrate 30–60 min prior to the scan. Use 100 mg only when the heart rate is >70 bpm. No β-blocker should be given for intrinsic heart rates <60.
- 20 or 18 G i.v. access antecubitally, supine position.
- Topogram/scan range: entire chest/base of heart to mid aortic arch (Fig. 23.1).
- Placement of ecg-leads.
- Immediately prior to the scan, application of 0.8 mg nitroglycerin orally, or alternatively 2.5 mg of isosorbide dinitrate (coronary and bypass dilatation).

Scan Parameters

See Table 23.1.

Tips and Tricks

1. Make sure i.v.-access is fully patent.
2. Attach ecg-leads after patient has lifted his/her arms above the head to avoid

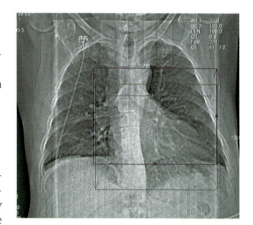

Fig. 23.1. Topogram. Arms above the head. The scan range should encompass the base of the heart as well as all bypass grafts. Generally it is sufficient to visualize the aortic origins of all venous grafts or arterial grafts used as free grafts; calcium scoring scan prior to the scan can be used as additional localizer for the contrast enhanced spiral, which is usually smaller than the nonenhanced scan. The carina is the upper border; the base of the heart is the lower border

dislocation. Follow the "rules" of each manufacturer for positioning (not a "normal" diagnostic ecg).
3. For 16- and 64-slice scanning, have the patient start to hold their breath about 5 s prior to scan (Valsalva maneuver will lead to decrease of heart rate). For 4-slice scanning the scan time will be considerably longer, so the breath hold should start with the scan.
4. Limit the scan range from the base of the heart to the mid-aortic arch. It is not necessary to scan the origin of the internal mammarian artery if that vessel is used as graft.

Table 23.1. Scan parameters

Parameters	4–8 slice scanners	10–16 slice scanners	32–64 slice scanners
Scanner settings			
Tube voltage (kV)	120	120	120
Rotation time (s)	0.5	0.375–0.5	0.33–0.4
Tube current time product (mAs)	150	140–160	150–180
Pitch corrected tube current time product (eff. mAs)	400	550–650	750–900
Collimation (mm)	1.00/1.25	0.625/0.75	0.6/0.625
Norm. pitch	0.375*	0.25*	0.2*
Recon. increment	1	0.8	0.4–0.6
Reconstr.-slice thickness (mm)	1.25	1.0	0.6–0.75
convolution kernel	standard/high res.	standard/high res.	standard/high res.
Specials	Retrospective ECG-gating	Retrospective ECG-gating	Retrospective ECG-gating
	ECG-pulsing for HR<60	ECG-pulsing for HR<70	ECG-pulsing for HR<80
Scan range	Base of heart to mid-ascending aorta	Base of heart to mid-ascending aorta	Base of heart to mid-ascending aorta
Scan direction	Caudocranial	Caudocranial	Caudocranial
Contrast media application			
Concentration (mg iodine/mL)	350–400	350–400	350–400
Mono/Biphasic	Biphasic	Biphasic	Monophasic
Volume (mL)	150	100	80
Injection rate (mL/s)	4.0, 2.5	4.0, 2.5	5.0
Saline chaser (mL, mL/s)	30, 2.5	30, 2.5	60, 5.0
Delay (s)	Test bolus	Test bolus	Test bolus or bolus tracking

* Pitch values as recommended for Siemens systems; values for other brands may be slightly different.

5. For good vessel opacification, use contrast media containing ≥350 mg iodine/mL.

Comments

Coronary artery bypass grafting (CABG) is one of the most common procedures for the treatment of symptomatic coronary artery disease (CAD). In excess of 570,000 procedures were carried out in the USA alone [1].

Early follow-up studies on treatment of CAD using CABG by Cameron and coworkers in 1995 indicated that CABG resulted in significant relief from the symptoms of CAD in the short term, as well as improved mortality rates in certain patient subgroups [2]. However, longer-term follow-up studies have demonstrated a significant recurrence of disease in patients between one and six years following treatment. Over 20% of treated patients presented with chest pain within one year of CABG, a figure that rises to higher than 40% at six years posttreatment. Furthermore, up to 25% of grafts were found to be occluded within five years of CABG [2,3]. Relapse is thought to occur either due to reoccurrence and progression of disease in the native vessels or as result of de novo disease in the bypass graft, with venous grafts proving apparently more susceptible than arterial grafts to de novo disease [4]. Early graft occlusion is also described in up to 23% of all patients and a large number of all patients develop angina pectoris within the initial three months [5].

Clearly then, one of the key issues for successful treatment management and securing improved mortality rates for symptomatic CAD patients is monitoring of graft patency and disease progression in both the distal runoff and the other native coronary arteries.

For the purposes of follow-up and monitoring, noninvasive techniques are preferable from both a patient care and cost perspective. Magnetic resonance imaging (MRI) and computed tomography (CT) are obvious candidates, and both have been used to successfully monitor graft patency. However, limitations in these imaging technologies have previously hindered the follow-up of preexisting disease.

Assessment of Graft Patency and Native Vessel Disease

At our institution, a standardized workflow is used for routine bypass CT exams: prior to the CT exam β-blockers are administered to regulate patient heart rate, if necessary. Before each contrast enhanced scan, the circulation rate is determined before administering IV, as described below. Only then is the diagnostic scan performed. Images are then postprocessed and reported.

Measurement of Circulation Time and Diagnostic Scan

To evaluate the circulation time, a test bolus is administered. The correct scanning delay is established by measuring CT attenuation values in the ascending aorta, taking the last slice with maximum contrast as circulation time. Alternatively, automated bolus detection can be used. This technique is especially suitable for >16-slice generation CT systems, since the scan time is only about 15 s. The rationale for not applying an automated bolus detection when using a CT system with 16 or less detectors is based on the subsequent difficulty of patient compliance to the breath hold command necessary to account for longer scan ranges and breath hold times between 22 and 27 s. Using a dual-head power injector, 80–150mL intravenous contrast agent plus a saline chaser bolus is injected. CT imaging starts at the diaphragm caudally to all cardiac structures and stops in the mid-ascending aorta cranial to all coronary ostia and the origin of all venous grafts. The contrast-enhanced scan is then acquired using the scan parameters given in the table. ECG-pulsing with reduced tube current during systole should be used whenever possible to minimize radiation exposure. It should not be used in patients with extra systoles and variable heart rate. Generally, we have found no substantial need to adapt scanning protocols for cardiac imaging of patients with prior CABG procedure in comparison to those with no bypass grafts present. The key adaptation being the extension of the scan range to include the ascending aorta. To date there is no conclusive data, whether the proximal part of IMA grafts, including its origin from the subclavian artery should be included in the scan range or not. Most centers prefer to limit the scan range to the proximal ascending aorta due to dose considerations.

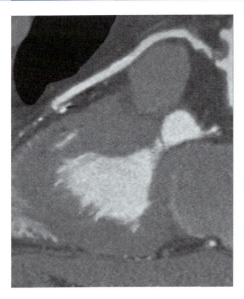

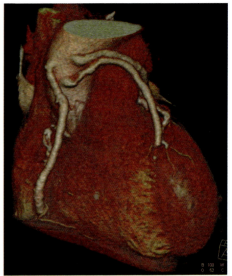

Fig. 23.2. Curved MPR of the venous graft onto the LAD of the same patient as in Fig. 23.2 proximally a high-grade lesion is present. Note that this lesion is difficult to see in the volume rendered image (Fig. 23.2). The distal anastomosis is preserved; the distal runoff is occluded. This postprocessing method can be used for demonstration of the diagnosis

Fig. 23.3. 3D volume-rendered image of a 64-slice scan: this is an excellent visualization method for global orientation and identification of single grafts, especially when multiple grafts are present. These images should however not be used for gauging bypass patency

Image Reconstruction

For image reconstruction, a preset reconstruction algorithm provided by each manufacturer can be used. Generally, the reconstruction window is set to start at 60% RR interval. If coronary segments show motion artifacts, an additional test series reconstructing single slices in 5% steps at a given z-position is recommended, ranging from 20 to 75% relative to the RR interval. The time point with the least motion artifacts is then chosen to reconstruct the entire stack of images of the MDCT scan. Typically we use a slice thickness of 0.6–1 mm with an increment of 0.4–0.8 mm and a medium smooth reconstruction kernel. Most vendors recommend specifically adapted bypass/cardiac kernels that should be used.

Visualization Techniques

Generally, advanced postprocessing techniques, such as 3D volume rendering and curved maximum intensity projections (curved MIPs), are too time-consuming for routine work and often of limited use for the physician reading cardiac images. Normal image interpretation techniques, such as double oblique MIPs or MPRs, yield fully diagnostic results. However, bypass grafts, especially sequential grafts, are considerably tortuous and therefore difficult to visualize in a single plane. Thus, curved MIP projections have proved to be an appropriate method to assess the entire graft and to illustrate the diagnosis appropriately (Fig. 23.2).

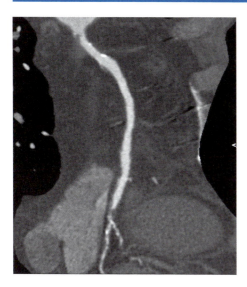

Fig. 23.4. Curved MPR of the venous graft onto the RCA of the same patient as in Fig. 23.2 and 23.3. The graft has a mild lesion proximally. The distal anastomosis shows a high-grade insertion stenosis, while the distal runoff is preserved

Also, in general practice, information about the precise number of the existing grafts and the exact location of distal anastomoses is often unavailable, and thus 3D volume rendering is helpful in many cases (Fig. 23.3).

Results from the Literature

As noninvasive bypass CTA is a relatively new multislice CT application, its use has not yet been introduced into mainstream cardiology. In order to assess the bypass supplied vessel to a full extent, not only the patency of the bypass graft itself, but also the distal runoff has to be evaluated (Fig. 23.4) [1]. This is especially challenging for 4-slice CT since temporal and spatial resolution may be sufficient to visualize the grafts itself, but not the distal runoff [6].

With the introduction of 16 slice scanners, very encouraging results were pub-lished by Schlosser et al. [7] as well as by Martuscelli et al. [8], yielding a sensitivity and specificity of >90% for graft assessment. These data suggest that the use of bypass CTA in the early postoperative phase in order to determine early bypass occlusion may be one indication. However, both studies did not investigate the visualization of the distal runoff, a clear limitation in order to gauge the clinical value of the method. With the introduction of >16-slice systems, there is reason to believe that these obstacles might be overcome.

References

1. Nieman K, Pattynama PM, Rensing BJ et al. (2003) Evaluation of patients after coronary artery bypass surgery: CT angiographic assessment of grafts and coronary arteries. Radiology 229:749–756
2. Cameron AA, Davis KB, Rogers WJ (1995) Recurrence of angina after coronary artery bypass surgery: predictors and prognosis (CASS Registry). Coronary Artery Surgery Study. J Am Coll Cardiol 26:895–899
3. Fitzgibbon GM, Kafka HP, Leach AJ et al. (1996) Coronary bypass graft fate and patient outcome: angiographic follow-up of 5,065 grafts related to survival and reoperation in 1,388 patients during 25 years. J Am Coll Cardiol 28:616–626
4. Loop FD, Lytle BW, Cosgrove DM et al. (1986) Influence of the internal-mammary-artery graft on 10-year survival and other cardiac events. N Engl J Med 314:1–6
5. Rifon J, Paramo JA, Panizo C et al. (1997) The increase of plasminogen activator inhibitor activity is associated with graft occlusion in patients undergoing aorto-coronary bypass surgery. Br J Haematol 99:262–267
6. Burgstahler C, Kuettner A, Kopp AF et al. (2003) Non-invasive evaluation of coronary artery bypass grafts using multi-slice computed tomography: initial clinical experience. Int J Cardiol 90:275–280
7. Schlosser T, Konorza T, Hunold P et al. (2004) Noninvasive visualization of coronary artery bypass grafts using 16-detector row computed tomography. J Am Coll Cardiol 44:1224–1229
8. Martuscelli E, Romagnoli A, D'Eliseo A et al. (2004) Evaluation of venous and arterial conduit patency by 16-slice spiral computed tomography. Circulation 110:3234–3238

24 Imaging of Coronary Stents

D. Maintz

Patient Preparation

- β-Blockage prior to the scan, target heart rate is 50-60 bpm (for details please see Chapter 21).
- 20 or 18 G i.v. access, supine position.

Patient Positioning

- Supine position, arms elevated.

Scan Range

- Base of the heart to carina (see Fig. 21.1).

Scan Parameters

See Chap. 21.

Introduction

Coronary artery stenting is the most frequent nonsurgical coronary revascularization procedure today. Approximately 537,000 stent implantations were performed in the USA in 2001 and 175,000 in Germany in 2002. In drug-eluting stents, a six-month in-stent restenosis rate of 0% was reported [1]. However, in nondrug eluting stents (which is still the majority), in-stent restenosis is a major clinical problem with a six-month restenosis rate ranging from 11 to 46% [2]. While invasive coronary angiography (ICA) remains the gold standard for coronary stent evaluation, noninvasive assessment of coronary stents would be highly desirable. Such an alternative to ICA would ideally have to address the three following clinical problems: (1) Stent occlusion (2) Stent restenosis (3) Disease progression in other coronary arteries.

A combination of beam-hardening and partial-volume artifacts causes artificial thickening of the stent struts during CT, the so-called "blooming" of stents. The same artifacts are responsible for the artificial lumen narrowing of stents. The magnitude of artifacts and consequently the degree of lumen narrowing depends on the type of stent, the stent diameter, and various scan and reconstruction parameters.

Stent Types

Stents can be classified according to their geometry (slotted tube, monofilament, multicellular, modular, helical-sinusoidal), underlying material (stainless steel, tantalum, cobalt-alloys, platinum, nitinol, titanium), modus of application (self-expandable, balloon-expandable), covering (phosphorylcholine, carbon), and drug elution (rapamycin, paclitaxel, actinomycin). Other features include flexibility, strut thickness, profile, radial stability, and shortening. The most important characteristics influencing radioopacity of stents are the material (atomic number, e.g., titanium=22, iron (steel)=26, cobalt=27, nickel=28, tantalum=73) and the relative amount of metal per stent area.

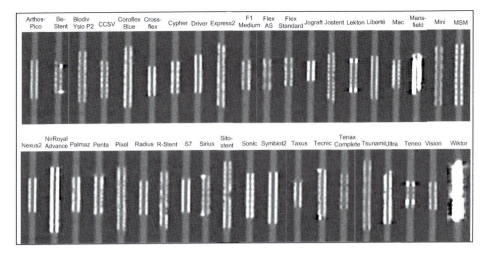

Fig. 24.1. Individual appearance of 40 different stents using 64-slice CT (in vitro experiment, lumen contrast 250 HU). The Wiktor and Mansfield stents are made from tantalum, the Radius and Symbiot stents are made from nitinol, the Arthos-Pico, Coroflex-blue, Driver, and Vision stents are based on cobalt–chromium alloys and all others are based on stainless steel

CT Imaging of Stents

Influence of Stent Type

Tantalum stents cause the most severe artifacts and are not suitable for lumen assessment in CT. Titanium and nitinolstents cause the weakest artifacts but they are rarely used for coronary arteries. Most coronary artery stents are based on stainless steel. The appearance of steel stents varies depending on the individual design (see Fig. 24.1).

Influence of Scanner Type

Results of 4-Slice CT

An in vitro study using 4-slice CT to assess 19 different stents showed that reliable lumen assessment was not possible [3]. The percentage of visible lumen ranged from 38–0%. Three patient studies have been published that report 100% correct assessment of stent patency (stent occluded or not occluded, decision based on the indirect sign of contrast in the vessel distal of the stent), but insufficient stent lumen visibility and stenosis assessment [4–6].

Results of 16-Slice CT

The introduction of 16-slice CT systems with increased spatial and temporal resolution effectuated improvement in general image quality and stent assessability. Stent lumen visibility assessed in two in vitro studies ranged from 80–0%, depending on the stent type and convolution kernel used (see Influence of Image Reconstruction) [7,8].

Reported results on stent stenosis assessment in vivo are scarce. One study found seven of nine significant stenoses in 22 patients and calculated a sensitivity of 78% and a specificity of 100%. Another study with 29 patients with left main coronary artery stents reported a correct detection of 4/4 significant stent stenoses.

Results of 64-Slice CT

The recent introduction of 64-slice CT offers a further increase of spatial and temporal resolution that might improve stent lumen assessment, however, there are no published data yet. Initial experience is encouraging, but results again vary depend-

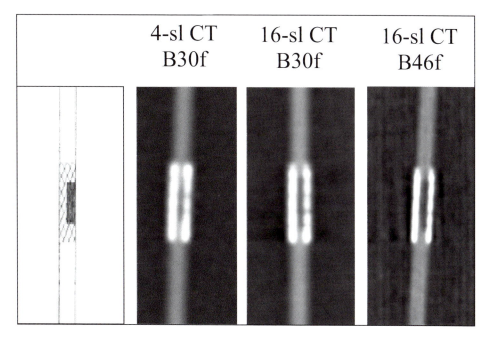

Fig. 24.2. Differences of lumen visibility and stenosis detection depending on the scanner type and the convolution kernel in an in vitro experiment. Schematic on the left shows location of the implanted stenosis. Note improved lumen visibility and stenosis delineation using 16-slice CT and B46f convolution kernel

ing on the stent type (see Fig. 24.1). In vivo studies are currently underway.

Influence of Image Reconstruction

The influence of image reconstruction algorithms on stent visualization is at least as important as the influence of the scanner type. In general, the sharper the kernel the higher percentage of the stent lumen becomes visible. However, using very sharp kernels the lumen attenuation might be artificially decreased. Therefore, stent-dedicated convolution kernels have been developed (e.g., B46f for Siemens) that have less overshoot in the low-frequency region of the modulation-transfer function and consequently offer more reliable lumen attenuation assessment. In vitro and in vivo studies have reported the superiority of a stent-optimized kernel (B46f) in comparison to the conventional medium-soft (B30f) convolution kernel (Fig. 24.2) [7–9]. The increase of image noise using a stent-optimized kernel can be retrospectively compensated for by smoothening filters [10].

Influence of Stent Diameter

The diameter of the stent is another important factor influencing the lumen visibility. The larger the stent diameter the higher the visible percentage of the lumen. Stents with a diameter of ≥3.5 mm can usually be evaluated (Fig. 24.3) [11].

3D Reconstructions

- MIP and VRT – used for localization of stent; not suitable for stent lumen assessment.
- MPR – used for stent lumen assessment.

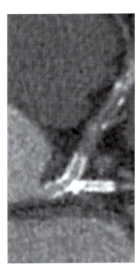

Fig. 24.3. Patient with one stent in the left main coronary artery and the proximal left anterior descending (LAD) coronary artery of >3 mm diameter and a second stent in the left circumflex coronary artery (LCx) of <2 mm diameter. Note the importance of a large stent diameter for lumen visibility. Images from a 64-slice CT, courtesy of A. Küttner, Tübingen

Indications/Considerations before Examining a Patient with a Stent

Stent assessment is not a generally accepted indication for a coronary CTA examination. However, considering the following special situations, a CTA might give helpful information about the stent patency and/or significant stent stenosis. (1) The stent type must be suitable for CT imaging (a catalogue of the appearance of different stent types in CT, as provided in Fig. 24.2, might be helpful for deciding). (2) The stent diameter should be >3 mm. (3) A 16-slice scanner or better a 64-slice scanner should be available if stent restenosis is the question of interest (stent occlusion may be diagnosed with a 4-slice scanner). (4) A stent-optimized convolution kernel must be available for image reconstruction. (5) General requirements that apply for standard CTA (contraindications, heart rate, etc.) must be considered.

References

1. Grube E, Silber S, Hauptmann KE et al. (2003) TAXUS I: six- and twelve-month results from a randomized, double-blind trial on a slow-release paclitaxel-eluting stent for de novo coronary lesions. Circulation 107(1):38–42
2. Antoniucci D, Valenti R, Santoro GM et al. (1998) Restenosis after coronary stenting in current clinical practice. Am Heart J 135(3):510–518
3. Maintz D, Juergens KU, Wichter T, Grude M, Heindel W, Fischbach R (2003) Imaging of coronary artery stents using multislice computed tomography: in vitro evaluation. Eur Radiol 13(4):830–835
4. Kruger S, Mahnken AH, Sinha AM et al. (2003) Multislice spiral computed tomography for the detection of coronary stent restenosis and patency. Int J Cardiol 89(2–3):167–172
5. Maintz D, Grude M, Fallenberg EM, Heindel W, Fischbach R (2003) Assessment of coronary arterial stents by multislice-CT angiography. Acta Radiol 44(6):597–603
6. Ligabue G, Rossi R, Ratti C, Favali M, Modena MG, Romagnoli R (2004) Noninvasive evaluation of coronary artery stents patency after PTCA: role of Multislice Computed Tomography. Radiol Med (Torino) 108(1–2):128–137
7. Maintz D, Seifarth H, Flohr T et al. (2003) Improved coronary artery stent visualization and in-stent stenosis detection using 16-slice computed-tomography and dedicated image reconstruction technique. Invest Radiol 38(12):790–795
8. Mahnken AH, Buecker A, Wildberger JE et al. (2004) Coronary artery stents in multislice computed tomography: in vitro artifact evaluation. Invest Radiol 39(1):27–33
9. Hong C, Chrysant GS, Woodard PK, Bae KT (2004) Coronary artery stent patency assessed with in-stent contrast enhancement measured at multi-detector row CT angiography: initial experience. Radiology 233(1):286–291
10. Seifarth H, Raupach R, Schaller S et al. (2005) Assessment of coronary artery stents using 16-slice MDCT angiography: evaluation of a dedicated reconstruction kernel and a noise reduction filter. Eur Radiol 15(4):721–726
11. Gilard M, Cornily JC, Rioufol G et al. (2005) Noninvasive assessment of left main coronary stent patency with 16-slice computed tomography. Am J Cardiol 95(1):110–112

25 Coronary Imaging at High Heart Rates

M. Hoffmann and A. Kuettner

Indications

- Coronary artery system: suspected coronary artery disease (CAD) [1–4] and coronary anomalies [5].
- Cardiac morphology scan: pericardial disease, congenital heart disease [6].
- Status of postcoronary therapy: follow-up after coronary artery bypass surgery (CABG) [7] or percutaneous coronary interventions (PCI) (stent imaging should only be considered in appropriate research settings).
- Postoperative phase after major cardiac surgery involving the coronaries, such as replacement of ascending aorta with reimplantation of the coronary ostia.
- Emergency scanning for possible involvement of coronaries, e.g., type A dissection.

Patient Preparation

If the conditions allow for heart-rate modification, monitor the ECG for 1 min prior to scan initiation. If the resting heart rate is stable and less than 75 bpm, no beta-blocker application is necessary. If the resting heart rate is unstable or greater than 75 bpm, slowly administer up to 20 mg metoprolol i.v. in 5 mg aliquots until the heart rate less than 75 bpm [8]. Image quality, using a voxel adapted multicycle reconstruction algorithm at a rotational speed of 0.4 s, is consistent up to 80 bpm. At higher heart rates, the scan may be initiated, but the rate of residual motion artifacts increases and image quality suffers [8].

In cases where the heart rate can not be controlled, such as acute perioperative phase or acute emergency (e.g., suspected aortic dissection), no special patient preparation may be possible and the scan protocol has to be adapted to this situation.

Patient Positioning

Supine, feet first, arms elevated, ECG electrodes positioned on anterior and lateral chest.

Topogram/Scan Range

For cardiac assessment, 0.5 cm below the Carina to diaphragm infracardially (≈13 cm). If necessary, expand the scan range to the diagnostic needs, such as ascending aorta/supraaortic branches (Fig. 25.1).

Table Scan Parameters

See Table 25.1.

Tips and Tricks

Phase selection for reconstruction is handled very differently using various vendor platforms. Most approaches rely on either absolute determination (milliseconds after or before an R spike) or relative (percentage) determination of the beginning of the reconstruction phase [9]. Other approaches using adaptive multi-cycle reconstruction provide percentages to determine the cen-

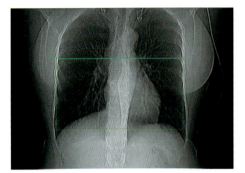

Fig. 25.1. Scan range for coronary artery scan. On an anteroposterior surview scan the cranial scan end is set 0.5 cm below the carina and extended to the diaphragmatic level of the heart as the caudal end. For a follow-up post-CABG, the cranial start has to be positioned in the thoracic aperture to cover the branching point of the mammary artery. Typical scan durations are 14 s for a coronary and 20 s for a post-CABG scan (40 detector rows)

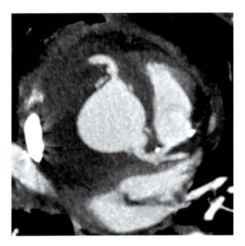

Fig. 25.2. Patient after ascending aorta replacement (aortic aneurysm) and reimplantation of coronary arteries. Both coronary ostia can be visualized without motion artifacts. The heart rate reached 143 bpm, but the average heart rate was 124 bpm (see *upper* ecg in Fig. 25.8). The R-R interval for reconstruction was 20%. Image aquired with a Siemens Sensation 64 System

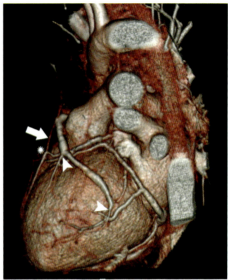

Fig. 25.3. Patient postcoronary artery bypass grafting. Volume rendering provides excellent anatomical overview with occluded mammary artery (*large arrow*). The distal anastomosis to LAD is elevated due to pedicle shortening. A large venous graft with sequential anastomoses to first diagonal branch (*arrowhead*) and a marginal branch (*arrowhead*) is opacified. The image, however, lacks accurate lumen delineation which is better seen on globe presentations (Fig. 25.4). Image aquired with a Philips Brilliance 40 System

ough knowledge of the phase positioning algorithm of your specific vendor is mandated before considering literature recommendations.

For initial reconstructions, one end-systolic phase (centered at 45% of the R-R interval) and one mid-diastolic phase in the diastasis (centered at 75% of the R-R interval) should routinely be acquired. Additional reconstructions are only necessary if no satisfactory image quality is provided by these two phases. For higher heart rates (>75 bpm) the optimal phase selection for reconstruction is end-systolic. Using physiological phase delays end-systole is consistently located at 40–50% of the cardiac cycle across a wide range of heart rates. If your platform uses non-physiologically adaptive phase settings you have to account for different heart rates manually.

ter of a phase window [10,11]. Even more complicated approaches account for the relative changes of systole and diastole over varying heart rates [10,11]. Therefore thor-

Table 25.1. Scan parameters

Parameter	10–16 slice scanners	32–64 slice scanners
Tube voltage (kV)	120	120
Rotation time (s)	0.37–0.42	0.33–0.37
Tube current time product (mAs)	>100	>140
Pitch corrected tube current time product (eff. mAs)	>500	>700
Collimation	0.75	0.625
Norm. Pitch	0.2–0.3	0.2
Reconstruction increment (mm)	0.5	0.3–0.5
Reconstr. Slice thickness (mm)	1	0.67–0.9
Convolution kernel	standard/high res.	standard/high res.
Scan direction	craniocaudal	craniocaudal
Contrast media application		
Concentration (mg iodine / ml)	400	400
Volume (ml / kg BW)	1,2	1,2
Injection rate ml/s	4	4
Scan delay	Bolus tracking (150 HU) + 6 sec	Bolus tracking (150 HU) + 6 sec

As a general rule, for heart rates of 75–85 bpm, 35–45% (this percentage determines the beginning of the phase reconstruction window) of the R-R interval is an optimal reconstruction phase, 85–95 bpm a 25–35% R-R interval seems to be most adequate and for heart rates > 95 bpm, a 15–25% R-R interval reconstruction yields results with the least motion artifacts present. However, this general rule is indicating only a trend, so that individual test series are necessary to individually determine the optimal time point for reconstruction (see Fig. 25.2). For scan initiation, automatic bolus triggering provides the most reliable results. Use a ROI in the descending aorta with a threshold of 150 HU and a scan initiation delay of 6 s.

Clinical Applications

As shown by multiple authors in single center studies in the past [1,2], noninvasive coronary CT angiography is suitable for ruling out CAD with a high negative predictive value. It should therefore be used as a gatekeeper for invasive coronary angiography to rule out disease in patients with equivocal clinical presentation not necessitating immediate intervention.

It may furthermore serve as an excellent adjunct for imaging suspected coronary anomalies or questionable disease of the proximal ostial part of the coronary tree, since it is superior for this purpose, even compared to conventional angiography [5]. Another application is imaging coronary artery bypass grafts with higher accuracy than that achieved by invasive angiography to detect graft patency [7]. Studies beyond 16 detector rows will be conducted to potentially extend this application and include imaging of the distal anastomotic site and the distal part of the grafted coronary artery (Figs. 25.3 and 25.4).

All these applications require robustness, which is still compromised for most

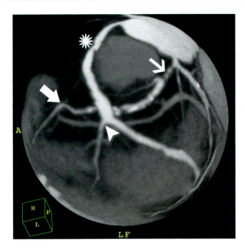

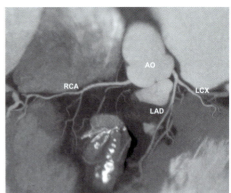

Fig. 25.4. D globe view of the same case as in Fig. 25.3. The sequential vein graft to first diagonal and a marginal branch is opacified with venous valve remnants (*asterisk*). Distal anastomosis to the diagonal branch (*arrowhead*). Proximal LAD shows a high-grade stenosis (*thin arrow*) and the tented region of distal anastomosis with the mammary pedicle (*thick arrow*). The globe view is generated by an MIP projection of centerline tracings on a spherical structure. This allows one to imitate classic projections of catheterization angiograms and renders suitable projections for the referring physician. Image aquired with a Philips Brilliance 40 System

Fig. 25.5. Sample 2D globe view with unfolded coronary tree. All three main branches are included (3 mm MIP projection). The image is generated after centerline placement in RCA, LAD and LCX. Soft plaque lesions are apparent in the mid-LAD and distal RCA. Image aquired with a Philips Brilliance 40 System

patients without sinus rhythm, although sufficient image quality for cases of atrial fibrillation have been reported sporadically [12]. Another critical issue is heart rate, with robust image quality available up to 80 bpm; image quality is substantially compromised beyond this threshold [8]. Therefore, beta-blocker application is still highly recommended.

Keeping these limitations in mind, the spectrum of indications for coronary or bypass imaging as is limited. Stent imaging or plaque assessment of early arteriosclerosis requires optimal image quality and thus should only be performed under conditions of low and stable heart rates. In the postsurgical or emergency situation the focus is limited to major pathology. In these cases "sufficient image quality" may be defined with different thresholds. If the principal luminal patency of a coronary artery or bypass graft is demonstrated, residual motion artifacts to some degree would be acceptable (see Fig. 25.7). For this application the minimum technical requirement is a CT scanner with at least 16 detector rows and gantry rotation times preferrally ≤400 ms.

Image Interpretation

The mainstay for diagnostic reading purposes is a thin-sliding MIP projection with variable slice thickness (typically in the range of 0.9–5 mm). The MIP projection is individually rotated around dynamically modified rotation centers. As this modality is not suitable for the generation of images for the referring physician, additional effort should be invested to generate curved MPR and MIP images or so-called globe images (Figs. 25.4 and 25.6). These allow a complete unfolding of the coronary tree in a single 2D plane (Fig. 25.6). 3D projections of the coronary tree allow accurate representations of the pathologic findings (Fig. 25.4). Segmentation is currently achieved with one single marker set in the midsection of the coronary branch of interest and auto-

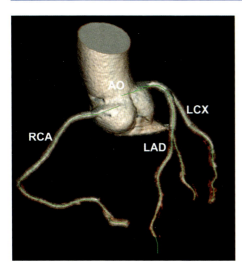

Fig. 25.6. To extract the coronary tree from the 3D volume acquisition, centerlines are threaded through the main vessel branches. This is achieved with a semiautomatic segmentation tool. Four detection points have to be set manually in the aortic root and the mid sections of the three major branches. The centerline is generated automatically on these anchor points. Currently, this method achieves reliable results in about 70% of the cases. Image aquired with a Philips Brilliance 40 System

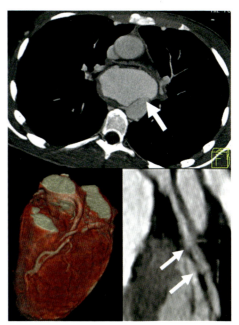

Fig. 25.7. 22-year-old male patient with acute aortic rupture (*single arrow*) and concurrent congenital coarctation. The ecg-gated study was performed to confirm the clinical suspicion of an aortic rupture. A previously performed non-gated single slice helical CT had merely diagnosed an aneurysm. Heart rate was greater than 120 bpm, the reconstruction interval was 15% R-R interval. Excellent image quality, especially of the left anterior descending artery in the VRT image (*lower left*). However the curved MIP-projection of the circumflex artery displays motion artifacts resembling coronary plaque, a very unlikely diagnosis in this case. Image aquired with a Siemens Sensation 64 System

matic extension as already achieved a high level of robustness, allowing one to handle both coronary arteries and bypass grafts (Fig. 25.6).

Dose Considerations

Retrospectively ECG-gated CT imaging is capable of irradiating a patient with significant amounts of radiation if inappropriate scan parameters are used. One inherent disadvantage of the method is, that only fractions of the applied dose within a cardiac cycle are used for high-resolution image reconstruction. This holds true for both single or multi-cycle reconstruction algorithms. To alleviate dose exposure, most manufacturers provide ECG-controlled tube current modulation which automatically reduces the dose to a minimum during phases not contributing to high resolution image reconstruction. Dose savings may amount up to 50% [13]. However phase selections after the scan are restricted to the very narrow window selected prior to scan initiation. In other words phases are selected based on the resting ECG prior to scan start and do not account for heart rate variations or arrhythma during the acquisition. This results in noise bands apparent on the reconstructions should heart rate variation exceed certain limits or in cases of premature contractions. Therefore, many centers prefer to use this feature only for stable low heart rates. Secondly, the algorithm works efficiently only at lower heart rates, so that the dose saving effect for heart rates >120 is marginal [13].

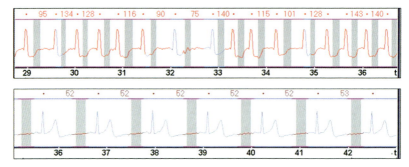

Fig. 25.8. Effectiveness of ecg controlled-dose modulation at various heart rates. The *lower* ecg trace shows a very efficient dose modulation (*pink line*) with a dose reduction of greater than 50% for low heart rates; the mean heart rate was 52 bpm. The *upper* ecg-trace shows a poor efficiency of the dose modulation with barely any dose reduction at high heart rates; the mean heart rate was 124 bpm

In conclusion, scanning at higher heart rates often is associated with an increase of the dose exposure (see Fig. 25.8). Thus a careful selection of patients is warranted. Clearly, in potentially life-threatening conditions the dose aspect should not be the clinicians first concern. If properly used, retrospectively ECG-gated imaging is a powerful tool to acquire potentially life-saving information even under unfavorable conditions.

References

1. Kuettner A, Trabold T, Schroeder S et al. (2004) Noninvasive detection of coronary lesions using 16-detector multislice spiral computed tomography technology: initial clinical results. J Am Coll Cardiol 44(6):1230–1237
2. Mollet N, Cademartiri F, Nieman K et al. (2004) Multislice spiral computed tomography coronary angiography in patients with stable angina pectoris. J Am Coll Cardiol 43(12):2265–2270
3. Hoffmann MHK, Shi H, Schmitz BL et al. (2005) Noninvasive coronary angiography with multislice computed tomography. JAMA 29(20):2471–2478
4. Kuettner A, Beck T, Drosch T et al. (2005) Diagnostic accuracy of noninvasive coronary imaging using 16-detector slice spiral computed tomography with 188 ms temporal resolution. J Am Coll Cardiol 45(1):123–127
5. Shi H, Aschoff AJ, Brambs HJ, Hoffmann MH (2004) Multislice CT imaging of anomalous coronary arteries. Eur Radiol 14(12):2172–1281
6. Boxt LM, Lipton MJ, Kwong RY, Rybicki F, Clouse ME (2003) Computed tomography for assessment of cardiac chambers, valves, myocardium and pericardium. Cardiol Clin 21(4):561–585
7. Schlosser T, Konorza T, Hunold P, Kuhl H, Schmermund A, Barkhausen J (2004) Noninvasive visualization of coronary artery bypass grafts using 16-detector row computed tomography. J Am Coll Cardiol 44(6):1224–1229
8. Hoffmann MHK, Shi H, Manzke R et al. (2004) Noninvasive coronary angiography with 16-detector row CT: Effect of heart rate. Radiology 2341031408
9. Pannu HK, Flohr TG, Corl FM, Fishman EK (2003) Current concepts in multi-detector row CT evaluation of the coronary arteries: Principles, techniques, and anatomy. RadioGraphics 23(90001):111–115
10. Hoffmann MHK, Shi H, Manzke R et al. (2005) Noninvasive coronary angiography with 16-detector row CT: effect of heart rate. Radiology 234:86–97
11. Vembar M, Garcia MJ, Heuscher DJ et al. (2003) A dynamic approach to identifying desired physiological phases for cardiac imaging using multislice spiral CT. Med Phys 30(7):1683–1693
12. Hoffmann MHK, Shi H, Schmid FT, Gelman H, Brambs H-J, Aschoff AJ (2004) Noninvasive coronary imaging with MDCT in comparison to invasive conventional coronary angiography: a fast-developing technology. Am J Roentgenol 182(3):601–608
13. Trabold T, Buchgeister M, Kuttner A et al. (2003) Estimation of radiation exposure in 16-detector row computed tomography of the heart with retrospective ECG-gating. Rofo 175(8):1051–1055

26 Diffuse Liver Disease

T. Helmberger

Indications

- Steatosis.
- Cirrhosis.
- Iron overload (hemodrom atosis).
- Hepatitis.
- Sarcoidosis.
- Portalvenous thrombosis.
- Budd–Chiari syndrome and venous congestion.

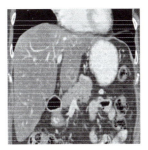

Fig. 26.1. Topogram. For better display, a coronal reformation is used. Be aware that in diffuse liver disease the form and longitudinal range of the liver can be highly variable

Patient Preparation

Supine, arms elevated, no oral contrast. Breath-hold imaging must be explained to the patient.

Scan Range

Level of diaphragm to lower rim of the liver/mid-level of kidney; hepatic contour normally visible on scout view (Fig. 26.1).

Table scan parameters

See Table 26.1.

Tips and Tricks

- In severe cases of diffuse liver disease (e.g., end stage cirrhosis and acute liver failure) the patient's cardiovascular situation can be impaired significantly. In these cases, the amount of delivered contrast has to be diminished as much as reasonably possible and the patient has to be monitored, especially

after the study. Otherwise, MRI is advisable.
- A wide variety of diseases are associated with diffuse parenchymateous changes of the liver that can be characterized by steatotic and/or fibro-cirrhotic changes. The pathological background may be metabolic–systemic, inflammatory–infectious, vascular, malignant, or due to other rarer entities (e.g., primary biliary cirrhosis) [1–3]. In general, the task of imaging is to identify secondary complications related to the underlying disease rather than to establish the diagnosis of diffuse liver disease.
- Since many diffuse liver diseases are associated with cirrhosis the portalvenous scan is essential to assess the status of the portal vein. With respect to nodular regeneration in cirrhosis with potential de-differentiation of a regenerating nodule to a hepatocellular cacinoma (HCC), characterized by arterial hypervascularization, an arterial dominant scan is justified in ambiguous cases. Nevertheless, it is generally accepted that MRI is by far superior

Table 26.1. Scan parameters for various multislice CT scanners

Parameters	4–8 slice scanners	10–16 slice scanners	32–64 slice scanners
Scanner settings			
Tube voltage (kV)	120	120	120
Rotation time (s)	0.5	0.5	0.5
Tube current time product (mAs)	124–300[*]	124–300[*]	124–300[*]
Pitch corrected tube current time product (eff. mAs)	155–250[*]	155–250[*]	155–250[*]
Collimation (mm)	2.5	1.25/1.5	0.6/0.625
Norm. pitch	0.8–1.2	0.8–1.2	0.8–1.2
Reconstr. increment (mm)	4–6	5–6, for recons. 1	5–6, for recons. 0.6
Reconstr.-slice thickness (mm)	4–6	5–6, for recons. 1.5–2	5–6, for recons. 0.75
Convolution kernel	Standard	Standard	Standard
Specials			
Scan range	Diaphragm to caudal hepatic surface	Diaphragm to caudal hepatic surface	Diaphragm to caudal hepatic surface
Scan direction	Craniocaudal	Caudocranial	Caudocranial
Contrast media application			
Concentration (mg iodine/ml)	300	300	300
Mono/Biphasic	Monophasic	Monophasic	Monophasic
Volume (mL)	120–150[*]	100–150[*]	100–130[*]
Injection rate (mL/s)	4.0–5.0	4.0–5.0	4.0–5.0
Saline chaser (mL, mL/s)	Optional	Optional	Optional
Delay (s)	Bolus tracking, portalvenous+50	Bolus tracking, portalvenous+55	Bolus tracking, portalvenous+60

[*] To be adapted to patient's weight and constitution.

in the characterization of diffuse liver disease and the detection of specific complications in diffuse liver disease compared to all other imaging methods [3–5].

Selected Pathologies

Steatosis of the liver is seen as the result of a spectrum of disorders such as alcoholism, severe hepatitis, hepatotoxic agents, or corticosteroids (Fig. 26.2). Steatosis can be reversible and may be silent, but it may also be associated with enlargement of the organ. CT features include the decreased attenuation of liver parenchyma in unenhanced and enhanced imaging. As a rule of thumb the attenuation of the liver is lower than that of the spleen or the kidneys.

Hepatic cirrhosis is most commonly caused by alcoholism or as a complication of hepatitis. The role of CT imaging here is

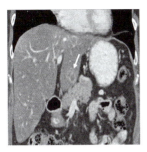

Fig. 26.2. Note the relatively low signal of the liver according to an increased storage of intracellular fat due to chemotherapy. Nevertheless, a residual metastasis from CRC is still visible (*arrow*) during arterial-phase imaging

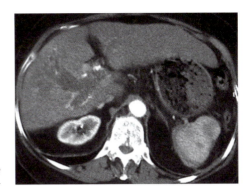

Fig. 26.3. Typical appearance of a portalvenous thrombosis

limited. However, CT can exclude alterations in hepatic size or shape, and especially exclude hepatocellular carcinoma, which may arise in cirrhotic livers more frequently. Typical signs of a cirrhotic liver are rounded lobular contours and the enlargement of the left and the caudate liver lobes.

Iron overloading of the liver is seen in various forms of hemochromatosis. Changes in the liver parenchyma lead to increased attenuation in unenhanced scans (>70 HU); however, this sign may also be seen, for example, in Wilson's disease.

While hepatitis is a frequent and important disease entity, the role of CT in hepatitis is limited, hence imaging findings are nonspecific. Sarcoidosis leads to an enlargement of the liver and spleen, and may also show multiple small hypodense nodules in both organs.

The most common causes for portalvenous thrombosis are local inflammation (such as pancreatitis and cholangitis) or local neoplasm. CT signs of portalvenous thrombosis are enlargements of the portal vein, lack of central portal vein enhancement but rim enhancing, and low attenuation in the affected vessels (Fig. 26.3). Indirect signs include alterations of hepatic blood supply detected by CT, such as transient attenuation differences of individual liver lobes.

The Budd–Chiari syndrome (occlusions of hepatic veins) is a thrombotic occlusion

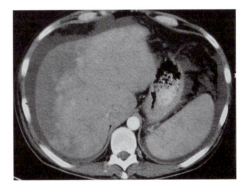

Fig. 26.4. CT appearance in Budd–Chiari syndrome. Inhomogeneous parenchymal contrast. Note the missing contrast in the inferior cava

of the venous outflow, and can be distinguished by careful observations of the hepatic veins in the venous phase, rather than being hypodense and leading to hepatic enlargement (Fig. 26.4).

In conclusion, diffuse liver disease with potential parenchymateous changes (e.g., alcoholism, infectious cirrhosis, Wilsons's disease, Budd–Chiari syndrome, hemochromatosis, etc.) and related complications (e.g., portalvenous thrombosis, collaterals in portal hypertension, hepatocellular carcinoma) can be detected by CT. Nevertheless, for improved characterization and detection of additional (hidden) lesions MRI is recommended.

References

1. Ros PR, Mortele KJ (2002) Hepatic imaging. An overview. Clin Liver Dis 6(1):1–16
2. Kemper J, Jung G, Poll LW, Jonkmanns C, Luthen R, Moedder U (2002) CT and MRI findings of multifocal hepatic steatosis mimicking malignancy. Abdom Imaging 27(6):708–710
3. Limanond P, Raman SS, Ghobrial RM, Busuttil RW, Saab S, Lu DS (2004) Preoperative imaging in adult-to-adult living related liver transplant donors: what surgeons want to know. J Comput Assist Tomogr 28(2):149–157
4. Mortele KJ, Ros PR (2001) Imaging of diffuse liver disease. Semin Liver Dis 21 (2):195–212
5. Valls C, Andia E, Roca Y, Cos M, Figueras J (2002) CT in hepatic cirrhosis and chronic hepatitis. Semin Ultrasound CT MR 23(1):37–61

27 Focal Liver Lesions

T. Helmberger

Indications

- Benign tumors
  - Simple cysts (and polycystic liver disease)
  - Parabiliary cysts
  - Hemangiomas
  - Focal nodular hyperplasia (FNH)
  - Hepatocellular adenoma
- Malignant tumors
  - Hepatocellular carcinoma (HCC)
  - Cholangiocarcinoma (CCC)
  - Metastasis
- Abscess

Patient Preparation

Supine, arms elevated, no oral contrast except if the biphasic hepatic protocol is incorporated into a whole-body scan for staging purpose. Bowel delineation by oral water or diluted contrast media is mandatory. Breath-hold imaging must be explained to the patient.

Scan Range

Level of diaphragm to lower rim of the liver/mid level of kidney (see previous chapter); the hepatic contour is normally visible on scout view (extent of scan range in case of whole body scan).

Table Scan Parameters

See Table 27.1.

Tips and Tricks

- According to the literature, most authors agree that an unenhanced scan adds no value to the biphasic scan and can be omitted (note: in follow-up studies after trans-arterial chemo-embolisation, unenhanced scanning can be helpful to display the lipiodol storage and distribution).
- To adapt the scan times individually to the patient's cardiovascular circulation times, a bolus tracking device should be used [1]. To gain a higher intravascular contrast 370 mg I/mL is recommended. If only contrast of 300 mg I/mL is available, sufficient attenuation can be achieved by increasing the volume to 150 mL and the flow rate up to 5.0 mL/s. Be aware of the risk of intra-extravascular fluid shift in circulatory instable patients [2].
- Flipping the scan direction from craniocaudal to caudocranial may be suitable in cases when the thorax has to be scanned additionally.
- In general, axial 4-mm slice thickness reconstructions will be diagnostically sufficient in most of the cases and are the best compromise between diagnostic accuracy and low noise and good image quality. Thinner reconstructions (1–2 mm) are recommended for secondary reconstructions (e.g., abdominal CT angiography) [3].

Anatomical Considerations

Most commonly, the liver segments are subdivided according to the surgical clas-

Table 27.1. Scan parameters for various multislice CT scanners

Parameters	4–8 slice scanners	10–16 slice scanners	16 slice scanners
Scanner settings			
Tube voltage (kV)	120	120	120
Rotation time (s)	0.5	0.5	0.5
Tube current time product (mAs)	124–300[*]	124–300[*]	124–300[*]
Pitch corrected tube current time product (eff. mAs)	155–250[*]	155–250[*]	155–250[*]
Collimation (mm)	2.5	1.25/1.5	0.6/0.625
Norm. pitch	0.8–1.2	0.8–1.2	0.8–1.2
Reconstr. increment (mm)	4–6	5–6, for recons. 1	5–6, for recons. 0.6
Reconstr.-slice thickness (mm)	4–6	5–6, for recons. 1.5–2	5–6, for recons. 0.75
Convolution kernel	Standard	Standard	Standard
Specials			
Scan range	Diaphragm to caudal hepatic surface	Diaphragm to caudal hepatic surface	Diaphragm to caudal hepatic surface
Scan direction	Craniocaudal	Craniocaudal	Craniocaudal
Contrast media application			
Concentration (mg iodine/mL)	300/370	300/370	300/370
Mono/Biphasic	Biphasic	Biphasic	Biphasic
Volume (mL)	100–150	100–150	100–150
Injection rate (mL/s)	4.0–5.0	4.0–5.0	4.0–5.0
Saline chaser (mL, mL/s)	Optional	Optional	Optional
Delay (s)	~20 and ~50	~25 and ~60	~25 and ~60

[*] To be adapted to patient's weight and constitution

sification proposed by Cuinaud in 1957, as shown in Fig. 27.1 (Cuinaud's classification of liver segments [4]).

Selected Focal Liver Lesions

In the group of benign tumors, cysts are easy to delineate. Simple cysts are common, occurring in 5–18% of the general population. They may be solitary or multiple and do not show enhancement after contrast administration. They are well circumscribed and feature a low density attenuation (usually <20 HU). Multiple hepatic cysts occur in patients with an autosomal dominant trait and polycystic kidney disease.

Hepatic hemangiomas are the most common benign lesions of the liver, detected in up to 7% of a normal population. Using CT, hemangiomas are sharply defined masses featuring a distinctive pattern of enhancement after contrast enhancement: this pattern is characterized by a slow sequential opacification beginning at the periphery of the lesion and proceeding towards the cen-

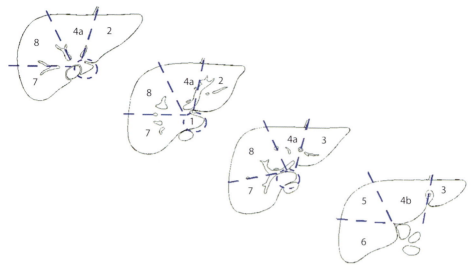

Fig. 27.1. Liver segments as subdivided according to the surgical classification

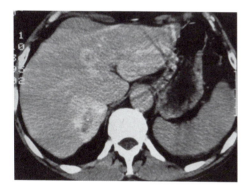

Fig. 27.2. Hemangiomas are sharply defined masses featuring a distinctive pattern of enhancement after contrast enhancement: this pattern is characterized by a slow sequential opacification beginning at the periphery of the lesion and proceeding towards the center

ter in about 60% of cases (Fig. 27.2). Fibrotic areas within the lesion that do not opacify are responsible for atypical contrast enhancement patterns. In almost all cases, an arterial dominant and a portalvenous contrast-enhanced scan allow one to assess diagnostically sufficiently the contrast behavior of a hemangioma.

Focal nodular hyperplasia (FNH) is the second most common benign tumor with preferred subcapsular location. A rela-

tively homogeneous enhancement during the arterial phase in contrast-enhanced CT is typically for this hypervasculatized lesion. The most prominent feature of the FNH is the central lower attenuation "scar" due to perivascular, central fibrosis, and is also visible in later phases of the contrast-enhanced scans. However, atypical features may be seen in a relatively high percentage of these lesions (ca. 30%), leading to a considerable overlap especially with the imaging features in hepatocellular adenomas.

Hepatocellular adenomas are relatively rare, usually solitary, and consist of normal hepatocytes. The CT (and MRI) appearance of hepatocellular adenomas are variable and nonspecific. Previous bleedings may lead to hypoattenuation, while hyperattenuation may also occur owing to more recent hemorrhage or large amounts of glycogen. Following contrast injection, adenomas often show substantial enhancement (Fig. 27.3).

Malignant Tumors

Hepatocellular carcinomas (HCC) are the most common malignant liver tumor and may be solitary or multifocal. The HCC is

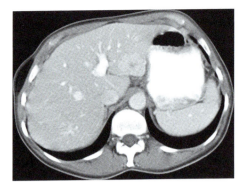

Fig. 27.3. Hepatocellular adenomas often show substantial enhancement

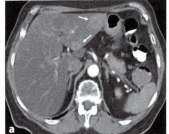

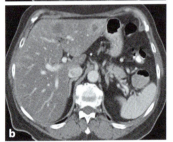

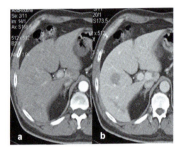

Fig. 27.4. Metastasis from colorectal cancer. The commonly hypovascularized lesion is only visible during the portalvenous scan (**b**). Note the pseudolesion in the caudate lobe due to early arterial enhancement (**a**). The suspected small metastasis could not be revealed in follow-up studies

Fig. 27.5. An increasing number of patients will be affected by one or more different primary malignancies and/or will undergo chemotherapy. As a consequence, metastases may present hyper- and hypovascularized patterns at the same time, necessitating biphasic study protocols. In the arterial-dominant scan (**a**) two different types of metastases are visible: a hypovascularized metastasis from CRC in segment 2, staying hypodense on the portalvenous scan (**b**), two metastases from breast cancer with rim-like hypervascularization are visible in segment 3 in the arterial-dominant scan (**a**, *arrows*), while the dorsally located lesion vanishes in the portalvenous scan

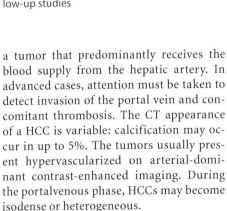

a tumor that predominantly receives the blood supply from the hepatic artery. In advanced cases, attention must be taken to detect invasion of the portal vein and concomitant thrombosis. The CT appearance of a HCC is variable: calcification may occur in up to 5%. The tumors usually present hypervascularized on arterial-dominant contrast-enhanced imaging. During the portalvenous phase, HCCs may become isodense or heterogeneous.

The cholangiocarcinoma (CCC) of the liver is much less common than the HCC and accounts for less than 10% of the primary malignant hepatic tumors. The typical appearance in contrast-enhanced CT is that of a poorly demarcated hypodense lesion, sometimes with elevated enhancement at the tumor margins.

Metastasis of extrahepatic tumors to the liver is a very common disease. Most metastases are hypovascularized relative to the normal hepatic parenchyma. Therefore, they present hypodense during the portalvenous phase. Nevertheless, the CT appearance of metastases is highly variable and sometimes difficult to differentiate from other lesions (Fig. 27.4). Calcifications may occur and are more frequently seen in metastases from mucinous tumors (e.g., colorectal carcinoma) or from ovarian cancer. If a carcinoid tumor is known, the

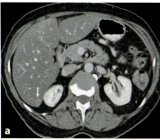

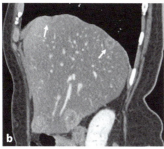

Fig. 27.6. Multiplanar reformations can be helpful for improved display of hepatic metastases especially in subcapsular/subdiaphragmatic localization (**a,b**, *arrows*)

hypervascularized metastases are best appreciated during the arterial phase, while the typical rapid washout and the tumor's anatomical relation to the hepatic vascularization can be best appreciated by a combined arterial-dominant and portalvenous scanning protocol (Fig. 27.5).

Abscesses of the liver can occur from ascending cholangitis (biliary origin), hematogenously, or from local infectious inoculation. Depending on the origin, the CT imaging features may vary. Usually there is a hypodense round or irregular lesion with little or no contrast enhancement in the portalvenous phase.

In conclusion, contrast-enhanced multislice CT is a commonly applied imaging modality in the evaluation of focal liver disease. Most primary (hepatocellular carcinoma) and about 20–25% of the secondary malignant lesions, as well as many benign lesions of the liver (e.g., hemangioma, hepatocellular adenoma, FNH) are hypervascularized, while many secondary malignant hepatic lesions are hypovascularized. To depict the more or less char-

acteristic vascularization patterns and to differentiate these lesions, a biphasic scan protocol after contrast injection is best suited.

Detection and characterization of hepatic lesions particularly in patients with malignancies is a crucial, highly clinically relevant diagnostic task. CT is widely accepted as the method of choice for this task. It is superior to ultrasound due to its user independency and reproducibility. In many malignancies it is appropriate to incorporate hepatic CT into a whole-body staging protocol with a short scanning time as clear advantage over MRI [3,5]. The high temporal and local resolution of multidetector CT enables multiplanar reformations (Fig. 27.6) enhancing the diagnostic accuracy [6–8], consequently CT-arterioportography is becoming less and less important partially due to the relatively high rate of false positive findings [9].

Even if CT of the liver and abdomen are diagnostically sufficient in a high number of cases, there will be equivocal cases mainly related to hepatic lesions that cannot be classified by CT. According to the recent literature, MRI is then recommended as a noninvasive tool in cases where biopsy is not advisable [7–9].

References

1. Itoh S, Ikeda M, Achiwa M, Satake H, Iwano S, Ishigaki T (2004) Late-arterial and portal-venous phase imaging of the liver with a multislice CT scanner in patients without circulatory disturbances: automatic bolus tracking or empirical scan delay? Eur Radiol 14(9):1665–1673
2. Engeroff B, Kopka L, Harz C, Grabbe E (2001) Impact of different iodine concentrations on abdominal enhancement in biphasic multislice helical CT (MS-CT). Rofo 173(10):938–941
3. Catalano C, Laghi A, Fraioli F, Pediconi F, Napoli A, Danti M, Passariello R (2002) High-resolution CT angiography of the abdomen. Abdom Imaging 27(5):479–487
4. Fischer, L, Cardenas C, Thorn M, Benner A, Grenacher L, Vetter M, Lehnert T, Klar E, Meinzer H P and Lamade W (2002) Limits of Couinaud's liver segment classification: a quantitative computer-based three-dimensional analysis. J Comput Assist Tomogr 26(6): 962–967

5. Foley WD, Mallisee TA, Hohenwalter MD, Wilson CR, Quiroz FA, Taylor AJ (2000) Multiphase hepatic CT with a multirow detector CT scanner. AJR Am J Roentgenol 175 (3):679–685

6. Itoh S, Ikeda M, Achiwa M, Ota T, Satake H, Ishigaki T (2003) Multiphase contrast-enhanced CT of the liver with a multislice CT scanner. Eur Radiol 13(5):1085–1094

7. Kopka L, Rogalla P, Hamm B (2002) Multislice CT of the abdomen--current indications and future trends. Rofo 174(3):273–282

8. Miles KA (2002) Functional computed tomography in oncology. Eur J Cancer 38(16):2079–2084

9. Vogl TJ, Schwarz W, Blume S, Pietsch M, Shamsi K, Franz M, Lobeck H, Balzer T, del Tredici K, Neuhaus P, Felix R, Hammerstingl RM (2003) Preoperative evaluation of malignant liver tumors: comparison of unenhanced and SPIO (Resovist)-enhanced MR imaging with biphasic CTAP and intraoperative US. Eur Radiol 13(2):262–272

28 MSCT Imaging of Biliary Tract Disease

M. Horger

Introduction

Imaging of the gallbladder and biliary tract has changed significantly over the past two decades due to advances in noninvasive imaging, especially through rapid development of modern cross-sectional imaging methods such as ultrasonography (US), computed tomography (CT), and recently magnetic resonance (MR) tomography.

Multidimensional imaging with near isotropic voxel, fewer artifacts, and a mean acquisition time of generally less than 20 s per series, which is compatible with breath hold techniques, provides exquisite anatomic data to the referring physician, pushing multidetector CT diagnostics into the center of the cross-sectional diagnostic tools of the radiologist together with US.

Indications

Indications for CT imaging in patients suspected of diseases of the biliary tract consist of:

1. Detection of level and cause of biliary obstruction in patients with jaundice.
2. Diagnosis of acute cholangitis and liver abscess.
3. Imaging of sclerosing cholangitis.
4. Detection of benign and malignant tumors of the biliary tract (adenomatous polyps, adenomyomatosis, biliary cystadenoma, hamartoma, cholangiocarcinoma, carcinoma of the gallbladder).
5. Evaluation of acute gallbladder disease (cholecystitis, empyema, Mirizzi syndrome, Bouveret's syndrome) in patients

who are not suitable (obese, meteorism) for US imaging.
6. Exclusion of extrinsic diseases with involvement of the biliary system.

Imaging Protocol

Immediately prior to scanning, the stomach and duodenum are distended with 500–1000 mL of water to serve as negative contrast to more clearly depict the gastric and duodenal walls. The use of high-attenuation contrast material should be avoided when using CT to evaluate potential biliary tract disease, because of related beam-hardening artifacts. Patients are positioned supine on the CT table. Usually, a topogram ranging from the level of the diaphragm down to the pelvic inlet will be performed. Scan parameters are listed in Table 28.1. Initial noncontrast scans are obtained of the upper abdomen to delineate the target volume to be scanned. Following rapid injection of 120–150 mL of nonionic contrast delivered via a power injector at 3–4 mL/s, the entire upper abdomen, including the liver and pancreas is scanned during a single breath hold at 0.7–1.00 mm following a 40-s injector delay. The late arterial injection is also valuable to detect subtle density changes in the liver parenchyma induced by perfusion abnormalities or mass effect. The liver portal vasculature is also more clearly depicted during this phase of scanning. Following late arterial-phase acquisition, venous-phase scanning is performed with a single breath hold at 70 s after the onset of IV bolus. This phase is essential to confirm liver metastases, portal vein occlusion, or diagnose primaries arising from the bili-

Table 28.1. Scanning parameters for abdominal imaging for three different MDCT scanners

Parameters	4–8 slice scanners	10–16 slice scanners	32–64 slice scanners
Scanner settings			
Tube voltage(kV)	120	120	120
Tube current time product (mAs)	250–300	250–300	230–260
Pitch corrected tube current time product (eff. mAs)	380–400	380–400	400–450
Collimation (mm)	1/2.5	1.25/1.5	0.6/0.625
Norm. pitch	0.65–0.75	0.65–0.75	0.57
Reconstr. increment (mm)	3	3, for recons 1	3, for recons 0.6
Reconstr.-slice thickness (mm)	3–5	3–5, for recons 1.5–2	3–5, for recons 0.75–1.5
Convolution kernel	Standard	Standard	Standard
Scan range	Diaphragm/ pelvic inlet	Diaphragm/ pelvic inlet	Diaphragm/ pelvic inlet
Scan direction	Craniocaudal	Craniocaudal	Craniocaudal
Contrast material application			
Concentration (mg iodine/mL)			
Mono/Biphasic	Monophasic/ biphasic	Monophasic/ biphasic	Monophasic/ biphasic
Volume (mL)	150 or 100/50	150 or 100/50	150 or 100/50
Injection rate (mL/s)	4.0 or 4.0/2.5	4.0 or 4.0/2.5	4.0 or 4.0/2.5
Saline chaser (mL, mL/s)	30/3.0	30/3.0	30/3.0
Delay (s)	40/70, eventually +180	45/70, eventually +180	50/70, eventually +180

ary tract. For detection of cholangiocarcinoma, late equilibrium perfusion phase (120–180 s) is beneficial. As an adjunct to interpretation of axial images alone, a variety of CT display techniques have been used to depict anatomical relation of pathologic changes to the underlying anatomy. These include maximum and minimum intensity projection, as well as volume-rendered images. Maximal intensity projection (MIP) images are most useful to display high-attenuation structures, such as vasculature or bile ducts, by CT-chlolangiography. Conversely, minimum intensity projection images aid in depicting low-attenuation structures, such as the bile duct, pancreatic duct, and hypoattenuating tumors. Both types of image display are often performed on a thin "slab" of stacked axial images. In addition to these techniques, curved planar reformations have proven to be quite useful in the display of the biliary system.

Suggestions
for Special Investigational Protocols

Unenhanced CT images increase the conspicuity of many common bile duct or gallbladder stones compared with intravenous contrast-enhanced images. They are also essential for determining the degree and dynamic of enhancement in inflammatory, or tumoral conditions.

Oral or intravenous administration of cholecystographic contrast material enables optimal visualization of the biliary tract in patients with no or mild cholestasis (bilirubin <1.8 g/L).

Sincalide, a cholecystokinin analogue, improves biliary opacification by causing contraction of the gallbladder and relaxation of Oddi's sphincter [1,2].

Normal Anatomy

The gallbladder is an oval-shaped organ situated in the gallbladder fossa between the right and left lobes of the liver. It is composed of following anatomical parts: fundus, body, neck, and cystic duct. The cystic duct joints the common hepatic duct to form the common bile duct. Size, form, and sometimes even location of the gallbladder can vary substantially. The normal wall thickness does not exceed 3 mm. The biliary tree is an arborized system consisting of subsegmental and segmental branches joining to form the right and left main ducts which then run together to form the main hepatic duct (MHD). The main hepatic duct joins with the cystic duct forming the main bile duct (MBD), which enters the head of the pancreas and then enters the duodenum through the sphincter of Oddi.

Diseases of the Biliary Tract

Biliary Obstruction

Imaging biliary obstruction means in the first line detection of dilated intra- or extrahepatic ducts. Intrahepatic duct dilatation is considered when the bile duct diameter exceeds 40% of the diameter of the adjacent intrahepatic portal vein. The diameter of the extrahepatic bile ducts should physiologically not exceed 9–10 mm on CT. There are several causes for bile duct obstruction, the most frequent being choledocolithiasis (Fig. 28.1), followed by ampullary stenosis, inflammation, and

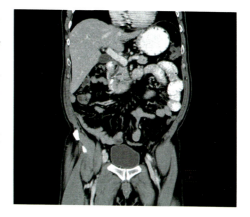

Fig. 28.1. 57-year-old male patient complaining about acute onset of right upper abdominal pain. MDCT (4-slice) coronal reformation image shows mild distension of the common bile duct and pancreatic duct (double duct sign) due to calcified stones in both ductal lumina, with extension down to the papilla major

tumor [3]. Determination of the cause and level of obstruction are both important for guiding further diagnostic and therapeutic intervention (Fig. 28.2a,b). Abrupt termination of the bile duct is a cholangiographic sign that has a high correlation with malignancy, whereas a gradually tapering duct generally represents a benign process. Although CT is not the method of choice to detect stones, it is able in many cases to reveal calcified gallbladder and duct stones (20% of all biliary stones), or even cholesterol stones, which appear of low attenuation compared with bile [4]. Precious diagnostic tools in detecting low attenuation bile duct stones are: the crescent-shaped bile duct lumen caused by contrast between low-attenuation bile and partial obstruction of the bile duct through slightly different low-attenuating stones; the focal-thickened distal common bile duct (>2 mm) due to associated inflammatory stricture; the target sign, representing central soft-tissue attenuation surrounded by water-attenuation bile, conspicuous especially on transaxial images; and the use of unenhanced CT with density measurements along the bile duct, in order to detect different intraductal attenuations.

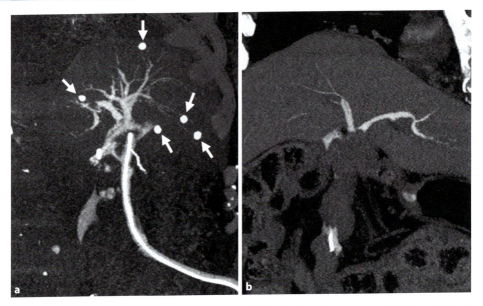

Fig. 28.2. 66-year-old male patient with jaundice, following bile duct surgery with hepatojejunal anastomosis. External bile drainage was laid intraoperatively. MIP reformation (**a**), and coronal MPR (16-slice MDCT) (**b**) from intravenous (IV) CT cholangiography shows local anatomy with three different anastomoses of the anterior and posterior branch of the right bile duct and the left bile duct. No opacification of the jejunal loop is seen. Small calcified intrahepatic granulomas are also visible (*arrowhead*)

Acute cholangitis, or chronic sclerosing cholangitis (PSC) are other nontumoral causes of bile duct obstruction. CT is in both cases indicated in order to demonstrate duct-wall thickening and wall enhancement. Acute cholangitis may be complicated by clustered liver abscesses, which are optimally depicted by CT. CT-guidance can also help in draining abscesses. In sclerosing cholangitis multifocal strictures of both intrahepatic and extrahepatic bile ducts lead to typical changes such as "pruning" (limited duct brunching), "beaded" appearance (alternation of strictures and dilatation of the bile ducts), and stone formation. Circular or focal mural thickening can help in the differentiation of cholangiocarcinoma (usually >5 mm), which is often related to PSC [5]. Particularly in these latter two pathological entities, it is mandatory to achieve optimal spatial resolution in order to depict discrete bile duct wall changes. While these diseases can also be visualized by means of US or MRI, it is the isotropic voxel technique that enables optimal multiplanar reformats of the biliary tree with excellent image quality. Using oral or intravenous cholecystographic contrast material, an even higher sensitivity of CT-diagnosis can be achieved. However, MRI remains an equally good diagnostic alternative in patients who are compliant.

Cholangiocarcinoma represents the most common tumor of the bile ducts. It can be classified as intrahepatic, or extrahepatic, with the hilar form (Klatskin) being most frequent (Fig. 28.3). Different growth appearances have been described histologically, most of them correlating well with the findings on cross-sectional imaging. The tumors are of less attenuation than liver on unenhanced CT, and do not strongly enhance after IV contrast material administration. Late enhancement (in the late equilibrium phase) is typical. Sometimes tumors show low attenuation simulating cystic masses if the tumor produces extensive mucin. However, delineation of

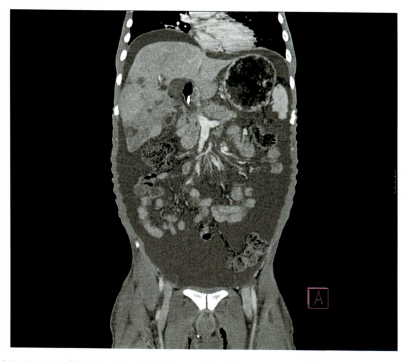

Fig. 28.3. 77-year-old male patient with known Klatskin tumor complaining about to have fever and chills over the last 48 h. Large intrahepatic tumor mass with necrosis and a few intrahepatic metastases were already known. The common bile duct was drained using a Teflon catheter. Coronal MPR (16-slice MDCT) shows intrahepatic low-attenuated abscesses, with related liver parenchymal perfusion abnormalities due to associated intrahepatic portal vein branch thrombosis. Ascites were also present around the liver

Klatskin tumors might sometimes be difficult on CT, requiring additional diagnostic techniques (US, MRI). Also suggestive for intrahepatic cholangiocarcinoma are the following: atrophy of liver parenchyma with retraction of the liver capsule; focal bile duct dilatation, peripherally from the tumor; altered liver parenchymal perfusion by tumor.

Gallbladder Diseases

CT plays, admittedly, a minor role in the diagnosis of acute cholecystitis because of the excellent experience with ultrasound diagnosis. There are, however, some known limitations with ultrasound, such as obesity and meteorism, which make CT valuable, particularly for exclusion of severe complications such as: empyema (CT density of the lumen >30 HU), gangrenous cholecystitis (mural necrosis, irregular or absent gallbladder wall enhancement, or intraluminal membranes), emphysematous cholecystitis (intraluminal or intramural air), gallbladder perforation (fluid collection surrounding the gallbladder) and xanthogranulomatous cholecystitis, which should be differentiated from tumor (low attenuation of the gallbladder wall on CT due to lipid-laden hystiocytes) [6]. CT also plays an important role in the differentiation of ordinary gallbladder stones from adenomatous polyps, showing enhancement even in tiny adenomas, where perfusion is difficult to demonstrate by Doppler.

Carcinoma of the gallbladder can be correctly diagnosed by all cross-sectional imaging methods (CT, US, MRI). However, CT is much more comfortable for whole-body staging (Fig. 28.4). Other rarer tumors such

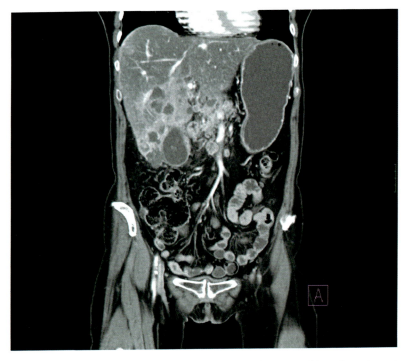

Fig. 28.4. 64-year-old female patient with gallbladder carcinoma and lymph node metastases. Coronal MPR (4-slice MDCT) shows thickening of the gallbladder wall with direct invasion of liver parenchyma and multiple liver metastases. Note also lymph node metastases in the liver portal and around the pancreas. The liver is low-attenuation due to steatosis hepatis. Good image contrast is achieved at the margins of tumor infiltration

as biliary cystadenoma/cystadenocarcinoma are mainly cystic, sometimes showing complex septations and soft-tissue nodularities. The larger these latter findings, the greater the chance of malignancy. Differentiation from hydatid cysts, hematoma, and abscesses is usually difficult. However, CT, as well as MRI, are able to demonstrate minimal enhancement of mural nodules of septa making tumor diagnosis more probable. Especially for exclusion of extraductal causes of duct obstruction, for instance by pancreas carcinoma invasion of the CBD, it is beneficial to perform CT or MRI diagnosis in order to achieve adequate information about tumor extension, vascular invasion, and to correctly stage the neoplasm and evaluate therapy options (Fig. 28.5).

There are also developmental abnormalities of the biliary system, which are also correctly diagnosed by CT such as: Caroli's disease, choledocal cysts, etc. [7].

In conclusion, the range of CT indications in abdominal diagnostics is widening every day, due to improvements in image resolution and shortening of acquisition times, making it one of the leading investigational methods. While in patients with acute complaints due to biliary disease US diagnosis successfully concurs with CT, the latter is more appropriately used for evaluation in patients with a wider differential diagnosis, a known history of chronic biliary disease, following surgery, or in patients with confusing clinical symptoms and signs.

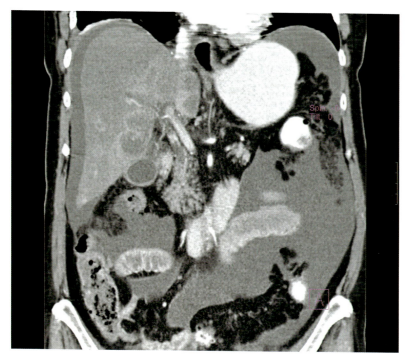

Fig. 28.5. 70-year-old female patient with jaundice. Coronal MPR (4-slice MDCT) reveals common bile duct thickening in the liver portal due to cholangiocarcinoma. Moderate distension of extrahepatic bile duct is seen. Note also ascites probably caused by peritoneal carcinomatosis

References

1. Fleischmann D, Ringl H, Schofl R (1996) Three-dimensional spiral CT cholangiography in patients with suspected obstructive biliary disease: comparison with endoscopic retrograde cholangiography. Radiology 198:861–868

2. Chopra S, Chintapalli K, Ramakkrishna K et al. (2000) Helical CT cholangiography with oral cholecystographic contrast material. Radiology 214:596–601

3. Co CS, Shea WJ, Goldberg H (1986) Evaluation of common bile duct diameter using high resolution computed tomography. J Comput Assist Tomogr 10:424–427

4. Neitlich JD, Topazian M, Smith RC, et al. (1997) Detection of choledocholithiasis: comparison of unenhanced helical CT and endoscopic retrograde cholangiopancreatography. Radiology 203:753–757

5. Campbell WL, Peterson MS, Federle MP, et al. (2001) Using CT and cholangiography to diagnose biliary tract carcinoma completing primary sclerosing cholangitis. AJR 177:1095–1100

6. Pickhardt PJ, Friedland JA, Hruza DS et al. (2003) CT, MR cholangiopancreaticography, and endoscopy findings in Bouveret's syndrome. AJR 180:1033–1035

7. Levy AD, Rohrmann Jr. CA, Murakata LA et al. (2000) Caroli's disease: radiologic spectrum with pathologic correlation. AJR 179:1053–1057

29 MSCT of the Upper Urinary Tract

U.G. Mueller-Lisse and E. Coppenrath

Indications

1. Differentiation of indeterminate or suspicious renal masses at IVU or ultrasound (e.g., cystic lesions, tumors, pseudotumors, calcifications, or arteriovenous malformations).
2. Oncologic indications, tumor detection in malignancies of unknown primary, tumor staging, and search for metastasis, follow-up.
3. Malignancy as the underlying cause of renal or ureteral obstruction.
4. Infectious disease (e.g., acute and chronic pyelonephritis, xanthogranulomatous pyelonephritis, tuberculosis, renal abscess).
5. Renal and ureteral calculus disease.
6. Renal trauma and macrohematuria.
7. Other indications (e.g., renal failure with hydronephrosis or renal vascular disease with ischemia, arterial stenosis, or venous thrombosis, and congenital anomalies) [1].

Patient Preparation

- Oral (e.g., water, tea) or intravenous (e.g., saline solution) hydration to physiologic hydration state (not in acute trauma patients and acute renal or ureteral colic).
- Appropriate pain medication in malignancy, trauma, and calculus disease.
- Serum creatine and thyroid parameters checked and appropriately treated prior to i.v. contrast administration.
- Antecubital intravenous line suitable for power injector pump at 2–3 mL/s (≥20 G).

Patient Positioning

Supine, head first, arms above head.

Topogram, Scan Range

Kidneys and adrenals only: diaphragm to iliac crest; caveat: pelvic kidney.
Entire upper urinary tract: diaphragm to symphysis pubis.

Scan Parameters

See Table 29.1. Scan series should be selected according to clinical indication.

Tips and Tricks

- Sudden change of urinary tract lumen along with wall thickening frequently indicates point of lesion [2].
- Unenhanced MSCT scans can be reduced to 30 mAs per slice to decrease radiation exposure (Fig. 29.1) [1,3].
- Postcontrast MSCT scans in the excretory phase (CT urography, CTU) can be reduced to 30–50 mAs per slice when indication for CTU is to determine ureteral course (Fig. 29.2).

Comments

According to statistics from the American Cancer Society, renal and urinary tract cancers are among the 10 most frequent malignancies affecting men and women. When tumors extend into the urinary tract,

Table 29.1. Scan parameters

Parameters	4–8 slice scanners	10–16 slice scanners	32–64 slice scanners
Scanner settings			
Tube voltage (kV)	120	120	120
Rotation time (s)	0.5	0.5	0.5
Tube current time product (mAs)	130–340	130–340	130–340
Pitch corrected tube current time product (eff mAs)	150–250, Low dose 30–50	150–250, Low dose 30–50	150–250, Low dose 30–50
Collimation (mm)	2.5	1.25/1.5	0.6/0.625
Norm. pitch	0.9–1.5	0.9–1.5	0.9–1.5
Reconstr. increment (mm)	3	3, for recons 1	3, for recons 0.6
Reconstr.-slice thickness (mm)	3–5	3–5, for recons 1.5–2	3–5, for recons 0.75–1
Convolution kernel	Standard	Standard	Standard
Contrast media application			
Concentration (mg iodine/mL)	300	300	300
Mono/Biphasic	Monophasic	Monophasic	Monophasic
Volume (mL)	100–120	80–110	80–100
Injection rate (mL/s)	2.5–3	2.5–3	2.5–3
Saline chaser (mL, mL/s)	Optional	Optional	Optional
Delay (s)	Portal venous 70 Nephrographic 80–100 Excretory 180–600	Portal venous 70 Nephrographic 80–100 Excretory 180–600	Portal venous 70 Nephrographic 80–100 Excretory 180–600

they most frequently present with macro-hematuria. While macrohematuria may be a sign of urinary tract malignancy, it is also associated with urinary calculus disease, trauma, arterial, or venous anomalies and malformations, and sometimes with infectious disease of the urinary tract. Currently, many renal tumors or tumor-like lesions are picked up by ultrasound in examinations of the upper abdomen originally performed for a different reason. CT is frequently applied to characterize and differentiate renal or ureteral masses that are indeterminate or suspicious at IVU or ultrasound [1].

Staging

CT is the imaging modality most frequently applied for staging of renal and urinary tract malignancies. It is particularly useful to determine macroscopic extent of primary tumor beyond the confines of the renal parenchyma or urinary tract linings, i.e., into renal sinus fat, perirenal fat, and periureteral or perivesical fat, and into adjacent structures (e.g., Gerota's fascia, renal veins, inferior vena cava) and organs (e.g., adrenal, uterus, prostate, rectum). Sensitivity and specificity vary between approximately 80 and 100% [1,4,5].

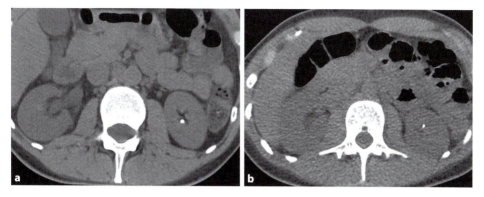

Fig. 29.1. a Nonenhanced CT scan for stone detection (standard dose protocol). **b** Low-dose CT scan for stone detection. Increase of noise, however, does not impede detection

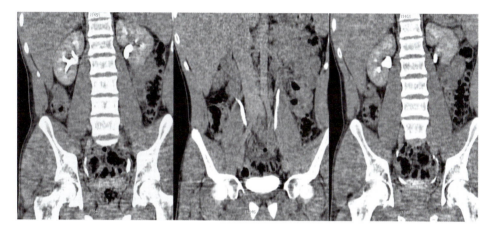

Fig. 29.2. Excretory phase of CT urography in the low-dose technique

CT Characteristics of Various Renal and Urinary Tract Lesions

Unenhanced scans of the urinary tract demonstrate calcifications within urinary calculi, renal cysts, and solid tumors, fat within solid tumors (implying angiomyolipoma, since macroscopic fat is exceptionally rare in renal cell carcinoma), water or urine within cystic lesions and urinoma, and extravasated blood in urinary trauma (increased density when compared with renal parenchyma) [1,3]. Renal arteries are best visualized within the first 15–25 s after i.v. contrast administration (arterial phase). However, unless specifically requested, renal CT arteriograms are not warranted in routine kidney protocols, due to the increase in radiation exposure. Differentiation of renal medulla and cortex is best in the corticomedullary phase (40–70 s after i.v. contrast administration), when the cortex shows high attenuation and the medulla shows low attenuation [1,6]. However, renal parenchymal lesions (e.g., cysts, solid tumors, abscesses, trauma) are best recognized and characterized in the portal venous (70–80 s after i.v. contrast administration), or even better, in the nephrographic phase (80–100 s after i.v. contrast administration) with its almost even attenuation throughout the renal parenchyma [1,4–7].

MSCT of lesions arising from or extending into the renal calices and pelvis (particularly, urothelial carcinoma or renal cell carcinoma) may benefit from strong contrast between soft tissue (low attenuation) and excretory products (high intraluminal attenuation of the urinary tract after i.v. contrast administration, with a delay of 3–5 min for the renal calices and pelvis, 5–10 min for the ureters, and 10–20 min for the bladder) [1,8].

MSCT Compared with other Radiologic Modalities in Renal and Urinary Lesions

When compared with magnetic resonance imaging (MRI), MSCT has the advantages of wider availability, shorter overall imaging time to complete an examination, and lower cost. On the other hand, MRI offers a wider range of soft-tissue contrasts, any number of sequence repetitions without restriction by considerations of radiation dose, and imaging in virtually any desired plane of view. Detection and staging of renal tumors is currently estimated to be of similar accuracy using MSCT and MRI [1,5]. Although less expensive, noninvasive imaging methods such as intravenous urography (IVU) and sonography are widely available, patients are oftentimes referred for definitive evaluation with CT when lesions are suspected in other studies. Ultrasound is an excellent modality for the evaluation of renal parenchyma, but hardly capable of demonstrating the ureters in European adults.

References

1. Mueller-Lisse UG, Mueller-Lisse UL (2004) MDCT of the kidney. In: Reiser MF, Takahashi M, Modic M, Becker CR (eds) Multislice CT, 2nd edn. Medical Radiology – Diagnostic Imaging. Baert AL, Sartor K (series eds). Springer, Berlin, Heidelberg, New York, pp 211–232
2. Rimondini A, Morra A, Bertolotto M, Locatelli M, Pozzi Mucelli R (2001) Spiral CT with multiplanar reconstruction (MPRS) in the evaluation of ureteral neoplasms: preliminary results. Radiol Med (Torino) 101:459–65
3. Tack D, Sourtzis S, Delpierre I, de Maertelaer V, Gevenois PA (2003) Low-dose unenhanced multidetector CT of patients with suspected renal colic. AJR Am J Roentgenol 180:305–11
4. Catalano C, Fraioli F, Laghi A, Napoli A, Pediconi F, Danti M, Nardis P, Passariello R (2003) High-resolution multidetector CT in the preoperative evaluation of patients with renal cell carcinoma. AJR Am J Roentgenol 180(5):1271–7
5. Hallscheidt PJ, Bock M, Riedasch G, Zuna I, Schoenberg SO, Autschbach F, Soder M, Noeldge G (2004) Diagnostic accuracy of staging renal cell carcinomas using multidetector-row computed tomography and magnetic resonance imaging: a prospective study with histopathologic correlation. J Comput Assist Tomogr 28(3):333–9
6. Cohan RH, Sherman LS, Korobkin M, Bass JC, Francis IR (1995) Renal masses: assessment of corticomedullary-phase and nephrographic-phase CT scans. Radiology 196:445–51
7. Willmann JK, Roos JE, Platz A, Pfammatter T, Hilfiker PR, Marincek B, Weishaupt D (2002) Multidetector CT: detection of active hemorrhage in patients with blunt abdominal trauma. AJR Am J Roentgenol 179:437–44
8. Caoili EM, Cohan RH, Korobkin M et al. (2002) Urinary tract abnormalities: initial experience with multi-detector row CT urography. Radiology 222: 353–60

30 Pancreas and Retroperitoneal Space

U. Baum and K. Anders

Indications

Pancreas

- Pancreatic tumors.
- Pancreatitis.
- Diffuse pancreatic changes.
- Pancreatic trauma.
- Postoperative changes.

Retroperitoneal Space

- Inflammation and abscess.
- Hematoma.
- Urinoma, cysts, lymphocele.
- Retroperitoneal tumors.

Patient Preparation

Oral Contrast

- Retroperitoneum, pancreatitis:
  1200 mL positive oral contrast, e.g., diluted iodinated contrast agent
- Pancreatic tumor:
  800 mL negative oral contrast, e.g., water, 15–20 min prior to the examination. Additional 300–500 mL given immediately before the scan, afterwards the patient has to rest in right lateral position (on the scanner table) for about 5 min to ensure sufficient filling of the duodenum.

Spasmolytic Drug

- 20–40 mg N-butyscopalamine i.v. or 1 mg glucagon i.v.

Patient Positioning

- Prior to the scan, rest in right lateral position for 5 min for patients with pancreatic tumors.
- Supine position during the scan.

Topogram/Scan Range

Topogram

- See Fig. 30.1.
- a.p.; complete abdomen.

Scan Range

- For indications of the different contrast medium phases, see Table 30.1.
- Precontrast scan: upper/whole abdomen.
- Late arterial phase (pancreatic parenchyma phase): upper abdomen.
- Portalvenous phase: whole abdomen.

Scan Parameters

See Table 30.2.

Tips and Tricks

- Advantages of negative oral contrast media are: better delineation of the duodenal wall, with the possibility to perform CT angiography without beam hardening artifacts caused by bowel contrast, as well as facilitating the detection of calcifications.

Table 30.1. Indications for the different contrast medium phases

	Precontrast	Early arterial phase	Pancreatic phase	Portalvenous phase
Pancreas				
Pancreatitis	+			+
Pancreatic tumors			+	+
Islet cell tumors		+		+
Diffuse pancreatic changes	+			+
Trauma/postoperative changes	+			+
Retroperitoneum				
Inflammation, abscess				+
Hematoma	+	(+)		+
Urinoma, cyst, lymphocele	+			+
Retroperitoneal tumors	(+)			+

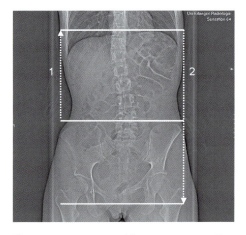

Fig. 30.1. Topogram with scan ranges. First scan (upper abdomen) during pancreatic parenchyma phase (scan delay: 35 s) with caudocranial scan direction. Second scan (whole abdomen) during portalvenous phase in craniocaudal scan direction

- Advantages of positive oral contrast media are: better delineation of abscesses, peripancreatic fluid collections, and pseudocysts.

- Detection of vascular infiltration: thin (2-mm) slices oblique coronal and oblique sagittal following the course of the vessels.
- An additional delayed scan 5–10 min after contrast injection should be performed in cases of suspected injury of the urinary tract.

CT Findings

Pancreas

Pancreatitis: Different Forms

In edematous or interstitial pancreatitis the CT appearance is characterized by an enlarged organ with decreased attenuation, blurring of the margins and thickening the Gerota's fascia, but with no perfusion defects. In the case of serous exsudative pancreatitis, CT exhibits fluid collections without a defined wall and peripancreatic fat necrosis, but no perfusion defects. Severe acute pancreatitis (extensive pancreatitis or fluid collections pancreatitis) is char-

Table 30.2. Scan parameters

Parameters	4–8 slice scanners	10–16 slice scanners	32–64 slice scanners
Scanner settings			
Tube voltage (kV)	120	120	120
Rotation time (s)	0.5	0.5	0.5
Tube current time product (mAs)	130–340[*]	130–340[*]	130–340[*]
Pitch corrected tube current time product (eff. mAs)	165–240	165–240	165–240
Collimation (mm)	Arterial 1/1.25 Portalvenous 2.5	0.625/0.75 1.25/1.5	0.6/0.625 1.2/1.25
Norm. pitch	0.8–1.4	0.8–1.4	0.8–1.4
Reconstruction increment (mm)	60–100% of slice thickness	60–100% of slice thickness	60–100% of slice thickness
Reconstr.-slice thickness (mm)	Arterial 3 Portalvenous 5 For recons.: 1.25	Arterial 3 Portalvenous 5 mm For recons.: 1	Arterial 3 Portalvenous 5 For recons.: 0.75
Convolution kernel	Soft/standard	Soft/standard	Soft/standard
Scan range	Arterial pancreas only/ venous whole abdomen	Arterial pancreas only/ venous whole abdomen	Arterial pancreas only/ venous whole abdomen
Scan direction	Craniocaudal	Craniocaudal	Craniocaudal
Contrast material			
Volume (mL)	100–120	100–120	100–120
Injection speed (mL/s)	4.0	4.0	4.0
Saline flush (mL, mL/s)	30, 4.0	30, 4.0	30, 4.0
Delay arterial (s)	35	35	40
Delay portalvenous (s)	70	70	70

[*] Adaptation to patient's weight necessary

acterized by an inhomogeneous, markedly enlarged, and poorly demarcated gland. Necrotic areas show a lack of enhancement of the parenchyma following contrast injection (Fig. 30.2). In contrast, chronic pancreatitis is suspected if atrophic parenchyma, calcifications and/or intraductal lithiasis is found.

Pancreatitis: Complications

Pseudocysts develop in 30% of acute pancreatitis. They are well encapsulated fluid collections of variable size with a detectable wall of nonepithelized granulation tissue. They are found intra- or extrapancreatic, calcifications are possible, septations are rare. An infected necrosis is suspected if

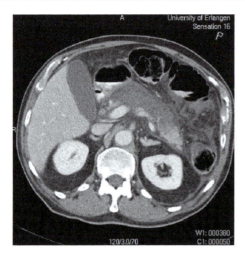

Fig. 30.2. Hemorrhagic necrotizing pancreatitis. The lesion is characterized by an inhomogeneous, markedly enlarged and poorly demarcated gland. Necrotic areas show no enhancement of the parenchyma

contrast medium enhancement is observed within the necrosis. A pancreatic abscess is characterized by liquid formation with an irregular rim enhancement and air inclusions. Care must be taken not to miss vascular complications that occur in terms of pseudoaneurysms or thrombotic occlusions.

Pancreatic Tumors: Cystic

Dysontogentic pancreatic cysts are typically sharply circumscribed, round or oval and without a visible wall. The appearance of pancreatic pseudocysts are described above. In microcystic serous adenoma the typical findings are multiple (>6) small cysts, 1–20 mm in size with serous fluid, hypervascular septa, multilobulated contour, and "sunburst" calcifications (15–40%). In contrast, the macrocystic mucinous adenoma consist of uni- or multilocular cystic mass, greater than 20 mm with mucinous fluid. They are multiloculated, have hyperattenuating septa (thicker and more irregular than of microcystic serous adenoma), lie most commonly in the body or tail and show peripheral calcifications. Macrocystic adenomas represent a premalignant lesion and should be resected. The cystadenocarinoma is the malignant variant of macrocystic mucinous adenoma (Fig. 30.3).

Intraductal papillary mucinous tumors (IMPT) show segmental or diffuse dilatation of the pancreatic duct with or without distal parenchymal atrophy, which is the typical finding in the main duct type, but sometimes intraductal papillae and/or calcifications can be recognized. A bulging papilla is found in 25% of the cases. The

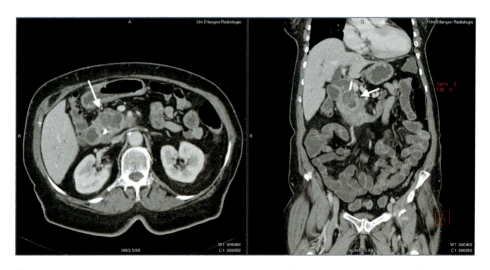

Fig. 30.3. Pancreatic cystadenocarinoma. Cystic mass with hyperattenuating septa. Dilation of the bile duct

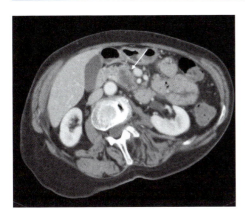

Fig. 30.3. Pancreatic adenocarcinoma. Inhomogeneous tumor of the pancreatic head with infiltration of the peripancreatic fat tissue, but without infiltration of the vessels

branch duct type is usually located in the uncinate process and characterized by a lobulated mass of clustered small cysts with central septations. The criteria of malignancy are a solid component, the dilatation of the pancreatic duct >10 mm, a bulging papilla, a diffuse or multifocal involvement, and an attenuating intraluminal content.

Pancreatic Tumors: Solid

Eighty percent of pancreatic carcinoma (adenocarcinoma) occurs in the pancreatic head, 15% in the body, and 5% in the tail. The typical CT-finding is a hypo- or isoattenuating mass during arterial phase and an isoattenuating lesion during the precontrast scan and portalvenous phase (Fig. 30.4). Dilation and abrupt cutoff of the pancreatic duct is found in 50% of the cases. In advanced stages, the peripancreatic fat planes are obliterated and the peripancreatic vessels are involved. Calcifications are rare (<2%).

Ninety percent of islet cell tumors are benign, 75% are hormonogenic. The diameter is usually smaller than 2 cm. In most cases the tumors can only be delineated in arterial phase images, calcifications can be observed in 20%. Other entities, such as solid papillary epithelial tumors, pleomorphic carcinomas, and lymphomas, are

rare. In metastases the CT-appearance depends on the vacularization of the primary tumors.

Retroperitoneal Space

Inflammation, Abscess, Haematoma, Urinoma, Cysts, Lymphoceles

Inflammations of the retroperitoneal space appear as an inhomogeneous mass with irregular configuration and irregular enhancement patterns. Abscesses are also delineable as inhomogeneous mass with an irregular configuration and rim enhancement, but are at times seen with liquid content and an air–liquid interface or small air/gas bubbles (Fig. 30.5).

Hematomas are easily seen using CT and have a mass appearance of varying size. The CT attenuation depends on the age and size of the bleeding. Sedimentation is possible. Sometimes active bleeding can be demonstrated on arterial phase or postcontrast scans as a high attenuation zone adjacent to a leaking vessel.

Urinomas present as fluid collection of urine within the perirenal fat after injuries of the urinary tract. Water-equivalent density values on precontrast or early CT scans, high contrast on late CT scans. True cysts of the retroperitoneal space are rare and exhibit water attenuation, thin wall, and no rim enhancement. Lymphoceles are more frequently observed after lymphadenectomy, kidney transplantation or gynecological surgery. Round or oval masses of water density without wall and without rim enhancement are seen here.

Primary Retroperitoneal Tumors

In retroperitoneal fibrosis a soft-tissue mass enveloping the aorta and vena cava is seen with an either sharply defined or indistinct margin. The posterior wall of the aorta is typically preserved. If a fibrous mass with fatty components is detected in the pelvis, a pelvic fibrolipomatosis should be considered.

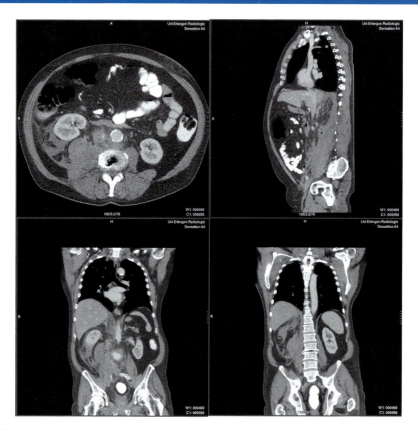

Fig. 30.5. Retroperitoneal abscess. Irregular enlargement and configuration of the right psoas muscle, streaky density changes in the retroperitoneal fat tissue. Air inclusions within the mass as a sign of infection

The most common mass in young children (50% are younger than 1 year, 90% are younger than 7 years) is the neuroblastoma. This is suspected if an inhomogeneous mass in the adrenal bed or paravertebral area, including areas of hemorrhage, necrosis, and calcifications, is seen. The differential diagnosis of the pediatric mass in the retroperitoneum is the rhabdomyosarcoma, featuring an inhomogeneous mass involving the urogenital tract or the muscles with intralesional hemorrhage and necrosis and strong enhancement.

Other entities include the teratoma with an very heterogeneous appearance with fat, soft-tissue, bone or teeth; lipoma with a well-circumscribed, homogenous mass of fat density without any soft tissue and without any enhancing component; liposarcoma, which is the second most common primary retroperitoneal tumor in adults, and is best described as a lipomatous mass with streaky densities, changes within of a lipomatous mass and sometimes with solid areas. A common lesion of the retroperitoneum is the malignant fibrous histiocytoma, showing an inhomogeneous mass with necrotic areas and intense contrast enhancement. Secondary retroperitoneal tumors, such as lymphadenopathy, must also be considered.

Comparison with other Imaging Modalities

Pancreas

The value of CT in management of severe acute pancreatitis is well established [1,2].

Magnetic resonance tomography has been shown to be as effective as CT in demonstrating the presence and extent of pancreatic necrosis and fluid collections. Both CT and MRI can be used to diagnose advanced chronic pancreatitis. But both have limitations in the recognition of earliest changes of chronic pancreatitis. For earliest changes, ERCP and pancreatic function tests remain more sensitive than CT and/or MRI (including MRCP).

With multislice CT it is possible to detect the pancreatic tumors and to provide information about the resectability of a tumor. Multiplanar reconstructions are very helpful to detect or to exclude vascular infiltration. The major limitation of CT is the poor sensitivity for detecting lymph node involvement. In different studies, the value of the different imaging modalities has been discussed. Soriano et al. [6] reported a prospective preoperative study comparing endoscopic ultrasonography, helical computed tomography, magnetic resonance imaging, and angiography. In this study spiral CT and endoscopic ultrasonography are the most useful individual imaging techniques in the staging of pancreatic cancer. Thus, helical CT as an initial test and EUS as a confirmatory technique seems to be the most reliable and cost-minimizing strategy [3–5].

Retroperitoneal Space

MSCT provides reliable imaging of the organs in the retroperitoneal space unaffected by bowel gas and also allows delineation of the facial planes and retroperitoneal compartments in arbitrary planes, making it an ideal tool for assessment of retroperitoneal disease. Ultrasonography is limited by a variety of patient-dependent, not to mention investigator-dependent, factors. In clinically stable patients MRI may be a useful modality for providing helpful and additional information in characterizing retroperitoneal abnormalities [1].

References

1. Szolar DH, Uggowitzer MM, Kammerhuber FH, Schreyer HH (1997) Benigne, nicht organgebundene Erkrankungen des Retroperitonealraumes. RöFo 167:107–121
2. Nishino M, Hayakawa K, Minami M, Yamamoto A, Ueda H, Takasu K (2003) Primary retroperitoneal neoplasms: CT and MRI imaging findings with anatomic and pathologic diagnostic clues. Radiographics 23:45–57
3. Robinson PJ, Sheridan MB (2000) Pancreatitis: computed tompgraphy and magnetic resonance imaging. Eur Radiol 10:401–408
4. Jacobs JE, Birnbaum BA (2001) Computed tomography evaluation of acute pancreatitis. Semin Roentgenol 36:92–98
5. Kalra MK, Maher MM, Mueller PR, Saini S (2003) State-of-the-art imaging of pancreatic neoplasms. Brit J Radiol 76:857–865
6. Soriano A, Castells A, Ayuso C, Ayuso JR, de Caralt MT, Gines MA, Real MI, Gilabert R, Quinto L, Trilla A, Feu F, Montanya X, Fernandez-Cruz L, Navarro S (2004) Preoperative staging an assessment of pancreatic cancer: prospective study comparing endoscopic ultrasonography, helical computed tomography, magnetic resonance imaging and angiography. Am J Gastroenterol 99:492–501

31 Gastrointestinal Tract

A.J. Aschoff

Indications

- Small bowel: tumors, bleeding, ischemia.
- Large bowel: bleeding, ischemia, diverticulitis.

Patient Preparation, Patient Positioning, Topogram/Scan Range

Do not use positive oral contrast. Instead have the patients drink 1.5 L water (the last 300–500 mL immediately before scanning on the CT table).

Bowel relaxation may achieve better image quality (e.g., 40 mg of Hyoscine-N-butylbromide (Buscopan, Boehringer Ingelheim, Germany) administered by i.v.).

Additional water is administered through a rectal enema tube immediately before examination for suspected colon pathology, e.g., diverticulitis (especially fistulae) (Fig. 31.1).

Supine scan position (arms elevated, feet first).

Scan from xyphoid through pubic symphysis.

Table Scan Parameter

See Table 31.1 (the given values are examples).

Tips and Tricks

The question of whether to use positive or negative contrast material for bowel disten-

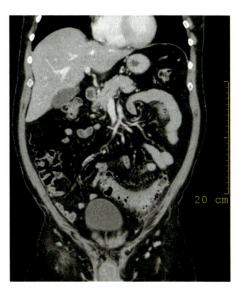

Fig. 31.1. Coronal reformation of venous phase scan depicting sigma diverticulitis

tion for MDCT of the gastrointestinal tract remains controversial. Some authors argue that positive contrast material is definitely indicated in cases of bowel obstruction and is also probably more advantageous for the delineation of the inner bowel wall layers in the case of pronounced hypoattenuation of the bowel wall. Water is probably more advantageous when assessing abnormal bowel wall enhancement in cases with absent or minor bowel wall thickening, especially if CT angiography is performed simultaneously [1]. We continuously achieve excellent results using water only.

In selected cases, modifying the protocol to perform a CT enteroclysis might improve sensitivity and specificity in depicting small bowel tumors or inflammatory changes,

Table 31.1. Scan parameters for gastrointestinal tract MD-CT

Parameters	4–8 slice scanners	10–16 slice scanners	32–64 slice scanners
Scanning parameters unenhanced/arterial venous			
Tube voltage (kV)	120	120	120
Rotation time (s)	0.5	0.375–0.5	0.33–0.5
Tube current (mAs)	200	200	200
Pitch corrected Tube current time product (eff. mAs)	220	160–200	220–240
Slice collimation (mm)	5 – 5	1.5 0.75 0.75	1.25 0.625 1.25
Norm. pitch	0.9 – 0.9	1.3 1.0 1.0	0.9 0.8 0.8
Reconstruction increment (mm)	6.5 – 3.2	5 1 1.5	1.5 0.4 1
Reconstruction thickness (mm)	6.5 – 6.5	2.5 2 3	3 0.8 2
Contrast material: indication (arterial and venous phase)			
Volume (mL) 300 mg I/mL 400 mg I/mL	 130 90	 – 90	 – 90
Injection speed (mL/s)	3	3.5	3.5
Saline flush (mL, mL/s)	40 3	30 3.5	30 3.5
Delay arterial (s)	–	30 (bolus track preferred)	30 (bolus track preferred)
Delay venous (s)	80	80	80
Contrast material: indication (single acquisition; venous phase only)			
Volume (mL)	110	90	90
Injection speed (mL/s)	3	3	3
Saline flush (mL, mL/s)	40 3	30 3	30 3
Delay (s)	60–80	60–80	60–80

such as in Crohn's disease [2]. Position an 8F nasojejunal tube into the duodenojejunal junction under fluoroscopic guidance. Infuse up to 2000 mL water at room temperature with a pressure-controlled pump at a rate of 150–200 mL/min.

Tumors

The most common gastrointestinal mesenchymal tumor is the gastrointestinal stromal tumor (GIST, synonyms: leiomyoma or leiomyosarcoma). GISTs may be found any-

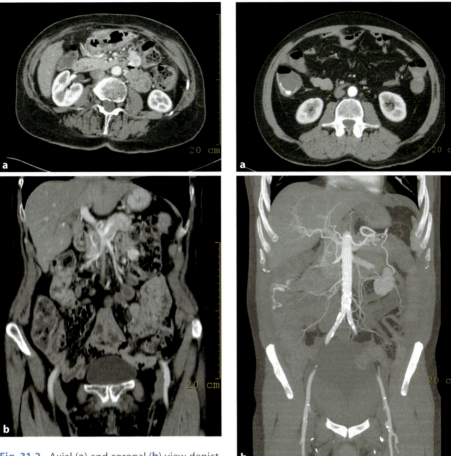

Fig. 31.2. Axial (**a**) and coronal (**b**) view depicting hypervasular gastrointestinal stromal tumor originating from proximal jejunum

Fig. 31.3. Axial CT (**a**) and coronal MIP (**b**) revealing active hemorrhage from angiodysplasia in the ascending colon

where in the GI tract, although the stomach is the most common site. MDCT may show hypervascular submucosal masses (Fig. 31.2).

GI Bleeding

Acute gastrointestinal (GI) bleeding is common with patients presenting with melena, hematemesis, or hematochezia. In addition to the established initial workup (endoscopy and barium studies), MDCT is beginning to establish itself for this indication (Fig. 31.3). It may be especially helpful in the workup of obscure bleeding (a recurrent bleeding in which no definite source has been identified through routine diagnostic examinations). Miller and coworkers reported their findings in 2004 using contrast-enhanced MDCT with water as an oral contrast agent to detect GI bleeding due to a number of etiologies [3]. Tew and coworkers even proposed MDCT as an alternative to first-line investigation to locate lower gastrointestinal bleeding before placing the patient under observation, performing embolization, or surgery [4].

Kuhle and Shiman experimentally determined that (conservatively) helical CT has the potential to depict active colonic

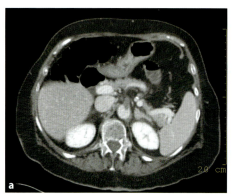

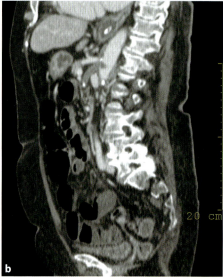

Fig. 31.4. Axial (**a**) and sagittal (**b**) view depicting thrombosis of superior mesenteric artery

hemorrhage at rates of 0.5 mL/min or even less [5].

Mesenteric Ischemia

Another relatively rare but important cause for acute abdominal pain is mesenteric ischemia. It may be caused by many conditions and may mimic various intestinal diseases. Bowel ischemia severity ranges from transient superficial changes of the intestinal mucosa to life-threatening transmural bowel wall necrosis. CT can demonstrate changes in ischemic bowel segments accurately, is often helpful in determining the primary cause of ischemia, and can demonstrate important coexistent findings or complications [1]. In a study by Taourel, each of the following findings had a specificity of more than 95% and a sensitivity of less than 30% for the diagnosis of acute mesenteric ischemia: arterial or venous thrombosis (Fig. 31.4), intramural gas, portalvenous gas, focal lack of bowel-wall enhancement, and liver or splenic infarcts [6]. When CT was used in the diagnosis of suspected acute mesenteric ischemia, the detection of at least one of these signs resulted in a sensitivity of 64% at a specificity of 92%.

References

1. Wiesner W, Khurana B, Ji H, Ros PR (2003) CT of acute bowel ischemia. Radiology 226:635–650
2. Boudiaf M, Jaff A, Soyer P, Bouhnik Y, Hamzi L, Rymer R (2004) Small-bowel diseases: prospective evaluation of multidetector row helical CT enteroclysis in 107 consecutive patients. Radiology 233:338–344
3. Miller FH, Hwang CM (2004) An initial experience: using helical CT imaging to detect obscure gastrointestinal bleeding. Clin Imaging 28:245–251
4. Tew K, Davies RP, Jadun CK, Kew J (2004) MDCT of acute lower gastrointestinal bleeding. AJR Am J Roentgenol 182:427–430
5. Kuhle WG, Sheiman RG (2003) Detection of active colonic hemorrhage with use of helical CT: findings in a swine model. Radiology 228:743–752
6. Taourel PG, Deneuville M, Pradel JA, Regent D, Bruel JM (1996) Acute mesenteric ischemia: diagnosis with contrast-enhanced CT. Radiology 99:632–636

32 CT Colonography

A.J. Aschoff

Indications

- The main clinical indication is the detection of colon polyps and tumorous lesions.
- Additional examination after incomplete colonoscopy.

Patient Preparation, Patient Positioning, Topogram/Scan Range

The most important prerequisite for successful CT colonography is a clean colon! Many different cleansing strategies obtain this goal. One example is described below in Tips and Tricks.

Bowel relaxation before rectal air insufflation achieves better pneumocolon (e.g., 40 mg of Hyoscine-N-butylbromide (Buscopan; Boehringer Ingelheim, Germany) administered by i.v.).

Room air (alternatively CO_2) is carefully insufflated through a rectal enema tube, e.g., using a manual balloon pump. The rectal balloon of the enema catheter is blocked to prevent air leakage. Filling is stopped when the patient expresses discomfort. Some centers use CO_2 for bowel distention. Since CO_2 is resorbed, it seems more comfortable for the patient in the time following the examination. However, a dedicated device for the insufflation of CO_2 is necessary.

Two scans are required: supine and prone positions (arms elevated, feet first).

Scan from xyphoid through pubic symphysis.

Scan Parameters

See Table 32.1 (the given values are examples).

Tips and Tricks

Bowel cleansing is important (Fig. 32.1)! The following is just one example for preparation; note that many different protocols may work.

Start two days prior to the examination with 10 mg of the suppository Bisacodyl (Laxbene, Merckel GmbH, Blaubeuren, Germany) followed by 5 mg of Bisacodyl the day before examination. From then on patients should drink one glass of fluids (coffee, tea, soup, etc.) every hour. At noon the day before CT colonography another 5 mg of Bisacodyl is taken and patients drink a glass of water every hour. Finally 1 L of polyethylene-glycol-based electrolyte solution (Delcoprep, DeltaSelect GmbH, Pfullingen, Germany) consisting of Na^+ (125 mmol/L), K^+ (10 mmol/L), Cl^- (35 mmol/L), HCO_3^- (20 mmol/L), SO_4^- (40 mmol/L) is taken orally 2.5 h prior to the examination.

Use the CT scout to evaluate air filling and proper distension of the colon. If pneumocolon seems insufficient, insufflate more air and obtain another CT scout.

Some prefer to do a quick analysis of the first scan using the axial source images and perform the second scan contrast enhanced if a suspect lesion is found.

In order to maintain a sufficient pneumocolon, we routinely administer more room air through the rectal tube after the patient has turned from supine to prone position before the second scan.

Table 32.1. Scan parameters for CT colonography

Parameters	4–8 slice scanners	10–16 slice scanners	32–64 slice scanners
Scanning parameters			
Tube voltage (kV)	120	120	120
Rotation time (s)	0.5	0.5	0.5
Tube current time product (mAs)	150–225	150–225	150–225
Pitch corrected tube current time product (eff. mAs)	120–150	120–150	120–150
Slice collimation (mm)	2.5	0.625/0.75	0.6/0.625
Norm. pitch	1.25–1.5	1.25–1.5	1.25–1.5
Reconstruction increment (mm)	1.5	0.5	0.5
Reconstruction thickness (mm)	3	1	0.75–1
Contrast material: indication	Unenhanced	Unenhanced	Unenhanced

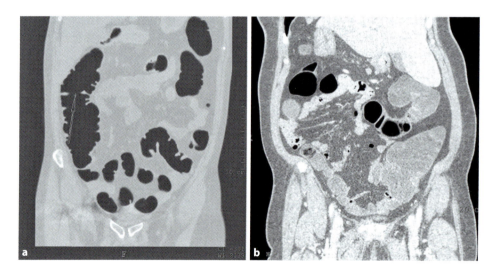

Fig. 32.1. Comparison of excellent bowel cleansing and sufficient pneumocolon (**a**) with unsatisfactory bowel cleansing (**b**) which renders sufficient pneumocolon and corresponding evaluation impossible

Image analysis: it should be noted that different vendors offer different fully automatic or semiautomatic analysis tools with FDA approval. However, one should not completely rely on these automatically computed results, but use axial and MPR reconstructions to verify the findings.

Virtual colonography was first described by Vining in 1994 [1]. The basic procedure has remained unchanged over the last 10 years (bowel cleaning, bowel distension, fast helical-CT, 2D and 3D postprocessing). The term CT colonography is preferred over virtual colonography [2]. Scanning patients in both the prone and supine position increases the sensitivity of polyp detection significantly [3].

The clinical background behind polyp screening is the well-known adenoma–carcinoma sequence. Polyps of more than 1 cm in size have a 10% risk over 10 years and of 25% risk over 20 years of becoming carcinomas [4].

Pickhardt and coworkers published the largest clinical study on CT colonography in 2003 [5]. A group of 1233 patients from three centers were examined with both CT colonography (slice thickness 1.5 or 2.5 mm) and conventional colonoscopy the same day. CT colonography was evaluated using 2D and 3D postprocessing. The authors calculated a sensitivity for the detection of polyps >10 mm in size of 93.8% (> 8 mm: 93.3%; >6 mm: 88.7%) and concluded that CT colonography with the use of a three-dimensional approach is an accurate screening method for the detection of colorectal neoplasia in asymptomatic average risk adults.

Dose issues are especially important in screening an asymptomatic population. One option to reduce dose is to scan either the prone or supine position with a reduced tube current, e.g., 50 mAs. Some authors are suggesting that even ultra-low-dose protocols with 10 mAs and an effective dose of less than 1 mSv are feasible [6].

Despite the excellent data presented by Pickhardt, it is still unclear whether CT colonography will establish itself for routine polyp screening; controversial data on this subject is still being published. In a recent study, Rockey and coworkers compared air contrast barium enema (ACBE), CT colonography (CTC), and colonoscopy in 614 patients and found that on a per-patient basis, for lesions 10 mm or larger in size (n=63), the sensitivity of ACBE was 48%, CTC 59%, and colonoscopy 98% (p<0.0001 for colonoscopy vs. CTC) [7]. The specificity was greater for colonoscopy (0.996) than for either ACBE (0.90) or CTC (0.96) as well and declined even further for ACBE and CTC when smaller lesions were considered.

Despite these studies, it is yet to be seen if CT colonography will really become a widespread clinically accepted alternative to conventional colonoscopy (Fig. 32.2).

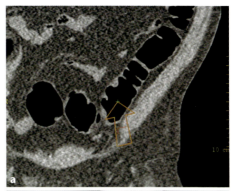
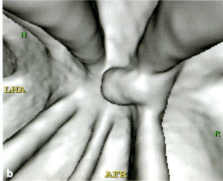
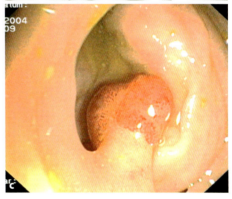

Fig. 32.2. Comparison of MPR (a), 3D virtual endoscopic (b) and real colonoscopic view (c) of a small polyp in the distal descending colon

References

1. Vining DJ, Gelfand DW (1994) Noninvasive colonoscopy using helical CT scanning, 3D reconstruction, and virtual reality. In: Annual meeting of the Society of Gastrointestinal Radiologists, 13–18 February 1994, Maui

2. Johnson CD, Hara AK, Reed JE (1998) Virtual endoscopy: what's in a name? AJR Am J Roentgenol 171:1201–1202

3. Fletcher JG, Johnson CD, Welch TJ, MacCarty RL, Ahlquist DA, Reed JE, Harmsen WS, Wilson LA (2000) Optimization of CT colonography technique: prospective trial in 180 patients. Radiology 216:704–711

4. Stryker SJ, Wolff BG, Culp CE, Libbe SD, Ilstrup DM, MacCarty RL (1987) Natural history of untreated colonic polyps. Gastroenterology 93:1009–1013

5. Pickhardt PJ, Choi JR, Hwang I, Butler JA, Puckett ML, Hildebrandt HA, Wong RK, Nugent PA, Mysliwiec PA, Schindler WR (2003) Computed tomographic virtual colonoscopy to screen for colorectal neoplasia in asymptomatic adults. N Engl J Med 349:2191–2200

6. Cohnen M, Vogt C, Beck A, Andersen K, Heinen W, vom Dahl S, Aurich V, Haeussinger D, Moedder U (2004) Feasibility of MDCT colonography in ultra-low-dose technique in the detection of colorectal lesions: comparison with high-resolution video colonoscopy. AJR Am J Roentgenol 183:1355–1359

7. Rockey DC, Paulson E, Niedzwiecki D, Davis W, Bosworth HB, Sanders L, Yee J, Henderson J, Hatten P, Burdick S, Sanyal A, Rubin DT, Sterling M, Akerkar G, Bhutani MS, Binmoeller K, Garvie J, Bini EJ, McQuaid K, Foster WL, Thompson WM, Dachman A, Halvorsen R (2005) Analysis of air contrast barium enema, computed tomographic colonography, and colonoscopy: prospective comparison. Lancet 365:305–311

VII Musculoskeletal

33 Musculoskeletal Imaging

F. Dammann

Indications

- Acute trauma.
- Posttraumatic follow-up (recalcification, pseudarthosis, intraarticular bodies).
- Inflammatory disease (chronic osteomyelitis, sequestration, fistulae).
- Soft tissue complications (fistulae, abscess, calcifications).
- Spine: vertebral disc protrusion and herniation, spondylolisthesis, arthrosis.
- Arthrography (capsular or cartilage damage).
- Congenital deformities.
- Bone and soft tissue tumors.
- MR contraindications.

Patient Preparation

No special preparation necessary; i.v. access if CM administration needed.

Patient Positioning

Depending on pathology and/or anatomical site, see comments.

Topogram/Scan Range

Depending on pathology and/or anatomical site, see comments.

Table Scan Parameter

- Cervical spine: see Table 33.1.

- Thoracic and lumbar spine, shoulder, and pelvis: see Table 33.2.
- Extremities, elbow, wrist, hand, knee, ankle, and foot: see Table 33.3.
- Three-dimensional reformations and soft tissue diagnosis: see Table 33.4.

Comments, Tips, and Tricks

Introduction

CT is accepted as the imaging modality of choice in most skeletal diseases when structural or spatial information of the affected bones and articulations is needed [1–3]. A special advantage of CT is its capability of a fast whole body examination that offers diagnostic information about all organ systems. When using the MSCT technique for whole-body evaluation, no additional CT examination is needed for musculoskeletal diagnosis in many cases. Specific image datasets that fulfill the requirements of musculoskeletal diagnosis can be calculated out of the primary raw dataset. However, best image quality is provided by focused musculoskeletal CT when optimized parameters are also applied for data acquisition.

Examination range, mAs setting, FOV, pitch, the type of image postprocessing (e.g., 3D reformations), and the i.v. application of contrast material depend on the clinical request. The examination of the extremity bones is not explicitly discussed in this chapter, but a CT protocol corresponding to the extremity joints (elbow, wrist, knee, and ankle) is recommended for these parts of the skeleton.

Table 33.1. Scan parameters for cervical spine. A thickness of 2 mm is recommended for standard axial slices. Additionally, a thin-slice dataset is calculated as a basis for multiplanar reformations

Parameters	4–8 slice scanners	10–16 slice scanners	32–64 slice scanners
Scanner settings			
Tube voltage (kV)	120	120	120
Rotation time (s)	<1	<1	<1
Tube current time product (mAs)	120–270	120–360	120–360
Pitch corrected tube current time product (eff. mAs)	150–300	150–300	150–300
Collimation (mm)	1.0–1.5	0,625–1.0	0.6–1.0
Norm. pitch	0.8-0.9	0.8–1.2	0.8–1.2
Reconstruction increment (mm)	2.0 for recons: 0.6	2.0 for recons: 0.5	2.0 for recons: 0.4
Reconstruction slice thickness (mm)	2–3 For recons: 1.0	2–3 For recons: 0.75–1	2–3 For recons: 0.6–0.75
Convolution kernel	Bone + standard	Bone + standard	Bone + standard
Contrast media application	no (facultatively)	no (facultatively)	no (facultatively)

Table 33.2. Scan parameters for thoracic and lumbar spine, shoulder, and pelvis. A small slice thickness and pitch is recommended. Increased values may be necessary when a large body range has to be examined.

Parameters	4–8 slice scanners	10–16 slice scanners	32–64 slice scanners
Scanner-settings			
Tube voltage (kV)	120	120	120
Rotation time (s)	<1	<1	<1
Tube current time product (mAs)	150–360	150–480	225–480
Pitch corrected Tube current time product (eff. mAs)	250–400	250–400	250–400
Collimation (mm)	1.0–2.0	0.625–1.5	0.6–1.2
Norm. Pitch	0.6–1.5	0.6–1.5	0.9–1.5
Reconstruction increment (mm)	2–3 For recons: 0.7	2–3 For recons: 0.6	2–3 For recons: 0.5
Reconstruction slice thickness (mm)	2.0 For recons: 1.0	2.0 For recons: 0.75	2.0 For recons: 0.6
Convolution kernel	Bone + standard	Bone + standard	Bone + standard
Contrast media application	no (facultatively)	no (facultatively)	no (facultatively)

Table 33.3. Scan parameters for bones and joints of the extremities (elbow, wrist, knee, and ankle). A slice thickness of maximum 1 mm is recommended for small bones especially when subtle trauma or pseudarthrosis has to be evaluated (reconstructions obligatory in angulated coronal and sagittal plane as well as anatomically adapted)

Parameters	4–8 slice scanners	10–16 slice scanners	32–64 slice scanners
Scanner-settings			
Tube voltage (kV)	120	120	120
Rotation time (s)	<1	<1	<1
Tube current time product (mAs)	30–135	30–144	30–144
Pitch corrected Tube current time product (eff. mAs)	50–150	50–150	50–150
Collimation (mm)	1.0–1.25	0.6–0.75	0.6–0.625
Norm. pitch	0.6–0.9	0.6–1.2	0.6–1.2
Reconstruction increment (mm)	0.6	0.5	0.4
Reconstruction slice thickness (mm)	2 For recons: 1.0	2 For recons: 0.75	2 For recons: 0.6
Convolution kernel	Bone–high res.	Bone–high res.	Bone–high res.
Contrast media application	no (facultatively)	no (facultatively)	no (facultatively)

Table 33.4. The calculation of additional image datasets out of the raw data is recommended for optimal image quality of multiplanar or 3D reformations and for soft-tissue evaluation

Parameters	4–8 slice scanners	10–16 slice scanners	32–64 slice scanners
Specials			
3D reformations (SSD, volume rendering)	Rec. incr.: 0.6 mm Rec. slice th.: 1.0 mm Kernel: (medium) soft	Rec. incr.: 0.5 mm Rec. slice th.: 0.75 mm Kernel: (medium) soft	Rec. incr.: 0.4 mm Rec. slice th.: 0.6 mm Kernel: medium (soft)
Soft tissue	Rec. incr.: 3–10 mm Rec. slice th.: 4–10 mm Convolution kernel: soft		

Scan Range

The scan range covers the entire extent of disease and also includes a sufficient part of nonaffected bone and/or related articulation to allow for a clear anatomical orientation and an appropriate surgical planning.

mAs

A standard or elevated mAs value is recommended for the evaluation of subtle fractures, osteoporotic bones, fracture healing, or soft tissue pathology. The mAs setting (and exposure dose, resp.) may be reduced when the information requested from CT is limited to the clarification of a complicated spatial position of fracture fragments or other bone deformations.

FOV, Pitch

The FOV should be set as small as possible since a high spatial resolution is crucial in skeletal CT. A small pitch factor improves the image quality within the z-axis and is recommended especially for the diagnosis of small anatomical structures. However, if a large scan range has to be covered, a higher pitch value may be required by the CT machine, depending on limitations of the heat capacity of the X-ray tube and/or the amount of raw data that is accepted for image processing.

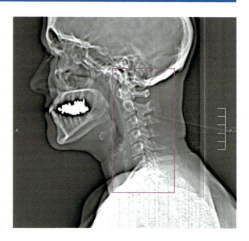

Fig. 33.1. Lateral topogram of the cervical spine. The CT examination of the entire cervical spine includes the skull base and the first thoracic vertebral segments

MPR, 3D Reformations

Multiplanar image reformation is a standard procedure in skeletal CT. The orientation of reformation planes should be anatomically adjusted in all three dimensions by the use of the MPR package of the CT software. Sagittal and coronal reformations are useful in almost all musculoskeletal examinations. Additional axially angulated slices can be helpful to achieve anatomically adopted images without the need of additional CT scans with angulated gantry or an uncomfortable patient positioning. Surface shaded display (SSD) or the volume-rendering technique (VRT) enable an intuitive understanding of the spatial information in trauma patients, congenital deformities, arthritis, or for the evaluation of posttherapeutic complications [2,4–7].

Contrast Material

The use of i.v. contrast material is indicated when bone affections go along with pathologic soft tissue changes, including diffuse or circumscript inflammatory disease, liquid retentions, abscesses, or solid soft-tissue tumors. For the diagnosis of fistulae or sequestration a direct CM injection into the cutaneous orifice of the fistula may be helpful to depict the localization and the extent of disease. In general MRI is the modality of choice for the diagnosis of musculoskeletal soft tissue affections due to the superior soft tissue contrast. However, musculoskeletal CT should include soft tissue evaluation with the use of i.v. contrast when MRI is contraindicated, useless due to metal artifacts, or in cases when CT is preferred over MRI for other reasons, such as shorter scan time.

A postmyelographic spinal CT is recommended for increased contrast when an intraspinal or intradural process, or other pathological narrowing of the CSF space is suspected.

Cervical Spine

Patient position is supine and head first, arms parallel to the body, shoulders down, using headrest. Remove dental prostheses, necklaces, etc. Scanner settings: see Table 33.1.

Orthogonal positioning of the patient's head simplifies the image interpretation. Sagittal and coronal MPR are obligatory. Axially angulated reconstructions perpen-

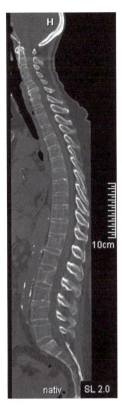

Fig. 33.2. Sagittal reformation of the entire vertebral spine (16-row MSCT, 100 mAs, coll. 0.75 mm, pitch 1.2, slice thickness 2 mm)

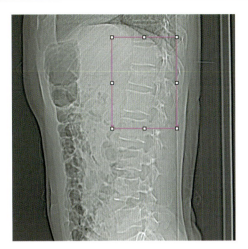

Fig. 33.3. Lateral topogram of a patient with acute fracture of the twelfth thoracic vertebral body. The topogram extends to the sacrum to enable an accurate classification of the anatomic level. The scan range includes the adjacent non-injured vertebral segments for surgical planning

dicular to the spine are recommended when a detailed evaluation of the intervertbral discs, the vertebral body, or vertebral arch is demanded. Trauma diagnosis includes the injured vertebral body (or bodies) as well as each noninjured adjacent segment cranially and caudally for surgical planning (Figs. 33.1 and 33.2).

Thoracic and Lumbar Spine

Standard patient position is supine and head first, arms elevated, legs elevated for comfort. Scanner settings: see Table 33.2.

A small pitch value (up to 1.0) is recommended for short scan ranges (e.g., up to three vertebrae) for increased image quality. The examination of large spine ranges often requires higher pitch values

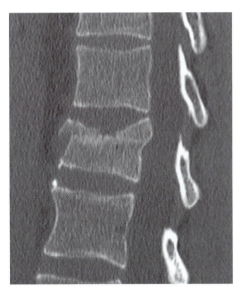

Fig. 33.4. Sagittal reformation shows compression fracture of the ventral part of the 12th vertebral body with involvement of the posterior surface as a sign of instability (16-row MSCT, 250 mAs, coll. 0.75 mm, pitch 0.9, slice thickness 2 mm)

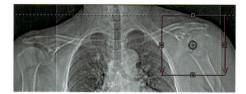

Fig. 33.10. Topogram of shoulder CT in acute trauma of the proximal humerus. A small field of view is recommended for optimal spatial image resolution

(Figs. 33.3 and 33.4). Scan range and MPR: see cervical spine.

Shoulder

Patient position: supine, head first, arms parallel to the body. Keep sufficient distance between gantry and shoulder, otherwise image quality may be reduced due to artifacts. Depending on the size of the patient a slightly lateral bending of the chest to the opposite side is recommended to increase the distance between shoulder and gantry. Scanner settings: see Table 33.2.

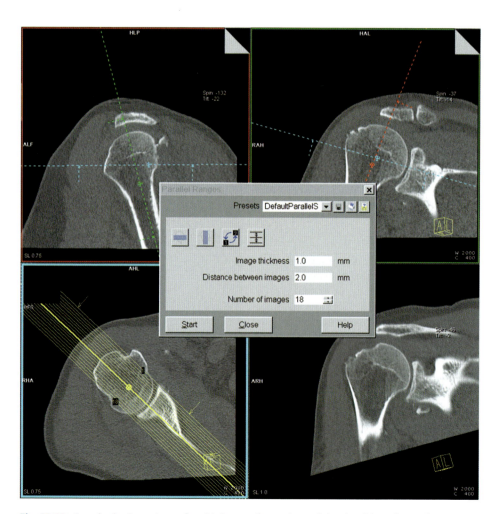

Fig. 33.11. Standard orientations of multiplanar reformations of the shoulder refer to the position of the scapula axis as the anatomical reference structure. Planning of semicoronal slices is shown in the left lower quadrant

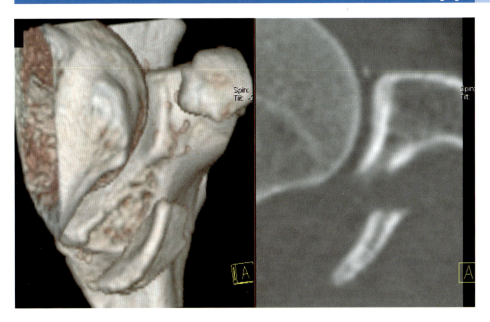

Fig. 33.12. VRT rendering and semicoronal reformation of the right shoulder show a large Bankart lesion at the antero-inferior glenoidal rim with displacement (16-row CT, 250 mAs, coll. 0.75 mm, pitch 0.9; 3D datasets: slice thickness 0.75 mm, increment 0.5 mm, kernel: medium soft for VRT and high for MPR)

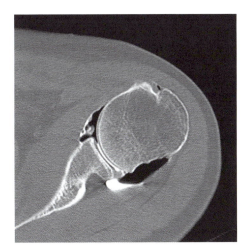

Fig. 33.13. Arthro-CT of the left shoulder. Articular capsule distended by air. Articular cartilage is delineated by covering of contrast material. Rupture and displacement of the anterior labrum (16-row CT, 250 mAs, coll. 0.75 mm, pitch 0.9, slice thickness 2 mm)

Scan range includes the acromioclavicular joint cranially and the inferior angle of the scapula caudally in the case of extended scapular trauma. For localized disease (affection of the humeral head or the glenoid process, also standard arthro-CT of the shoulder) the caudal extension of the scan is limited to the infraglenoid bursa. MPR images include semicoronal slices parallel to the scapular axis and perpendicularly oriented semisagittal slices. Double contrast arthro-CT is indicated for the evaluation of the glenoid labrum, the glenohumeral ligaments, and the fibrous capsule (Figs. 33.10–33.13).

Elbow

Patient position: prone, head first. Affected arm elevated and the other arm parallel to the body. A slight angulation of the elbow is recommended to simplify the image interpretation. Do not angulate the forearm parallel to the gantry, otherwise an increased

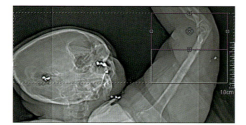

Fig. 33.8. Topogram for planning elbow CT in a patient with chronic osteomyelitis of the humerus and limited mobility of shoulder and elbow following complex trauma. Examination range depends on the clinical region of interest

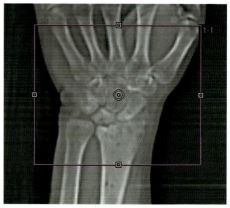

Fig. 33.5. AP topogram of the wrist in a patient with posttraumatic arthrosis. Scan range includes a part of the metacarpal bones and the distal radius to allow for the evaluation of the entire functional compartment

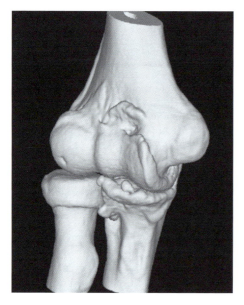

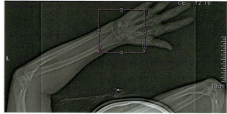

Fig. 33.6. Topogram of focused scaphoid bone CT with the patient's forearm slightly inclined. As a result, the long axis of the scaphoid bone is positioned parallel to the scan plane

Fig. 33.9. SSD of the elbow in a long term follow-up after elbow luxation. A central defect within the capitulum surface, severe arthrotic deformation of the humeroulnar joint and osseous articular bodies are clearly depicted (16-row CT, 90 mAs, coll. 0.75 mm, pitch 0.9; 3D dataset: slice thickness 0.75 mm, increment 0.5 mm, kernel medium soft; SSD threshold 220 HU)

the forearm, respectively. 3D reformations are often very helpful due to the limited anatomical clearness of slice images at the elbow (Figs. 33.8 and 33.9).

Wrist/Hand

Patient position: prone, head first. Affected arm elevated and the other arm parallel to the body. For wrist and general hand CT, a position of the forearm perpendicular to the gantry is recommended to simplify the image interpretation. As an exception, in scaphoid CT for the diagnosis of acute scaphoid fracture or pseudarthosis, a hand position with the long axis of the scaphoid

image noise will reduce the image quality notably. Scanner settings: see Table 33.3.

Sagittal reformations are angulated parallel to the humerus and ulna (and/or radius, resp.). For coronal images two separate image sets are recommended with an orientation parallel to humerus or parallel to

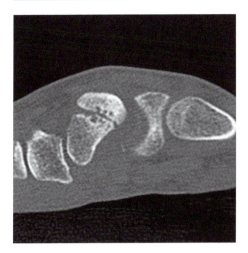

Fig. 33.7. Direct high-resolution scan of the scaphoid bone (patient position: see Fig. 33.6) showing a posttraumatic pseudarthrosis. 16-row CT, 90 mAs, coll. 0.75 mm, pitch 1.0, slice thickness 0.75 mm

bone adjusted parallel to the scan plane (patient position to be verified on topogram), a very small FOV (max. 50 mm), an image thickness of 1 mm, and a high or ultrahigh kernel is recommended to achieve high image resolution.

In addition to coronal and/or sagittal reformations 3D images are often very helpful to understand the spatial relationships of bones, fragments, or articulations in trauma patients or congenital deformities (Figs. 33.5–33.7).

Pelvis

Standard patient position is supine and head first, arms elevated. If the examination includes hip and femur a feet-first position may be necessary, depending on the patient size and table movement range. Scanner settings: see Table 33.2.

Axial and coronal reformations are most advantageous. In trauma patients sagittal reformations of the hips, coronary angulated reformations of the sacrum and/or the femoral neck, and 3D reformations (SSD, VRT) are very helpful for surgical planning and postoperative follow-up. Soft tissue im-

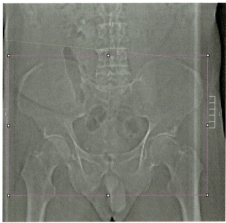

Fig. 33.14. AP topogram of the pelvis. Scan range includes iliac crest and pelvic floor

ages (Table 33.4) are frequently used to di-

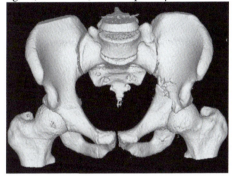

Fig. 33.15. SSD of a pelvic fracture with involvement of the left acetabulum (16-row CT, 250 mAs, coll. 0.75 mm, pitch 1.2)

agnose hematoma or inflammatory disease as a complication of pelvic bone affection (Figs. 33.14 and 33.15).

Knee

Patient position is supine and feet first. Arms may rest parallel to the body. Scanner settings: see Table 33.3. Examination range varies with the extent of disease. A conventional radiograph can be helpful for planning. An intermediate or low mAs setting can frequently be applied at knee CT

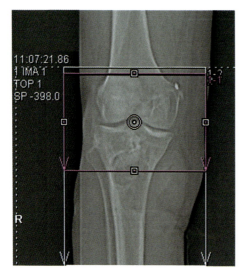

Fig. 33.16. AP topogram of the knee. Scan range depends on clinical request. Figure demonstrates example of a standard (small) range and an extended range that was applied in this case because posttraumatic sequestration within the proximal tibia had to be evaluated

with the exception of the presence of plaster casts or orthopedic metal devices. Coronal, sagittal, and 3D reformations are frequently more helpful than the primary axial slices (Fig. 33.16 and 33.17).

Ankle/Foot

Patient position is supine and feet first. To simplify the image interpretation a 90-degree angulation of the ankle is recommended and can be achieved by using a wood block and fixation of the feet. Scanner settings: see Table 33.3.

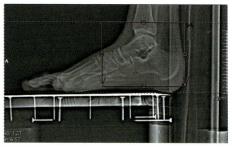

Fig. 33.18. Lateral topogram of the ankle and foot. Foot positioning is supported by a wooden block. Scan range depends on clinical request and includes the ankle and the tarsal bones in this case

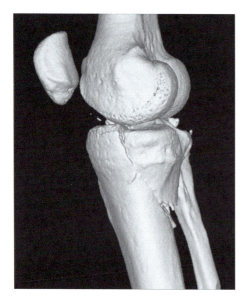

Fig. 33.17. Mediolateral SSD view of a tibial depression fracture with displacement of a large dorsal fragment (16-row CT, 90 mAs, coll. 0.75 mm, pitch 0.9; 3D dataset: slice thickness 0.75 mm, increment 0.5 mm, kernel medium soft; SSD threshold 220 HU)

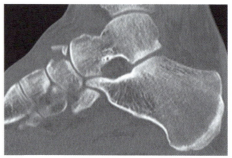

Fig. 33.19. Fracture at the dorsal surface of the navicular bone. Sagittal reformation (16-row CT, 90 mAs, coll. 0.75 mm, pitch 0.9, slice thickness 2 mm)

Sagittal and coronal reformations are recommended as a standard in evaluating the ankle and the bones of the foot. 3D reformations are also very helpful due to the complex three-dimensional relationship of pathologic findings to the anatomical structures and may also be used to diagnose soft tissue involvement (Figs. 33.18–33.19).

References

1 Hipp JA, Springfield DS, Hayes WC (1995) Predicting pathologic fracture risk in the management of metastatic bone defects. Clin Orthop 312:120–135
2 Watura R, Cobby M, Taylor J (2004) Multislice CT in imaging of trauma of the spine, pelvis and complex foot injuries. Br J Radiol 77(1): S46–S63
3 Buckwalter KA, Farber JM (2004) Application of multidetector CT in skeletal trauma. Semin Musculoskelet Radiol 8:147–156
4 Choplin R, Buckwalter KA, Rydberg J, Farber JM (2004) CT with 3D rendering of the tendons of the foot and ankle: Technique, normal anatomy, and disease. RadioGraphics 24:343–356
5 Pretorius ES, Fishman EK (1999) Volume-rendered three-dimensional spiral CT: Musculoskeletal applications. RadioGraphics 19:1143–1160
6 Rieker O, Mildenberger P, Rudig L, Schweden F, Thelen M (1998) 3D CT of fractures: comparison of volume and surface reconstruction. Rofo Fortschr Geb Rontgenstr Neuen Bildgeb Verfahr 169:490–494
7 Kiuru MJ, Haapamaki VV, Koivikko MP, Koskinen SK (2004) Wrist injuries; diagnosis with multidetector CT. Emerg Radiol 10:182–185

VIII Trauma

34 Trauma Imaging

R. Kottke and A. Kuettner

Indications

Rapid assessment of patients with major trauma and suspected life-threatening injuries. When attempting to rationale the most appropriate examining strategy, please refer to the text below. The following chapter will include discussion of:

- Minor and blunt chest trauma;
- Minor and blunt abdominal trauma;
- Head trauma;
- Spinal trauma;
- Penetrating trauma.

Patient Preparation

I.v. access, supine position. Topogram/scan range: apex of the lungs to symphysis pubis, extend to upper thigh when major injury with vascular complication or perforation is suspected. Include skull and cervical spine when appropriate (Fig. 34.1).

Table Scan Parameters

See Table 34.1.

Tips and Tricks

- Even though time is critical, obtain as much clinical information as possible. The scanning protocol can be adjusted accordingly.
- Make sure i.v.-access is sufficiently patent; an 18-G needle or larger is desirable for all arterial scanning protocols.

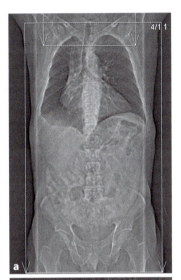
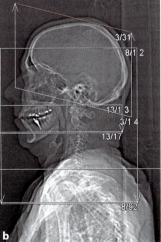

Fig. 34.1. Topogram. **a** Arms above the head. Scan range apex of lungs to symphysis pubis. One single spiral contains all compartments of abdomen and thorax for blunt chest and thoracic trauma. **b** Lateral topogram for head scan containing the cervical spine. Arms are parallel to body

Table 34.1. Scan parameters

Parameters	4–8 slice scanners	10–16 slice scanners	32–64 slice scanners
Scanner settings			
Spirals[a]	Single spiral/ (postscan)	Thorax/ abdo+pelvis/ (postscan)	Thorax/ abdo+pelvis/ (postscan)
Scan direction	Craniocaudal	Craniocaudal	Craniocaudal
Tube voltage (kV)	140[b]	120	120
Tube current time product (mAs)	125–170[b]	170–200	170–200
Pitch corrected tube current time product (eff. mAs)	90–120	120–140	120–140
Collimation (mm)	1.0, 2.5	0.75, 1.5	0.6, 1.2
Norm. pitch	1.4	1.4	1.4
Rotation time (s)	0.5	0.5	0.33
Reconstruction			
Slice thickness (mm)	1.25/5	1.0/5	-/5[c]
Increment (mm)	1.0 /5	0.8/5	-/5[c]
Convolution kernel	standard/bone	standard/bone	standard/bone
Secondary reconstructions	MPR spine 2/2	MPR spine 2/2	MPR spine 2/2
Specials		Bolus triggering[d]	Bolus triggering[d]
I.v. contrast (monophasic)			
Amount (mL)	120–150	120–150	120–150
Injection rate (mL/s)	2.0–3.0	2.0–3.0	2.0–3.0
Saline chaser (mL, mL/s)	60/2.0–3.0	60/2.0–3.0	80/2.0–3.0
Delay (s)	35 periph. (30 central)	Bolus triggered[d]/70	Bolus triggered[d]/70

[a] If there is suspicion of injuries to the head or neck, a native CT scan will be done first. For protocols, see the respective chapters. In severe abdominal trauma a delayer scan (postscan) of the abdomen and pelvis at 3–5 minutes to exclude damage to the urinary tract should be done.
[b] Tube current of 4-slice scanners may be limited after preceding scans of head and neck. Increase of voltage improves image quality.
[c] Coronal and sagittal reconstructions should be performed, either from thin axial slices or directly from the raw data if possible.
[d] Premonitoring scan (20 mAs), place ROI in aortic arch, set triggering at 100 HU, check at 1.5 s intervals.

- Secure all cables and tubing, especially the respiratory tube, before scanning since a high table feed will occur.
- Allow sufficient length of all lines, tubes, and cables for table movement during scanning.

Rationale

Not every patient arriving in the emergency room is always a poly-traumatized patient requiring a total body scan. Since the true condition of the patient it is not always clear before scanning the patient, some rationale should be given to choose the appropriate examining strategy. By the same token, if there is any doubt, it is rather advised to examine too much than not enough. Some clinical conditions require a rapid diagnosis to facilitate immediate treatment after arrival to the emergency department to achieve a favorable clinical outcome [1]. A standardized diagnostic algorithm is very helpful, thus even when time is critical, obtain as much clinical information as possible before the scan. The scan protocol can be adapted accordingly (e.g., high pitch, one spiral only, etc.).

CT is the most sensitive modality for the diagnosis of cerebral, thoracic and abdominal injuries at an early clinical stage. Ultrasound is fast and sensitive for diagnosing free abdominal fluid, however, it cannot rival CT for other acute indications. In thoracic trauma, CT is markedly superior to conventional chest radiographs for the detection of traumatic complications [2].

These protocols are intended for the examination of patients with major trauma and potentially life-threatening injuries of one or more organ systems.

The aim should be to make a state-of-the-art examination allowing all diagnoses to be made from one examination with no need for doing further scans later, e.g., of the spine. Therefore, the scan range has to cover all possible questions, and the scanning technique should facilitate adequate postprocessing, e.g., sagittal and coronal reconstructions.

Basic Radiological Management of Major Trauma Patients

After the initial clinical assessment and stabilization of circulatory functions, a focused abdominal US scan is performed to detect free fluid and a plain chest film (optional) is usually recommended. If possible, the next diagnostic step is a contrast-enhanced CT-scan providing a comprehensive assessment of all vital organ systems within a short period of time (10–15 min) [3,4].

Thin collimation with almost isotropic resolution permits high-quality multiplanar reconstructions (MPR) making conventional radiographs largely redundant in this scenario. A short acquisition time reduces respiratory and gross movement artifacts. The proposed protocols are intended for the examination of patients with major trauma and potentially life-threatening injuries of one or more organ systems. The aim should be to make a state-of-the-art examination allowing a comprehensive diagnosis to be made from one examination with no need for repeat scans, e.g., of the spine, afterwards [5].

Exam Strategies

Minor and Blunt Chest Trauma

If the mechanism of trauma can be sufficiently assessed to be limited to the thorax and at the same time plain chest films cannot rule out fractures or vascular injuries, the decision towards a contrast-enhanced chest CT should be made. If in doubt as to whether possible injury is limited to the thorax, extend the investigation to a thoraco-abdominal scan.

The following pathologies are of primary focus: thoracic aortic dissection or rupture, intramural hematoma, pneumothorax, pleural effusion including hemothorax, pericardial effusion including pericardial bleeding, parenchymal lung injuries, sternal and rib fractures, as well as spinal injuries. Also check for position of tubes and lines (Fig. 34.2).

Minor and Blunt Abdominal Trauma

If the mechanism of trauma can be sufficiently assessed to be limited to the abdomen and at the same time ultrasound and/or plain films cannot rule out parenchymal or vascular injury, the indication for a contrast enhanced abdominal CT should be made. If in doubt as to whether possible injury can be limited to the abdomen, ex-

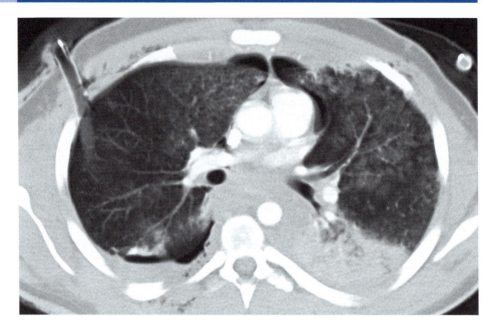

Fig. 34.2. Axial reconstructions (5/5). Contusion of the lungs, serial rib fractures, bilateral pneumothorax with chest drains

tend the investigation to thoraco-abdominal scan.

The following pathologies are of primary focus: injuries of the spleen, liver, gallbladder, kidneys, pancreas, bowel, mesentery, and diaphragm. Retro- and intraperitoneal hemorrhage has to be differentiated from other fluids, e.g., urine after intraperitoneal bladder rupture (an additional postscan can be helpful to identify leaks/injuries of the urogenital complex). Sites of active arterial bleeding have to be identified using an arterial phase. Fractures may also be the cause of significant bleeding, e.g., pelvic fractures, and should be assessed with regard to this. If possible, the source of all arterial or venous bleeding should be definitively identified. Look for free abdominal air indicating bowel perforation (Fig. 34.3).

Head Trauma

There is substantial debate whether a CT scan of the head is mandatory in each and every case to rule out significant intracra-

nial pathology, such as haemorrhage, herniation, or cervical spine injuries. We advise the use of an adapted "Canadian CT head rule [6,7]." The cervical spine should always be included in the scan range when performing a head CT on a high-risk patient.

A head scan is absolutely mandatory under the following conditions, with major head injury defined as:

- Glasgow Coma Sore 13–15 and obvious penetrating skull injury, obvious depressed fracture or acute focal neurological deficit;
- Glasgow Coma Sore 13–15 and unstable vital signs associated with major trauma or seizure before assessment in the emergency department.

A CT scan may be omitted for a patient presenting with minimal head injuries defined as:

- Head trauma, Glasgow Coma Sore 13–15 with no obvious skull injury, and no witnessed loss of consciousness, amnesia, or disorientation.

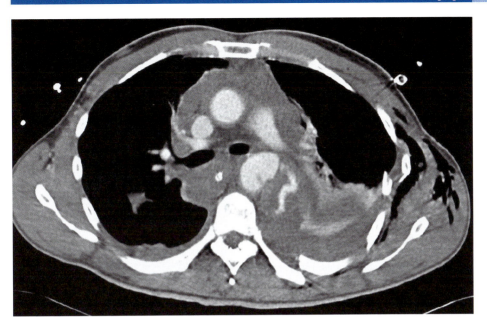

Fig. 34.3. Aortic dissection (type B) with arterial bleed from descending aorta, hemothorax, serial rib fractures

A CT scan should be performed in patients with minor head injury defined as head trauma with Glasgow Coma Sore 13–15 with witnessed loss of consciousness, amnesia, or disorientation, and if at least one of the following conditions is additionally present:

- Glasgow Coma Score <15 at 2 h after injury;
- Suspected open or depressed skull fracture;
- Any sign of basal skull fracture (haemotympanum, "raccoon" eyes, cerebrospinal fluid otorrhoea/rhinorrhoea, Battle's sign);
- Vomiting (≥ two episodes);
- Age ≥65 years;
- Amnesia before impact (>30 min);
- Dangerous trauma mechanism (pedestrian struck by motor vehicle, occupant ejected from motor vehicle, fall from height >3 ft or five stairs).

Spinal Trauma

The assessment of spinal injuries in blunt trauma (head, chest, abdomen or combined) should always be reconstructed from the initial CT data sets. An additional or primary, isolated noncontrast enhanced scan of the whole spine to solely rule out spinal injury is obsolete.

An exemption of this rule may be an isolated trauma, where initial plain films cannot safely rule out spinal damage, but a contrast enhanced CT scan seems unnecessary. In this case a noncontrast CT scan of the spinal region in doubt may be indicated. The second exemption might be an unclear pathology seen on the reconstructed images from the primary dataset. In this case a second high-resolution CT scan of that particular region might be indicated.

Penetrating Trauma

Always scan the entire compartment, at least the entire chest, or entire abdomen;

in case of doubt, scan both (see chest and abdominal trauma).

Examination Protocol

If there is suspicion of head trauma, an unenhanced CT-scan of the head will usually be done first to exclude intracranial intraparenchymal (ICB) or subarachnoidal (SAH) bleeding, which are otherwise not safely detectable. Before the patient is moved, attention should next be focused on clearing the cervical spine. This can be done by a dedicated examination, or by reconstructing the spine from a spiral examination of the neck vessels. If there is no clinical suspicion of injuries to the arms or shoulder girdle, both arms can be repositioned above the head for the following thoracic and abdominal scans, thus reducing artifacts [1].

After the injection of i.v.-contrast medium, scanning of the chest and thorax is recommended in the arterial phase, while the examination of abdomen and pelvis can be recommended in different phases, depending on the question asked. Scanning in the arterial phase is obligatory if an arterial laceration or dissection is suspected. Scanning in the portalvenous phase ensures optimal contrast for the visualization of the parenchymal organs, and helps to exclude traumatic laceration of the spleen, the kidneys, or the liver.

With 16- and 64-row scanners the arterial spiral can be extended in the caudal direction for coverage of the upper legs, if required. In severe abdominal trauma, a postscan of the abdomen and pelvis to look for injuries to the urinary tract should be done [1]. However, a prerequisite for a high-quality reconstructions (MPR, 3D, VRT) is always a narrow collimation. For the diagnosis of fractures to the spine, MPRs (sagittal/coronal planes) of the thoracic and lumbar spine are used. In pelvic fractures 3D reconstructions are helpful to demonstrate the extent and position (Fig. 34.4).

In conclusion, CT is the most sensitive and most complete modality for the diag-

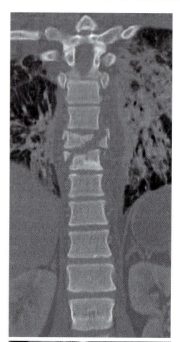

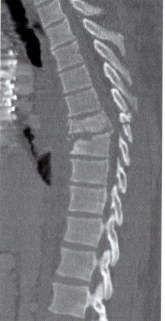

Fig. 34.4. MPR (2/2) of the thoracic spine in coronal and sagittal planes. Fracture of thoracic vertebra 7 and 8 with perivertebral hematoma

nosis of cerebral, thoracic, and abdominal injuries at an early clinical stage. Ultrasound is fast and sensitive for diagnosing free abdominal fluid, but it cannot rival CT for other acute indications. In thoracic trauma, CT is markedly superior to a conventional chest X-ray for the detection of traumatic complications.

References

1. Novelline RA, Rhea JT, Rao PM, Stuk JL (1999) Helical CT in emergency radiology. Radiology 213(2):321–339
2. McLaughlin JS, Shama Z, Hirsch E, Khazei, AH, Attar S, Cowley A (1969) Cardiovascular dynamics in human shock. Am Surg 35(3):166–176
3. Leidner B, Adiels M, Aspelin P, Gullstrand P, Wallen S (1998) Standardized CT examination of the multitraumatized patient. Eur Radiol 8(9):1630–1638
4. Rieger M, Sparr H, Esterhammer R, Fink C, Bale R, Czermak B, Jaschke W (2002) Moderne CT-Diagnostik des akuten Thorax- und Abdominaltraumas. Radiologe 42:556–563
5. Roos JE, Hilfiker P, Platz A, Desbiolles L, Boehm T, Marincek B, Weishaupt D (2004) MDCT in emergency radiology: is a standardized chest or abdominal protocol sufficient for evaluation of thoracic and lumbar spine trauma? Am J Roentgenol 183(4):959–968
6. Stiell IG, Wells GA, Vandemheen K et al. (2001) The canadian CT head rule for patients with minor head injury. Lancet 357:1391–6
7. Schlegel PM, Walter MA, Kloska SP et al. (2005) Is the canadian CT head rule for minor head injury applicable for patients in germany? Rofo 177(6):872–876

IX CT-Guided Interventions

35 CT-Guided Abscess Drainage

A.H. Mahnken

Introduction

Percutaneous CT-guided drainage has become a standard procedure for patients with infected or symptomatic fluid collections. This technique is not only suited for the treatment of abscesses, but all types of pathologic fluid collections in nearly every organ system including biloma, urinoma, hematoma, etc. Although most lesions can be approached with ultrasound-guidance, CT-guidance is well established for all fluid collections and in particular those that are not amenable to ultrasound or fluoroscopy-guided puncture. In deep pelvic or subphrenic regions, and especially in the chest, CT is often superior to other imaging modalities for guiding drainage catheters. As percutaneous drainage is a highly effective procedure with a low complication rate requiring only a short hospital stay, this technique is preferable to surgical techniques if sufficient access to the fluid collection can be established.

Indications

There is a variety of underlying diseases leading to abscesses and other fluid collections that can occur in all regions of the body. Thus, indications for percutaneous drainage in general can be classified as follows:

- To obtain a diagnostic sample for microbiologic, laboratory, or cytological analysis.
- To drain the fluid from an infectious and/or symptomatic lesion.

- To treat a symptomatic collection by instilling a sclerotic agent.

Minimally invasive therapy of abscesses is the main reason for percutaneous drainage, with abscesses generally requiring a combination of drainage and antibiotics. Exceptions are small abscesses <3 cm, which sometimes resolve with antibiotic therapy alone [1]. However, the latter often requires needle aspiration to obtain material for culture. Further important indications for drainage include symptomatic fluid collections causing pain or obstruction of the bowel or the ureter.

There are no absolute contraindications to CT-guided drainage as long as there is a safe access route to the lesion. Relative contraindications for percutaneous drainage include disordered coagulation state and inability to cooperate. These problems, however, can be managed pharmaceutically if necessary.

Scan Parameters

See Table 35.1.

Anatomy and Access Route

It is sound principle to choose the safest and most effective route to the lesion. Any noninvolved structure should be avoided. Damage to the spleen and the intestines in particular must be carefully prevented. The pleural recess should be avoided if at all possible [2]. The latter, however, is associated with an increased risk for pneumothorax, pleurisy and pleural empyema.

Table 35.1. These scan parameters are applicable for sequential localizer scans. Diagnostic scans, as well as abscessograms, should be performed using examination protocols for the corresponding anatomic region

Parameters	4–8 slice scanners	10–16 slice scanners	32–64 slice scanners
Scanner settings	Sequential	Sequential	Sequential
Tube voltage (kV)	120	120	120
Tube current (mAs)	70–150	60–120	40–80
Collimation (mm)	2.5	1.5	0.6
Norm. pitch	n.a.	n.a.	n.a.
Reconstr.-slice thickness (mm)	2.5	4.5	6.0
Convolution kernel	standard/ soft	standard/ soft	standard/ soft
Specials	Use same table position	Use same table position	Use same table position
	Real time imaging with fluoroscopy	Real time imaging with fluoroscopy	Real time imaging with fluoroscopy
	Slice combination may be helpful	Slice combination may be helpful	Slice combination may be helpful
Scan range	Adapted to the skin entry of the needle	Adapted to the skin entry of the needle	Adapted to the skin entry of the needle
Scan direction	n.a.	n.a.	n.a.
Contrast media application	Optional	Optional	Optional
Concentration (mg iodine/ml)			
Mono/Biphasic			
Volume (mL)			
Injection rate (mL/s)			
Saline chaser (mL, mL/s)			
Delay (s)			

Upper Abdomen

The majority of pathologic fluid collections can be drained with a reasonably straightforward access (Fig. 35.1). If a lesion can not be approached directly without affection of noninvolved structures a transhepatic approach is considered to be safe. In some circumstances a transgastric approach may be considered, although this approach should be used for fine needle aspiration biopsy only. A transpleural approach for drainage of fluid collections is only acceptable if no transabdominal route is available and should be absolutely avoided in patients suffering from abscess.

Pelvis

Pelvic fluid collections are typically approached via transabdominal or trans-

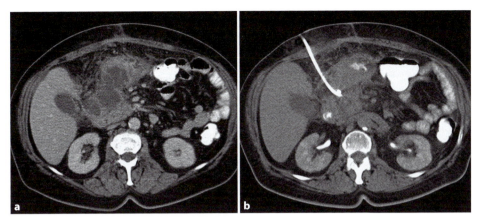

Fig. 35.1. CT-guided drainage of an infected pancreatic pseudocyst. CT scan after oral and i.v. contrast material shows a hypodense lesion originating from the pancreas with surrounding edema of the mesenteric fat (**a**). After drainage the fluid collection is completely resolved indicating sufficient percutaneous drainage (**b**)

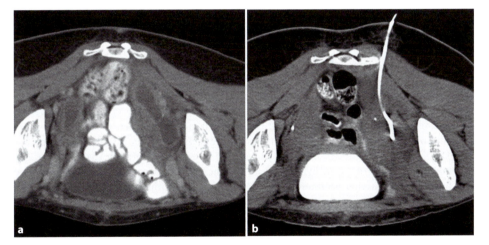

Fig. 35.2. Both-sided pelvic abscess in a male 43-year-old male patient. Axial CT image obtained with oral and intravenous contrast material shows thick-walled abscesses on the left and on the right side (**a**). A 10-F drainage catheter was deployed via a transgluteal approach into the lesions on the right side (**b**). The approach was chosen as close to the sacrum as possible to avoid sciatic nerve injury

gluteal access (Fig. 35.2) [3]. However, alternatives like the transperineal approach are available. Transrectal or transvaginal access routes are normally used with ultrasound guidance, especially since dedicated ultrasound probes are available.

Chest

CT permits access to all thoracic regions using a direct approach (Fig. 35.3). However, the optimal skin entry point has to be chosen to avoid crossing of pleural fissures [4], as the latter results in an increased risk of pneumothorax.

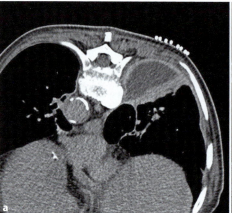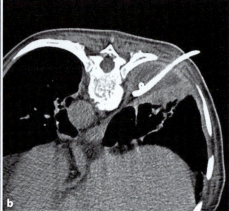

Fig. 35.3. Pleural empyema before (**a**) and after CT-guided percutaneous drainage (**b**). The skin entry point in the *x-y* direction was highlighted using radiopaque markers

Patient Preparation

CT-guided drainage can generally be performed under local anesthesia. Sometimes, however, additional sedation or even general anesthesia is needed. Prior to any drainage, a preinterventional diagnostic workup with up-to-date coagulation status including platelet count has to be performed (Quick > 50%, pTT < 50 s, platelets ≥ 70,000 µL). Warfarin has to be replaced by i.v. Heparin. In rare cases, further preinterventional workup might be required. Furthermore, an intravenous access is mandatory for i.v. medication or contrast material application. In suspected infectious collections i.v. administration of a broad-spectrum antibiotic is recommended. Administration of antibiotics immediately (<1 h) prior to the intervention does not interfere with microbiologic examination of fluid aspirated from the collection [5].

Patient positioning is crucial for the success of the puncture. Various positions may be necessary, depending on the region of the lesion and the approach. The arms (at least one) have to be elevated above the head to ensure sufficient image quality without streak artifacts. In all cases the patient's position has to be stable and comfortable, as this position has to be preserved during the entire procedure.

Technique

A fine needle (19–22G) may be sufficient in the case of a diagnostic aspiration biopsy, otherwise pigtail- or J-catheters with side holes are used. The size of the catheter has to be matched to the viscosity of the fluid with increasing lumen diameters in more viscous fluids. It is essential to place the side holes of the catheter inside the lesion, especially in abscesses. If not, dispersal of infectious or other material (e.g., biliary) to other sites of the body will be fostered.

Basically, there are two different puncture techniques, the coaxial Seldinger or the direct Trocar technique. While operator preferences are usually a matter of personal experience, the Trocar technique may be recommended in straightforward situations, while the coaxial technique is often used in more complex settings to reduce the risk of puncture related complications.

Seldinger Technique

The coaxial Seldinger technique starts with the insertion of a hollow needle into the fluid collection. This needle can be used for aspiration biopsy. A guide wire is placed through the needle and thereafter the needle is withdrawn and a catheter is placed over the wire and positioned in the fluid collection. Serial dilatation of the puncture tract prior to catheter placement is often necessary. An important advantage of the Seldinger technique is the use of thin needles for the first puncture; with a consecutively reduced risk of puncture related complications. Further, the coaxial technique allows one to direct the wire to the exact position planned for the catheter deployment. But, in comparison to the direct Trocar technique, it is more time consuming.

Trocar Technique

The direct Trocar technique uses a catheter mounted on a sharp Trocar, that is, directly placed in the target lesion. This technique is easy and fast to handle and holds only little risk of dissemination of hazardous material. Potentially painful serial dilatation of the puncture tract can be avoided, but this technique instantly results in a large puncture tract and repositioning of the needle may be difficult.

Puncture Procedure

Ideally, a recent (contrast-enhanced) CT-study of the lesion should be made available for planning the procedure. In many cases a nonenhanced study preceding the puncture will be sufficient for evaluation of a safe access. Whenever possible a needle path that can be imaged in one plane should be chosen, as the complexity of the puncture increases with a double angulated puncture path. Gantry tilting may be helpful to find an optimal approach without leaving the scan plane. Prior to the intervention the angle for the puncture, the minimum distance to the target and the maximum safe distance from the cutaneous entry point have to be marked. The entry point of the needle is indicated by the laser positioning device on the skin, while the location in the x-y plane can be determined from anatomical landmarks or radiopaque markers attached to the skin (Fig. 35.3a).

Two different techniques are available for monitoring the intervention and determination of the needle position: sequential localizer scans or (near) real-time imaging with CT fluoroscopy.

Localization Scans

While the needle approaches the lesion, control scans are required to check the catheter position. In general, single scans will be sufficient to monitor the exact needle position. In more complex situations short spirals may be required. Applying this imaging technique, MSCT offers the advantage of simultaneous acquisition of multiple sections within a single scan. This allows for direct control if a needle deviates in a caudal or cranial direction from the target. Duration of the procedure will be shortened if a foot switch for starting a scan and an additional display monitor are available in the examination room.

CT Fluoroscopy

In contrast to sequential localization scans CT fluoroscopy allows for real-time imaging and therefore continuous needle tracking. However, CT-fluoroscopy results in an increased radiation exposure, even if low dose settings are used. Thus, this technique should only be used in critical phases of a procedure. To avoid direct radiation exposure to the hand of the radiologist, the use of special needle holders is advantageous [6].

Postinterventional Management

Image documentation has to be performed if the drainage is in place, ideally before and after aspiration of the fluid.

After decompression of a fluid collection, irrigation is useful in the case of an abscess, except for lung abscesses in which irrigation is contraindicated. This technique effectively liquefies thick debris. It is crucial to perform irrigation with lesser vol-

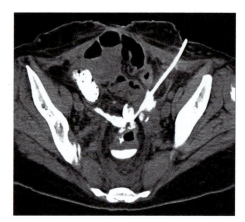

Fig. 35.4. 54-year-old male patient with a post-surgical pelvic abscess. The abscessogram shows contrast material in the abscess as well as in the rectum, proving the presence of a fistula

bidity as compared to surgery. Overall, curative percutaneous abscess drainage can be achieved in more than 80% of patients. Partial success occurs in 5–10% of patients. Another 5–10% experience recurrence and a similar rate of failure was reported. Complications are seen in approximately 10% of patients, with the highest complication rate in chest procedures (2–10%). Complications include bacteremia, septic shock, hemorrhage, bowel injury, and pneumothorax [7].

Tips and Tricks

- If a direct approach is not available, modulation of respiration or modification of patient positioning may be helpful.
- Displacement of the bowel by saline or air injection is a very effective technique to widen the access route.
- Passage of the bowel for fine-needle aspiration (19–22G) is generally safe. Passage of the colon, however, should be avoided, as colonic flora will contaminate the specimen.
- The table should be positioned as low as possible to offer enough space for the needle and interventional maneuvers in the gantry opening.
- As the needle is a high contrast object, the use of low-dose scan parameters is feasible for control scans.

Comparison of US-, CT-, and MR-Guidance

umes of fluid than previously drained from the abscess to avoid intracavitary pressure and consecutive bacteremia. Antibiotic cover is recommended for this procedure. Additional compounds like urokinase or N-acetylcystein can be added to the irrigation solution, but 0.9% saline without any additives will suffice in most patients.

In the case of septated lesions or suspected fistula an "abscessogram" with injection of diluted contrast material (1:10) via the drainage catheter will be helpful. In septated lesions this technique helps decide if additional drainage catheters are required to reach all areas of an abscess. An abscessogram is capable of depicting communications with structures like the pancreatic duct, the bowel, or the genito-urinary system (Fig. 35.4).

Finally the catheter has to be fixed to the skin with a tolerance to allow for motion compensation. Especially in large catheters, suture is well suited for fixation. To avoid clogging and consecutively exchanging of a catheter, regular saline flushing of the catheter is mandatory.

Results

Percutaneous drainage is considered cost effective with reduced mortality and mor-

Percutaneous drainage can be performed with ultrasound (US)-, fluoroscopy-, CT-, and magnet resonance (MR)-guidance. Ultrasound and fluoroscopy are often used for imaging guided drainage. Both techniques offer real-time imaging allowing for online monitoring of the catheter application. Moreover, these techniques are cheap and therefore widely accepted drainage procedures. However, in complex anatomic situations or in areas with a limited acoustic window, as well as in the chest, US imaging is disadvantageous as compared to CT or MRI.

CT and MRI provide excellent imaging of fluid collections in all parts of the body. Both techniques are independent of the acoustic window. MR imaging shows high tissue contrast even without administration of contrast material. Although CT is generally preferred to MR-guidance, both techniques are suited for drainage procedures. Both techniques allow multiplanar imaging for puncture planning, but direct acquisition of multiplanar images is only possible with MR imaging, whereas a delayed reconstruction of multiplanar images is needed with CT data. Real-time imaging is possible with both techniques using CT or MR fluoroscopy. Radiation exposure is the main drawback of CT, while MR imaging is limited due to the relatively long duration of MR-guided intervention as well as its limited availability and high cost.

References

1. Gervais DA, Brown SD, Connolly SA, Brec SL, Harisinghani MG, Mueller PR (2004) Percutaneous imaging-guided abdominal and pelvic abscess drainage in children. Radiographics 24:737–754

2. McNicholas MM, Mueller PR, Lee MJ, Echeverri J, Gazelle GS, Boland GW, Dawson SL (1995) Percutaneous drainage of subphrenic fluid collections that occur after splenectomy: efficacy and safety of transpleural versus extrapleural approach. AJR Am J Roentgenol 165:355–359

3. Harisinghani MG, Gervais DA, Maher MM, Cho CH, Hahn PF, Varghese J, Mueller PR (2003) Transgluteal approach for percutaneous drainage of deep pelvic abscesses: 154 cases. Radiology 228:701–705

4. Ghaye B, Dondelinger RF (2001) Imaging guided thoracic interventions. Eur Respir J 17:507–528

5. Harisinghani MG, Gervais DA, Hahn PF, Cho CH, Jhaveri K, Varghese J, Mueller PR (2002) CT-guided Transgluteal Drainage of Deep Pelvic Abscesses: Indications, Technique, Procedure related Complications, and Clinical Outcome. RadioGraphics 22:1353–1367

6. Froelich JJ, Wagner HJ (2001) CT-fluoroscopy: Tool or gimmick? Cardiovasc Intervent Radiol 24:297–305

7. Bakal CW, Sacks D, Burke DR, Cardella JF, Chopra PS, Dawson SL, Drooz AT, Freeman N, Meranze SG, Van Moore A Jr, Palestrant AM, Roberts AC, Spies JB, Stein EJ, Towbin R (2003) Society of Interventional Radiology Standards of Practice Committee. Quality improvement guidelines for adult percutaneous abscess and fluid drainage. J Vasc Interv Radiol 14:S223–225

36 CT-Guided Diagnostic Punctures

A. Wallnöfer, T. Helmberger and M.F. Reiser

Indications

Suspicious lesions in parenchymal organs, soft tissue and bone that can not be clarified by any other non-invasive method.
- Lung
- Mediastinum
- Liver
- Pancreas
- Retropentoneum
- Kidnea and Adrenals
- Bone

Tips and Tricks

- Document where the needle tip is when taking the probe (by additional scan).
- CT fluoroscopy is recommended for moving organs (lower lung, liver, pancreas), whereas spinal and pelvic punctures do not necessitate fluoroscopy.
- In necrotic tumors it is important to get samples from the solid tumor parts.
- For most parenchymal organs true-cut needles are used, while for lung biopsies aspiration needles ("Chiba needles") are preferred by most centers.
- In subcapsular lesions with an increased risk of a punch hole by direct puncture a transparenchymal access path should be chosen.

Introduction

Computed tomography was first used for diagnostic punctures in 1975 [1,2]. CT-guided procedures have been established in the meantime due to improved tissue contrast and resolution in crucial anatomical localisations resulting in increased precision and decreased procedure-related complication rates.

General Contraindications

Since CT-guided punctures are elective procedures, conditions that may endanger the patient have to be avoided. Besides an unintended injury to an organ, the major risk of any percutaneous procedure is bleeding. Therefore, a sufficient coagulation status is essential. Quick values should not be below 50–60%, the international normalized ratio (INR) should not be more than 1.5 and the platelet count should be at least 60,000–80,000/mm^3 [3].

In general, anticoagulation therapy must be stopped early enough in advance. If cumarine, heparin, or the more modern substances ticlopidine and clopidogrel are used for anticoagulation, the coagulation parameters have to be checked before a procedure is planned [4,6]. If low-dose acetyl salicylic acid (typically 60–100 mg) was administered, normal platelet function can be expected after pausing for a few days [5].

Needles for Biopsy

In general, three types of needles can be used:

- Fine needles (Chiba-needle type) with diameters from 0.64 to 1.07 mm (23–19 G) for cytological aspiration specimens
- True-cut needles with diameters of 1.27–2.77 mm (18–12 G) for tissue samples

Table 36.1. Scan parameters (given values are examples)

Parameters	4–8 slice scanners	10–16 slice scanners	32–64 slice scanners
Scanning parameters			
Tube voltage (kV)	120	120	120
Rotation time (s)	0.5	0.5	0.5
Tube current time product (mAs)	30	30	30
Pitch corrected tube current time product (eff. mAs)	30	30	30
Slice collimation (mm)	5	5	5
Norm. pitch	None	None	None
Reconstruction increment (mm)			
Reconstruction thickness (mm)	5	5	5
Reconstruction kernel	Soft	Soft	Soft
Contrast media	Variable	Variable	Variable

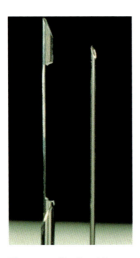

Fig. 36.1. Cutting biopsy needle with the Tru-Cut principle; demonstration of probe groove

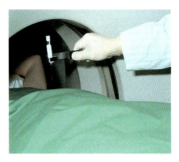

Fig. 36.2. For reduction of hand radiation exposure, when available usage of needle holder

- Large-core needles with diameters of 2.11–3.40 mm (14–10 G) for bone biopsies (Jamshidi-needle type)

The needle diameter chosen for a specific anatomical target should represent a compromise between sufficient sample size and as low as possible complication rate. For most parenchymal organs true-cut needles are used, while for lung biopsies aspiration needles (Chiba needle) are preferred by most centers. However, due to the small sample size, aspiration needles only allow cytological diagnostics. Automated aspiration systems do not overcome this limitation [7]. If the needle has to travel a long distance, needle bending can be a problem due to the resulting deviation of the needle tip. Beside biopsy, Chiba needles can also be used for the minimal-invasive injection and instillation of various substances and drugs as in neurolysis or interstitial pain therapy.

In contrast to aspiration needles half-, or fully-automated true-cut needle biopsy systems produce large core samples enabling

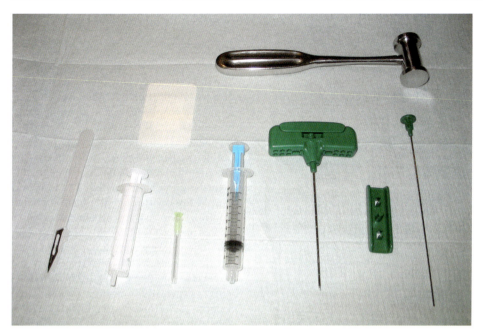

Fig. 36.3. Example of a large lumen bone biopsy needle from Somatex 14 G/2.00 mm and 10-cm length. Aspiration syringe and sterile hammer

intact cellular and tissue structures, even for immuno-histochemical staining. Even if the punch hole of true-cut needles is significantly larger than of aspiration needles, there is no significantly higher complication rate known.

To assure a diagnostically valuable result several probes are necessary. Therefore, it is advisable to take at least three probes from a fan-shaped covered area (Fig. 36.1).

In some locations the use of a needle holder for the biopsy needle is helpful and avoids complications, such as high radiation to the investigator's hands (Fig. 36.2).

In contrast to soft-tissue biopsy, more rigid and stable needles are used for bone biopsies, which allows one to drill the needle trough the bone (corticalis). The stiffness requirements of these needles necessitate larger sizes (e.g., 10–14 G) in comparison to soft-tissue biopsy needles (Fig. 36.3).

Procedure

CT-guided biopsy procedures can be performed online or offline under CT-fluoros-copy guidance. Based on preinterventional imaging, the target and entry site of the biopsy needle have to be defined. It is useful to mark the skin at the entry site with a waterproof or radiopaque marker using the gantry built-in laser light as reference. The access route from the skin entry site to the target has to be planned carefully to avoid unintended injury to the structures that are between the entry site and target. After preparation (cutaneous disinfections, local anesthesia, general analgo-sedation if necessary, local incision) the biopsy needle is advanced in- or off-plane, depending on the localization of the target and the related anatomical accessibility. The needle path, with attention on the needle tip, must be monitored, either by subsequent single-slice imaging or by online fluoro-scopic scanning. A 5-mm collimation for both imaging types is generally sufficient to maintain a sufficient image quality and an adequate control of the needle tip. Due to partial volume effects, thicker collimation is not recommended since the needle tip cannot be exactly determined in a 10-mm slice.

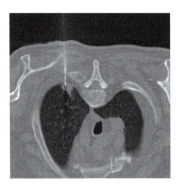

Fig. 36.4. Positioning of an 18-G needle cutting biopsy in the suspicious lung round lesion from dorsal paravertebral. Histology: highly differentiated adenocarcinoma

In contrast to offline control CT fluoroscopy allows online visualization of the needle tip during needle advancement, which also facilitates double oblique access routes and the compensation for breathing-dependent motion of the target and needle. Additionally, joystick control of the CT couch motion allows very rapid promotion of the procedure. Nevertheless, even using optimally reduced scan parameters, CT-fluoroscopy results in increased radiation exposure to the patient and interventional radiologist since the exposure dose correlates directly with the fluoroscopy time. Therefore, radiation protection is a critical and mandatory issue [8,9].

New technical developments, such as dose modulation by switching off the radiation beam during a specific part of the rotation (e.g., HandCARE, Siemens Medical System, Germany), will help to reduce the radiation exposure especially for the interventionist. Reductions of up to 30% for the patient and up to 70% for the interventionist seems possible using this technique. Nevertheless, the most important factor to keep the radiation exposure as low as possible is to keep the fluoroscopic time as short as possible.

Due to the excellent positioning control, the overall complication rate of CT-guided punctures e.g., 0.1–1.5% for abdominal punctures, in comparison to other invasive procedures is very low [10].

Special Indications

Lung

The indication of a lung biopsy is, the need of a histological or microbiological evaluation of a suspicious lesion when no other method is suitable.

The local anesthesia (LA) has to incorporate the parietal pleura without passing through the pleura folds. Once the target is identified, the biopsy needle has to be advanced rapidly through the pleura folds to minimize the risk for an extended injury to the pleura resulting in pneumothorax. Spiking the target with the tip of the biopsy needle increases the confidence that the target is not missed while getting the probe. This is especially important in subpleural lesions. Nevertheless, the likelihood of a negative sample is higher for smaller lesions.

The procedure is finished with a control scan to monitor probable immediate complications as parenchymal bleeding or pneumothorax.

Depending on the clinical situation, a control X-ray of the chest is recommended 2–24 h after the procedure.

Pneumothorax after transthoracic biopsy occurs with a frequency of 20% [11] to 40% [12], while the need for a chest tube ranges from 2% [11] to 17% [12]. The general complication rate, including bleeding, infection, injury of nerves, vessels, or adjacent organs, is about 10% [13]; the total mortality rate is about 0.02% [14] (Fig. 36.4).

Mediastinum

Due to the vascular structures within the mediastinum, not all areas of the mediastinum can be biopsied percutaneously. Planning the access route has to incorporate the parasternal subpleural (fat) spaces that can be expanded by injecting saline and creating access ways to the retrosternal mediastinal parts. By doing so, pneumothoax can be avoided in almost all cases.

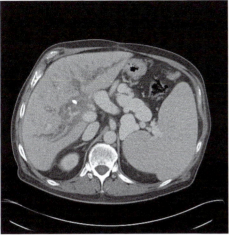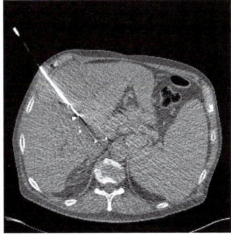

Fig. 36.5. Presentation of a central space occupying lesion in liver hilum after liver transplantation. Puncture of this lesion under CT fluoroscopy with a 16-G biopsy needle. Histology: posttransplantation lymphoproliferative disorder (PTLD)

Liver

In cases where imaging is nondiagnostic and the differentiation of a lesion is essential for further treatment, planning histological proof is mandatory and in general a percutaneous biopsy indicated.

The planning of the procedure encloses the evaluation of the costo-diaphragmatic recess to avoid a transpleural or transpulmonary access route. To prevent damage of the liver capsule – similarly to lung biopsies – the needle should be advanced rapidly through the capsule. In subcapsular lesions with an increased risk of a punch hole by direct puncture, a transparenchymal access path should be chosen. Due to the capsular enervation crossing of the falciform ligament, the hilus or the gallbladder bed should be avoided.

While sensitivity, specificity, and overall accuracy of CT-guided liver biopsies are very high with 91.1, 100, and 93.3%, respectively [19], minor and major complications in hepatic biopsies are very rare. Tumor seeding along the needle track in biopsies of malignancies is reported in the literature to range from 0.003–0.009% [15,16] to 1.6–3.4% [18,17] (Fig. 36.5).

Pancreas

A biopsy of the pancreas is indicated in cases where surgical exploration is excluded and palliative therapy is planned, or a potential tumor has to be differentiated from inflammation.

Due to the retroperitoneal localization of the pancreas, the biopsy is technically demanding. Different access routes are possible: (1) transperitoneal with or without crossing the stomach, duodenum, or liver, (2) transretroperitoneal, paracaval. Usually 16–18 G needles are used, however, 20–22 G needles are recommended when using the transgastric or transduodenal access route. Using the latter routes, fasting for at least six hours is advisable to avoid secondary infections. Pancreatic head and tail are sometimes better approached via a retroperitoneal route. The instillation of saline or air can be helpful to prepare the access path. The sensitivity reaches – depending on the used technique – up to almost 100% [20–23], the complications rate ranges from 0.5–3% [24,25], and tumor seeding is reported between 0.003 and 0.009% [15].

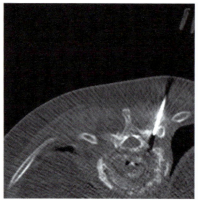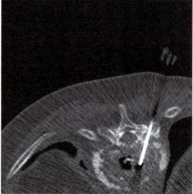

Fig. 36.6. Known spondylodiscitis, probe removal for microbiological evaluation with a 10-G bone marrow biopsy needle

Retroperitoneum

Typical indications are retroperitoneal masses, enlarged lymph nodes, or a bulky mass suspicious of lymphoma. Planning the delineation of the paraspinal vessels and the ureteres will avoid unintended injuries.

In lymphomas the sensitivity of the biopsy sample is about 90% and the specificity more than 97% [26] with a negligible complication rate.

Kidney and Adrenals

The indication for a renal or adrenal biopsy is rarely given. A typical example is the suspicion of lymphoma or metastatic disease. In the suspicion of pheochromocytoma one must be aware of the potential of a hypertensive crisis and has to be prepared for the treatment of such an occurrence.

In general, the left adrenal is more accessible than the right one. It can be also reached via a transhepatic path.

Bone

Suspicion of malignancy and infection may raise the indication for a bone biopsy. When the corticalis has to be incorporated within the specimen or solid bone has to be crossed to reach the target lesion, typically a Jamshidi-like needle is used which is stable enough to cross solid bone. In osteolytic lesions, a true-cut needle is often sufficient. Due to the high algesia of the periosteviro ample anesthesia is mandatory, as well as absolute sterility to avoid secondary bone infection.

The diagnostic specificity in osteolytic lesions is 80–90% [27] while osteoplastic and mixed lesions are correctly sampled with 70–80% [27]. Bone biopsies are very safe procedures with an over all complication rate of about 1% (Fig. 36.6).

References

1. Haaga J, Alfidi R (1976) Precis biopsy localization by computed tomography. Radiology 118:603–607
2. Dondelinger R (1995) A short history of nonvascular interventional radiology. J Belge Radiol 78:363–370
3. Günter R, Adam G, Keulers P, Klose K, Vorwerk D (1996) CT-gesteuerte Punktionen. Interventionelle Radiologie. Thieme, Stuttgart, pp 605–634
4. British Committee for Standards in Haematology (1998) Guidelines on oral anticoagulation, 3rd edn. Br J Haematol 101:374–378
5. Herth FJ, Becker HD, Ernst A (2002) Aspirin does not increase bleeding complication after transbronchial biopsy. Chest 122:1461–1464
6. Hittelet A, Deviere J (2003) Management of anticoagulants before and after endoscopy Can J Gastroenterol 17:329–332

7. Hopper KD, Abendroth CS, Sturtz KW, Mattews YL, Shirk SJ (1992) Fine-needle aspriation biopsy for cytopathologic analysis: utility of syringe handles, automated guns, and the nonsuction method. Radiology 185:819–824

8. Mellenberg DE, Sato Y, Thompson BH, Warnock NG (1999) Personel exposure rates during simulated biopsies with a real-time CT scanner. Acad Radiol 6:687–690

9. Seifert H, El-Jamal A, Roth R, Urbanczyk K, Kramann B (2000) Reduzierung der Strahlenexposition von Patienten mit ausgewählten interventionellen und angiographischen Maßnahmen. Fortschr Röntgenstr 172:1057–1064

10. Neuerburg J, Gunther RW (1991) Percutaneous biopsy of pancreatic lesions. Cardiovasc Intervent Radiol 14:43–49

11. Muehlstaedt M, Bruening R, Diebold J, Mueller A, Helmberger Th, Reiser MF (2002) CT/Fluoroscopy-guided transthoracic needle biopsy: sensitivity and complication rate in 98 procedures. J Comput Assist Tomogr 26:191–196

12. Cox JE, Chiles CC, McManus CM, Aquino SL, Choplin RH (1999) Transthoracic needle aspiration biopsy; variables that affect risk of pneumothorax. Radiology 212:165–168

13. Cardella JF, Bakal CW, Bertino RE et al. (1996) Quality improvement guidelines for image-guided percutaneous biopsy in adults: Society of Cardiovascular and Interventional Radiology Standards of Practice Committee. J Vasc Intervent Radiol 7:943–946

14. Klein JS (1997) Transthoracic needle biobsy: an overview. J Thorac Imaging 12:232–249

15. Smith EH (1991) Complications of percutaneous abdominal fine-needle biopsy. Radiology 178:243–258

16. Livraghi T, Torzilli G, Lazzaroni S, Olivari N (1997) Biopsia percutanea con ago sottile delle lesioni focali. In: Torzilli G, Olivari N, Livraghi T, Di Candio G (eds) Ecografia in Chirurgia. Paletto Editore, Milan, pp 167–190

17. Kim SH, Lim HK, Lee Wj, Cho JM, Jang AJ (2000) Needle-tract implantation in hepatocellular carcinoma: frequency and CT findings after biopsy with a 19.5 gauge automatied biopsy gun. Abdom Imaging 25:246–250

18. Durand F, Regimbeau JM, Belghiti J, Sauvanet A, Vilgrain V, Terris B et al. (2001) Assessment of the benefits and risk of percutaneous biopsy before surgical resection of hepatocellular carcinoma. J Hepatol 35:254–258

19. Wutke R, Schmid A, Fellner F, Horbach T, Kastl S, Papadopoulos T, Hohenberger W, Bautz W (2001) CT-gesteuerte perkutane Schneidbiopsie: effektive Genauigkeit, diagnostischer Nutzen und effektive Kosten. Fortschr Röntgenstr 173:1025–1033

20. Rodriguez J, Kasberg C, Nipper M et al. (1992) CT-guided needle biopsy of the pancreas : A retrospectiv analysis of diagnostic accuracy. Am J Gastroenterol 87:1610–1613

21. DelMaschio A, Vanzulli A, Sironi S et al. (1991) Pancreatic cancer versus chronic pancreatitis: diagnosis with CA 19-9 assessment, US, CT, and CT-guided fine needle biopsy. Radiology 178:95–99

22. Brandt KR, Charboneau JW, Stephens DH, Welch TJ, Goellner JR (1993) CT- and US-guided biopsy of the pancreas. Radiology 187:99–104

23. Zech CJ, Helmberger T, Wichmann MW, Holzknecht N, Diebold J, Reiser MF (2002) Large core biopsy of the pancreas under CT fluoroscopy control: results and complications. J Comput Assist Tomogr 26:743–749

24. Aideyan OA, Schmidt AJ, Trenkner SW et al. (1996) CT-guided percutaneous biopsy of pancreas transplants. Radiology 201:825–828

25. Jennings PE, Donald JJ, Coral A et al. (1989) Ultrasound-guided core biopsy Lancet 1:1369–1371

26. Demharter J, Muller P, Wagner T, Schlimok G, Haude K, Bohndorf K (2001) Percutaneous core-needle biopsy of enlarged lymph nodes in the diagnosis and subclassifiction of malignant lymphomas. Eur Radiol 11(2):276–283

27. Duda SH, Johst U, Krahmer K, Pereira P, König C, Schäfer J, Huppert P, Schott U, Böhm P, Claussen CD (2001) Technik und Ergebnisse der CT-gesteuerten perkutanen Knochenbiopsie. Orthopäde 30:545–550

37 CT-Guided Ablation Therapy

S. Clasen and P.L. Pereira

Indications for Ablation Therapy

- Primary and secondary liver tumors
- Osteoid osteoma
- Renalcellcarcinoma
- Primary and secondary lung malignancies
- Osserus and soft-tissue tumors

Comments

Percutaneous thermal ablation including radiofrequency (RF) ablation, laser interstitial thermotherapy (LITT), microwave (MW) ablation, high-intensity focussed ultrasound (HIFU), and cryoablation are minimal invasive therapy options in the treatment of hepatic and nonhepatic tumors. CT-guided RF ablation gained importance in the potential curative therapy of primary and secondary liver tumors and is a well-established treatment of benign osteoid osteoma. Currently new fields of image-guided RF ablation are represented by primary and secondary malignancies of the lung, renal cell carcinoma, and the treatment of symptomatic osseous and soft-tissue tumors.

Thermal ablation procedures destroy tumor tissue with either heat or cold in a circumscribed area. The RF ablation is the most widespread thermal ablation therapy. The principle of RF ablation is an induction of frictional heat caused by the movement of ions. Therefore a high-frequency electrical current (375–480 kHz) is applied leading to a coagulation of the tissue. The electric current is closed between two electrodes. Most currently available RF devices are monopolar in that there is a single "active" electrode positioned in the target tissue and dispersive electrodes (grounding pads) placed on the body surface. In bipolar and multipolar RF devices the electrodes are placed in the target tissue and no grounding pads are required. In bipolar RF ablation, the electric circuit is closed between two RF electrodes placed in or at the periphery of the tumor. A design of two electrodes located on different shafts or on the same shaft is possible. In multipolar RF ablation more than two electrodes are combined allowing a consecutive activation of every possible pair of electrodes. There are also variations in the design of the RF electrodes like multitined expandable electrodes, internally cooled electrodes, and perfusion electrodes.

Patient Preparation and Positioning

Image-guided ablation therapy can be performed under general anesthetic or under local anesthetic in combination with conscious sedation. General anesthesia should be performed at the patients request and in the treatment of osteoid osteoma or in painful osseous and soft tissue tumors. An i.v. access is necessary for medication application and contrast media capable for a flow of 3 mL/s. Sufficient blood coagulation tests are mandatory (quick test > 50%, platelets > 50,000 µL). When a monopolar RF system is used an adequate placement of grounding pads prior to the intervention is obligatory. Therefore, depending on the RF device used, one to four grounding pads should be placed at equidistant sites from the target tissue. Usually, grounding pads are placed on the thighs and the back of the patient and orientated with the lon-

Table 37.1. Scan parameters

Parameters	4–8 slice scanners	10–16 slice scanners	32–64 slice scanners
Scanner settings			
Tube voltage (kV)	120	120	120
Rotation time (s)	1	0.5	0.5
Tube current time product (mAs)	190–270	45–80	45–100
Pitch corrected tube current time product (eff. mAs)	150–180	60–80	60–80
Slice collimation (mm)	1.0, 2.5	0.75, 1.5	0.6, 1.2
Norm. pitch	1.25–1.5	0.75–1	0.75–1.2
Reconstr.-slice thickness (mm)	5	5	5
Convolution kernel	Standard	Standard	Standard
Specials			
Scan range	Liver and adjacent parts of lung and abdomen	Liver and adjacent parts of lung and abdomen	Liver and adjacent parts of lung and abdomen
Scan direction	Craniocaudal	Craniocaudal	Craniocaudal
Contrast media application			
Concentration (mg iodine/mL)	370	370	400
Mono/Biphasic	Monophasic	Monophasic	Monophasic
Volume (mL)	60–80	60–80	60–80
Injection rate (mL/s)	3.0	3.0	3.0
Saline chaser (mL, mL/s)	No	No	30/3.0
Delay (s)			

gest surface edge facing the RF electrode. A bipolar or multipolar RF system does not require grounding pads. Patient positioning in supine or prone position depends on the supposed transcutaneous approach. An elevation of the right or left flank might be necessary in order to facilitate the positioning of the electrode by displacing vulnerable organs. It has to be ensured that the patient can stay in the supposed position over the time necessary for the intervention. The topogram should include the target tissue and the adjacent anatomic structures. For example, the CT scan before hepatic ablation therapy should include the whole liver and the adjacent parts of the lung and abdomen.

Scan parameters

See Table 37.1.

Tips and Tricks

Before patient positioning, the supposed approach should be defined based on previous images to avoid repositioning after the first CT scan. While patient and table positioning, ensure that there is enough space between patient and CT gantry for applicator insertion. Therefore it might be necessary to lower the table for easier ventral access. Or an RF applicator not longer than the required length should be chosen.

Use reduced amounts of contrast medium since several series for planning, positioning, and controls after RF application will be necessary.

Indications for Image-Guided Ablation Therapy

Primary and Secondary Liver Tumors

Surgical segmental resection and liver transplantation for hepatocellular carcinoma (HCC) are the gold standard therapies in the treatment of primary and secondary liver malignancies. Due to technical and functional reasons, curative surgery is possible in only 10–25% of patients. Therefore, minimal invasive ablation therapy is a promising and rapidly evolving technique in inoperable patients or patients who refused surgery. Because of its efficiency and relatively easy use, RF ablation is the most widespread ablation modality beyond all image-guided thermal therapies. RF ablation increasingly gains importance in the treatment of primary and secondary hepatic malignancies [1]. However there are no uniform indications validated up to now and no large prospective randomized studies comparing RF ablation with the gold standard surgery. In the following, the indications for RF ablation of HCC and colorectal metastases (CRM) as recommended by the German working group on image-guided tumor ablation are given (www.drg.de).

Recommendation for therapy:
- Hepatocellular carcinoma (HCC)
  - Child A and B; Child C only in selected cases.
  - Maximum diameter: 6 cm.
  - Maximum number: 3 tumors per liver lobe.
  - Absence of extrahepatic tumor manifestations.
- Smaller tumors (< 3 cm) can be treated by a sole RF ablation.
- In larger tumors (3–6 cm) a transcatheter arterial chemoembolization (TACE) should be performed before RF ablation.

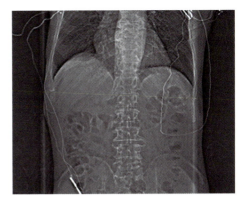

Fig. 37.1. Topogramm of a CT scan before a hepatic ablation therapy. The scan includes the liver and the adjacent parts of the thorax and abdomen

- Colorectal metastases (CRM)
  - Multifocal: maximum diameter 3.5 cm.
  - The number of metastases is not limited if a complete ablation of all metastases is possible.
  - Unifocal: maximum diameter 5 cm (overlapping RF ablations are necessary).
  - Absence of extrahepatic tumor manifestations; extrahepatic tumors without progression or an option for a sufficient therapy (e.g., pulmonary or bone metastases) are not a strict contraindication.

For metastases other than colorectal (Fig. 37.2), no clear indications are defined so far. In a potentially curative therapy concept, a complete ablation of all metastases has to be intended (Fig. 37.3 and 37.4). An ablation therapy is also applicable as a symptomatic therapy, for example, an ablation of neuroendocrine metastases can relieve related clinical symptoms. The indication for an image-guided ablation therapy should be based on an interdisciplinary consensus. If necessary, an ablation therapy can be a part of a multimodal therapy in combination with chemotherapy and/or surgery.

A potential contraindication for a hepatic RF ablation is a tumor location close to

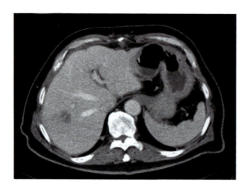

Fig. 37.2. Colorectal metastasis before radiofrequency ablation showing a low attenuation in a portal phase

the liver hilus due to the risk of a secondary bile duct stenosis. Another critical location is a subcapsular RF ablation adjacent to stomach, adrenal gland or bowel. In these cases it should be tried to distance/displace the adjacent organ, or a laparoscopic approach should be considered. Due to perfusion-mediated tissue cooling a complete ablation of tumors adjacent to large vessels is difficult.

Osteoid Osteoma

Osteoid osteoma is a benign but painful tumor, and has a characteristic radiological appearance. The therapy options are surgical, conservative (medical), and percutaneous ablation therapy. Pain relief can be achieved by long-term application of nonsteroidal antiinflammatory medication, but is associated with gastrointestinal side effects. Traditional surgical treatment can be difficult because of intraoperative problems to identify the exact tumor location and thus may lead to recurrence. CT-guided percutaneous RF ablation of osteoid osteoma can be performed with a high rate of success and minimal morbidity (Fig. 37.5). Surgical treatment should be preferred if the osteoid osteoma is in the vicinity of the spinal cord or nerves. Image-guided percutaneous RF ablation can be considered as the treatment of choice for most osteoid oste-

omas located in the appendicular skeleton and pelvis [2].

Radiofrequency Ablation in Lung and Kidney

RF ablation of renal cell carcinoma and pulmonary malignancies is a new field of ablation therapy. Preliminary results show that RF ablation in lung and kidney is safe and feasible [3,4]. The evaluation of long-term efficacy is necessary and based on further results the indications may be defined. Currently, image-guided thermoablation is being investigated in patients who are not surgical candidates.

Indications in primary lung malignancies might be a localized primary tumor without pathological lymph nodes (N0) in inoperable patients due to comorbidity or a symptomatic ablation, e.g. to relief paraneoplastic symptoms. Surgical metastasectomy is a potentially curative procedure [5]. The most important prognostic factor is that resection has to be complete and thus ablation therapy should have the same intention.

Renal cell carcinoma (RCC) in patients with single kidney, synchronous primary malignancies (e.g., Hipple-Lindau's disease), and comorbidity are candidates for minimal invasive nephron-sparing surgery or percutaneous ablation therapy. There is an easy percutaneous approach to dorsal and lateral parts of the kidney, where most RCCs are located. Currently, the best indication for percutaneous RF ablation is an exophytic tumor with a maximum diameter of 3 cm [4].

Symptomatic Treatment of Osseous and Soft-Tissue Tumors

RF ablation can provide an effective palliation of localized, painful lytic metastases involving bone [6]. This is an additional therapy option if standard treatments like radiation, chemotherapy, and oral medication fail. RF ablation can be helpful in the palliative treatment of osseous or soft tis-

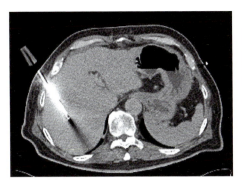

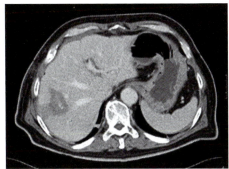

Fig. 37.3. Image shows a nonenhanced CT scan to control placement of the radiofrequency electrode

Fig. 37.4. This enhanced CT scan shows the zone of coagulation without enhancement in the portal phase. The high attenuation in the centre of the coagulation is caused by carbonization around of the electrode tip. Lateral to the zone of coagulation there is wedge-shaped area of reduced liver perfusion. The coagulation of the needle track causes the ventro-lateral hump of the zone of coagulation. The needle track has a slightly caudocranial orientation and therefore only a part of the linear zone of coagulation is included in the shown image

sue neoplasms if surgery is not possible and chemotherapy is not effective. Possible indications are pain relief and decompression of vascular and neuronal structures. The indication of an ablative therapy as palliative treatment is an individual decision and a careful evaluation is mandatory.

CT-Guided Radiofrequency Ablation

The procedure of a CT-guided ablation therapy will be described by means of a CT-guided RF ablation of hepatic malignancies. After patient preparation and positioning we perform a native and contrast enhanced (i.e., arterial and portal phase) multislice CT for the planning of the procedure. An arterial and portal phase is routinely performed in hypo- and hypervascular tumors to have a delineation of arteries and veins. We use a reduced amount of contrast media (60–80 mL) compared to a diagnostic dual phase CT of the liver. The reason is that repetitive application of contrast media might be necessary to ensure correct placement of the RF electrode or to rule out a complication. After selection of an appropriate approach we mark the supposed cutaneous access with a grid or barium paste and verify the position in a control CT scan. Placement of the RF electrode can either be performed under CT fluoroscopy or with repetitive single slices in the biopsy mode. When an angulation in the craniocaudal

direction is required, a multiplanar reconstruction along the electrode shaft is helpful to guide the electrode placement. After correct placement, a high-frequency electrical current is applied leading to heat production in the surrounding of the electrode tip caused by molecular friction. The induced coagulation necrosis shows a low-density occupation in an unenhanced CT. An additional central high attenuation caused by carbonization around the electrode tip may occur and formation of air bubbles as a side effect is possible. On enhanced CT the coagulation is nonenhancing with the best delineation in a portal phase. The coagulation may have an enhancing rim related to hyperemia from thermal injury [7]. This is more typically on an arterial dominant phase. The zone of coagulation could be accompanied by an adjacent peripheral-based wedge-shaped area of altered liver perfusion [7]. For complete tumor ablation, a repositioning of the RF electrode may be necessary for an overlapping ablation. After supposed complete tumor ablation the needle track is coagulated while the RF electrode is removed. For this reason, the

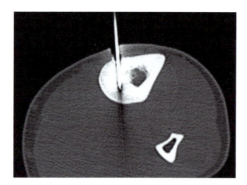

Fig. 37.5. CT scan in biopsy mode to verify placement of the radiofrequency electrode inside the nidus of an osteoid osteoma located in the tibia

risk of a tumor cell seeding or bleeding from the electrode tract should be minimized. The ablation track may be visible as linear zone of coagulation on further imaging. After ablation therapy we perform a dual-phase CT of the liver and the adjacent parts of thorax and abdomen to exclude a complication like an active bleeding. An exact prediction of the extent of coagulation immediately after ablation therapy is not possible due to an ongoing process of thermal injury. The differentiation of reactive hyperemia and residual tumor may be difficult and therefore further follow-up is necessary.

Comparison between CT, MR, and US guidance

Image-guided ablation therapy can be performed under CT, magnetic resonance (MR) or ultrasound (US) guidance. The ideal qualities of an image technique are clear delineation of tumor and the surrounding anatomy, real-time imaging, multiplanar capabilities, and monitoring of treatment effects. Ultrasound offers real-time imaging and therefore a fast applicator placement is possible. The disadvantage is that a monitoring of treatment effects is very difficult due to air bubbles produced by vaporization thus preventing a clear delineation of the tumor after application of RF energy.

Thus a repositioning of the RF electrode can hardly be visualized. A pathologic correlation of ultrasound images and pathologic specimen showed discrepancies and therefore the echogenic response should be viewed only as a rough approximation of the area of induced tissue necrosis. The final assessment of ablation should be deferred to an alternative imaging technique [8]. CT and MR imaging provide a sensitive detection of liver lesions and, compared to US, a better evaluation of posttherapeutic effects. MR images show a high tissue contrast even without administration of contrast media. A clear delineation of liver lesions on CT images is often limited to a time window after application of contrast media.

For MR imaging there is a more distinct contrast between the signal of the tumor tissue and the posttherapeutic zone of coagulation on T2-weighted MR images compared to changes of density on CT images. Therefore MR imaging provides better monitoring of treatment effects in parenchyma, e.g., liver and kidney. The drawback is that MR-guided ablation therapy is time consuming. CT guidance is superior in the treatment of osteoid osteoma and pulmonary malignancies due to the better visualization of lung tumors and small bone lesions. CT and MR imaging both offer the possibility of muliplanar images. However, a direct acquisition of multiplanar images is only possible with an MR scanner, whereas delayed reconstruction of muliplanar images is required with data from multislice CT. Near real-time imaging using CT or MR fluoroscopy is possible. The exposure to X-ray radiation during CT fluoroscopy is a disadvantage compared to MR fluoroscopy.

Multislice CT is suited for the possible indications of image-guided ablation therapy. MR imaging is an alternative for image-guidance. The decision about a certain imaging technique has to consider the individual situation like tumor size and location, possible contraindications for contrast media, and the interventionalists preference with the different modalities of image guidance.

References

1. Decadt B, Siriwardena AK (2004) Radiofrequency ablation of liver tumors: systematic review. Lancet Oncol 5(9):550–560
2. Rosenthal DI, Hornicek FJ, Torriani M, Gebhardt MC, Mankin HJ (2003) Osteoid osteoma: percutaneous treatment with radiofrequency energy. Radiology 229(1):171–175
3. Chhajed PN, Tamm M (2003) Radiofrequency heat ablation for lung tumors: potential applications. Med Sci Monit 9(11):ED5–ED7
4. Lui KW, Gervais DA, Arellano RA, Mueller PR (2003) Radiofrequency ablation of renal cell carcinoma. Clin Radiol 58(12):905–913
5. Pastorino U, Buyse M, Godehard F et al. (1997) JB for the International Registry of Lung Metastases. Long-term results of lung metastasectomy. Prognostic analyses based on 5206 cases. J Thorac Cardiovasc Surg 113(1):37–49
6. Goetz MP, Callstrom MR, Charboneau JW, Farrell MA, Maus TP, Welch TJ, Wong GY, Sloan JA, Novotny PJ, Petersen IA, Beres RA, Regge D, Capanna R, Saker MB, Gronemeyer DH, Gevargez A, Ahrar K, Choti MA, de Baere TJ, Rubin J (2004) Percutaneous image-guided radiofrequency ablation of painful metastases involving bone: a multicenter study. J Clin Oncol 22(2):300–306
7. Limanond P, Zimmerman P, Raman SS, Kadell BM, Lu DS (2003) Interpretation of CT and MRI after radiofrequency ablation of hepatic malignancies. AJR Am J Roentgenol 81(6):1635–1640
8. Leyendecker JR, Dodd GD 3rd, Halff GA, McCoy VA, Napier DH, Hubbard LG, Chintapalli KN, Chopra S, Washburn WK, Esterl RM, Cigarroa FG, Kohlmeier RE, Sharkey FE (2002) Sonographically observed echogenic response during intraoperative radiofrequency ablation of cirrhotic livers: pathologic correlation. AJR Am J Roentgenol 178(5):1147–1151

38 Vertebroplasty

R.T. Hoffmann, T.F. Jakobs and T.K. Helmberger

Indications and Contraindications

Indications

Symptomatic vertebral hemangioma. Painful osteolytic vertebral body tumour (particularly metastases and multiple myeloma) and painful fracture of osteoporotic vertebral body refractory to conservative analgetic treatment. The aim is the stabilization of the fractured vertebral body and, due to the stabilization, an effective pain treatment [1].

Relative Contraindications

Patients under 60 years of age – no long-term data regarding used cement. Osteoplastic metastases. More than 3–5 vertebral bodies affected. Tumorous lesions with epidural extension due to possible epidural overflow and spinal cord compression [1].

Absolute Contraindications

Septicemia. Hemorrhagic diathesis. Non-symptomatic vertebral body fractures. Prophylactic vertebroplasty [1].

Patient Preparation

Patients must be informed and must have signed an informed consent form at least 24 h prior to intervention. Further patient preparation includes an i.v. line, premedication (if necessary), and local anesthesia. Blood coagulation parameters must be available and must not be older than 72 h. Before performing the procedure we strongly recommend scanning the region of interest in order to plan an optimal access route, to choose the correct needle length, and to avoid harming nerve and vascular structures next to the targeted vertebral body.

Patient Positioning

For thoracic and lumbar levels, the patient is best positioned in the prone position. For cervical levels, the patient has to be positioned in the supine position.

Topogram and Scan Range

CT fluoroscopy is especially recommended for needle positioning and cement instillation.

Table Scan Parameters

Depend on the scanner used for intervention.

Tips and Tricks

- A 15-G needle should be used for cervical spine and a 10-G needle is recommended for thoracic and vertebral spine.
- If the PMMA cement is cooled before mixing (both the powder and the fluid monomer), the time period in which the cement can be used is prolonged, because the cement remains in a fluid phase longer (6–8 min).

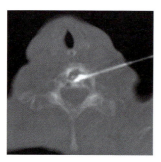

Fig. 38.1. Anterolateral approach. The needle is inserted latero-dorsal to the carotid artery in the prone position of the patient. The carotid artery should be palpated during the subcutaneous passage of the needle. The needle travels through the sternocleidomastoid muscle. Care should also be taken not to injure the vertebral artery, lying behind to the shown site of needle entry to the vertebral body

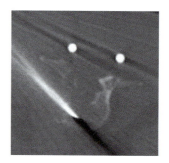

Fig. 38.2. Posterolateral approach. May serve as an alternative to the transpedicular approach in the lumbar spine (when a central needle position is not achievable with the transpedicular approach). Patient in prone position. In the posterolateral approach the needle travels through the intercostals space, the iliopsoas muscle, and enters the vertebral body laterally. Care has to be taken not to enter the pleural space

Comments

Since percutaneous vertebroplasty (VP) was first described by Galibert et al. in 1984 [2] the interest in this treatment option has grown and many technical improvements have been made. Percutaneous VP has become a widely accepted procedure with an increasing number of published studies.

Percutaneous VP has to be performed under stringent sterile conditions using sterile needles, applicators, surgical gloves, and cutaneous disinfection.

The procedure itself is normally performed under local anesthesia only and, if necessary, in combination with an intravenous analgo-sedation using, for example, Midazolam (Dormicum®) and Piritramid (Dipidolor®). General anesthesia is generally not necessary, but may be considered when planning multiple heights.

After selecting the access route and height on the previously performed CT scan, the local anesthesia should be injected under CT-fluoroscopic control to administer the anesthesia along the selected route and to reliably anesthetize the deep layers of skin and periost. After local anesthesia, a small skin incision by a scalpel has to be made to enable the 10–15-G needle to penetrate the skin.

Depending on the height that has to be treated, different approaches are recommended. On the cervical level, the optimal approach is anterolateral (Fig. 38.1), while on the lumbar level the posterolateral (Fig. 38.2) or – most often used – the transpedicular approach (Fig. 38.3) should be chosen. In the thoracic spine, a transpedicular approach is sometimes possible, but an intercostovertebral (Fig. 38.4) approach should be the first choice.

The advancement of the VP needle can be safely guided under CT-fluoroscopic control. Ideally, the needle tip is placed in the anterior third to fourth of the vertebral body, close to the midline. Using this needle position, contralateral access is normally not necessary to obtain a good cement distribution within the vertebral body [3]. Cortical perforation often requires the use of a surgical hammer. When the needle is optimally positioned, the stylet has to be removed from the needle and the cement can be prepared. The PMMA cement has to be administered during its toothpaste-like phase using either small (2–5 mL) syringe or a pressure syringe (e.g., Optimed, Karlsruhe, Germany). The injection of the cement has to be carefully controlled either under fluoroscopy or under CT fluoroscopy. The injection of the cement has to be

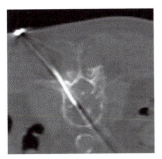

Fig. 38.3. Transpedicular approach. The most frequently used approach on the lumbar spine. CT-guidance is straightforward. When using a huge needle, fractures of the pedicular process may occur. Therefore, CT-fluoroscopic control of the advance of the needle is mandatory

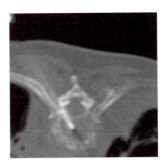

Fig. 38.4. Intercostovertebral approach. This is the most common approach used on the thoracic spine. Risks are minimal, however, careful advancement of the needle under fluoroscopic control is necessary

stopped immediately if the mixture starts to pass into the disc space or the paravertebral tissue. Special care has to be taken to avoid cement into the epidural space, since this may cause severe neurological deficits and thus major complications. The distribution of the cement can be controlled by moving and rotating the needle. A good result is obtained if there is cement within at least 30–50% of the vertebra (about 3 to 7 mL) [4]. A complete filling of the treated vertebra has to be avoided regarding to a possible fracture of the neighboring vertebra due to the increased strength of the adjacent treated vertebral body.

After injection of the cement, it is suggested that the trocar be repositioned within the needle to press any remaining cement out of the needle and to avoid unwanted cement distribution along the access pathway. After finishing the procedure, the patient should have a single intravenous broad spectrum antibiotic treatment to avoid infection. A regional CT scan should be done to document the distribution of the cement and to rule out any complications.

Possible Complications [5]

- The most common serious complications are cement leakage toward the epidural veins, epidural space, and neural foramina. The most serious complication is leakage towards the epidural space with a consecutive spinal cord compression leading to severe neurological deficits, such as paraplegia (if in thoracic or lumbar heights) or even paresis of the upper and lower limbs (cervical spine). In severe cases, the patient has to undergo an orthopedic or neurosurgical intervention. Cement leaks into the adjacent disk do not usually have clinical consequences; however, these leaks may increase the risk of a collapse of the neighboring vertebra. This leakage may be missed by CT-fluoroscopic control, and may necessitate fluoroscopic control or a spiral CT to investigate the adjacent vertebral bodies. Leaks into paravertebral veins can lead to pulmonary cement embolism, which is not normally clinically apparent, but can cause, in the worst cases, death or failure of the right ventricle.
- The second-most reported complication is infection. For this reason strict sterility during intervention is mandatory. Prophylactic antibiotic treatment during the procedure may be considered.
- The occurrence of temporal pain after the procedure is normal and should disappear within 24 h after intervention. Postprocedural pain is proportional to the administered amount of cement and is often observed after "good packing" of the vertebra.

- Allergic reactions and hypertension occur far less often after VP as compared to orthopedic surgery, due to the smaller volume of cement used.

References

1. Hoffmann RT, Jakobs TF, Wallnöfer A, Reiser MF, Helmberger TK (2003) Percutaneous vertebroplasty: indications, contraindication and technique. Radiologe 43:709–717

2. Galibert P, Deramond H, Rosat P, Le Gars D (1987) Preliminary note on the treatment of vertebral angioma by percutaneous acrylic vertebroplasty. Neurochirurgie 33:166–168

3. Ganghi A, Dietemann JL, Guth S, Steib JP, Roy C (1999) Computed tomography (CT) and fluoroscopy-guided vertebroplasty: Results and complications in 187 patients. Sem Intervent Radiol 16(2):137–142

4. Barr JD, Barr MS, Lemley TJ, McCann RM (2000) Percutaneous vertebroplasty for pain relief and spinal stabilization. Spine 8:923–928

5. Ganghi A, Guth S, Imbert JP, Marin H, Dietemann JL (2003) Percutaneous Vertbroplasty: Indications, Technique and Results. Radiographics 23:e10–e10

Subject Index